Statistics for Biology and Health

Series Editors:
M. Gail
K. Krickeberg
J. Samet
A. Tsiatis
W. Wong

Per Kragh Andersen • Lene Theil Skovgaard

Regression with Linear Predictors

With 171 illustrations by Therese Graversen

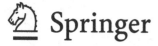 Springer

Per Kragh Andersen
University of Copenhagen
Dept. Biostatistics
Øster Farimagsgade 5
DK-1014 Copenhagen K
Denmark
p.k.andersen@biostat.ku.dk

Lene Theil Skovgaard
University of Copenhagen
Dept. Biostatistics
Øster Farimagsgade 5
DK-1014 Copenhagen K
Denmark
l.t.skovgaard@biostat.ku.dk

Series Editors

M. Gail
National Cancer Institute
Bethesda, MD 20892, USA

A. Tsiatis
Department of Statistics
North Carolina State University
Raleigh, NC 27695, USA

K. Krickeberg
Le Chatelet
F-63270 Manglieu, France

W. Wong
Department of Statistics
Stanford University
Stanford, CA 94305-4065, USA

J. Samet
Department of Preventive Medicine
Keck School of Medicine
University of Southern California
1441 Eastlake Ave. Room 4436, MC 9175
Los Angeles, CA 90089

ISBN 978-1-4614-2627-1   ISBN 978-1-4419-7170-8 (eBook)
DOI 10.1007/978-1-4419-7170-8
Springer New York Dordrecht Heidelberg London

Springer is part of Springer Science+Business Media (www.springer.com)

Preface

This is a book about *regression analysis*, that is, the situation in statistics where the distribution of a response (or outcome) variable is related to explanatory variables (or covariates). This is an extremely common situation in the application of statistical methods in many fields, and *linear* regression, *logistic* regression, and *Cox proportional hazards* regression are frequently used for quantitative, binary, and survival time outcome variables, respectively.

Several books on these topics have appeared and for that reason one may well ask why we embark on writing still another book on regression. We have two main reasons for doing this:

1. First, we want to highlight *similarities* among linear, logistic, proportional hazards, and other regression models that include a *linear predictor*. These models are often treated entirely separately in texts in spite of the fact that all operations on the models dealing with the linear predictor are precisely the same, including handling of categorical and quantitative covariates, testing for linearity and studying interactions.
2. Second, we want to emphasize that, for any type of outcome variable, multiple regression models are composed of simple building blocks that are added together in the linear predictor: that is, t-tests, one-way analyses of variance and simple linear regressions for quantitative outcomes, 2×2, $2 \times (k+1)$ tables and simple logistic regressions for binary outcomes, and 2- and $(k+1)$-sample logrank tests and simple Cox regressions for survival data. This has two consequences. All these simple and well known methods can be considered as special cases of the regression models. On the other hand, the effect of a single explanatory variable in a multiple regression model can be interpreted in a way similar to that obtained in the simple analysis, however, now valid only for the other explanatory variables in the model "held fixed". Note the important point that addition of simple terms in the linear predictor will imply an assumption of no *interaction*; that is, the effect of an explanatory variable is the same for all values of other explanatory variables in the model. This is an assumption that often needs careful consideration as part of the analysis.

In Chapter 1 the basic ideas are set up and the examples to be used throughout the book are introduced. Chapter 2 presents a review of background material on probability distributions and the principles of statistical inference. In Chapter 3 the simple building blocks for categorical explanatory variables are introduced for the three main types of outcome variables. Chapter 4 deals with one quantitative explanatory variable, first when a linear effect can be assumed and, next, certain models with a nonlinear effect of the covariate (still described by a linear predictor, however) are introduced. A very common example of such a nonlinear effect is a polynomial.

Having presented the building blocks, Chapter 5 discusses multiple regression models (i.e., models with several explanatory variables). We focus on models with two covariates and introduce the concepts of confounding and interaction ("effect modification"). In Chapter 6 we discuss model building strategies, in particular selection of explanatory variables for answering a specific research question and illustrate the strategies by thorough analyses of three specific examples.

Whereas Chapters 3 through 6 primarily deal with examples of linear models for quantitative outcomes, logistic models for binary data, and Cox models for lifetimes, Chapter 7 presents a number of other regression models with a linear predictor. These include the logistic models for ordinal and multinomial data, Poisson-type models for counts as well as alternative models for quantitative, binary, and lifetime data. Chapter 8 briefly mentions a number of extended models all involving a linear predictor. These include multivariate models with more than one response variable per individual, for example repeated measurements and other types of correlated outcomes, and models with covariate measurement errors. The multivariate models include random effect models and marginal models. The treatment of these topics is by no means meant to be exhaustive but to serve mainly as a warning that models more complicated than the ones treated earlier in this book occur quite frequently and will produce erroneous conclusions if not analyzed properly. The book is concluded with four appendices summarizing notation, the use of logarithms, some recommendations, and simple programming, respectively.

It is important to notice that some sections of the book are more difficult to read than others, simply because of the varying level of complexity for the different methods we wish to cover.

The book is based on our personal experience as teachers, consultants, and researchers in biostatistics for more than three decades and all data examples are based on this.

Our intended readers are primarily researchers from scientific areas where statistics is being *applied* to analyze numerical data, for example, fields such as medicine, public health, dentistry, agriculture, and so on. For that reason we do not expect readers to have a strong background in mathematics. We limit the amount of mathematical formulas used, and we avoid the use of Greek letters in formulas altogether. We do, however, expect readers to have some familiarity with basic statistical terms but, to set a common level, Chapter 2 gives an overview of the necessary concepts. Although we have mainly written the book for applied scientists it is our hope that readers with a more mathematical background who wish to enter the field of biostatistics will also benefit from studying the book. We intend to provide a book that can both serve as a reference source and a course textbook. For the last purpose, chapters conclude with a series of exercises all dealing with data analysis.

The mainstream of our text presents aspects of the methods that are important for building regression models, yet we have in some places found it natural to add brief discussions of related concepts that are less important for regression analysis. Such digressions are marked in the text as *Digression* and also include some historical and more technical remarks.

An applied statistical text such as the present book, obviously includes a large number of practical examples, and computational aspects are crucial. We have chosen *not to* base the presentation of examples in the book on a single piece of software. Instead, the book is accompanied by Web pages documenting examples by including computer code for the computations in R and SAS. It is our intention to supplement the Web pages with code in STATA as well but we have chosen not to include SPSS code because it is our impression that most users of this program use the menu interface rather than writing program code. In addition, a brief appendix (Appendix D) includes very simple and "raw" commands for fitting the basic types of regression models in R, SAS, and STATA.

It has been our ambition that the Web pages should be user-friendly with facilities for making an entry based on both book chapters and on the different examples. The pages can be found at

www.biostat.ku.dk/~linearpredictors

We would like to thank our medical colleagues who have granted us permission to use their data as illustrations. We also wish to thank colleagues at the Department of Biostatistics, University of Copenhagen, Denmark, for creating a friendly and productive working environment. In particular, we thank Ørnulf Borgan, Bendix Carstensen, Saskia le Cessie, Thomas Gerds, Niels Keiding, Kajsa Kvist, Maja Olsbjerg Larsen, Henrik Ravn and Willi Sauerbrei for comments, advice, assistance or encouragement. Part of the manuscript was written during a week-long workshop in Oberwolfach, Germany, and we wish to thank Mathematisches Forschungsinstitut, Oberwolfach, for hospitality during that week.

Last, but definitely not least, our most sincere thanks go to Therese Graversen. Not only did she design the accompanying Web pages and produce all the graphics in the manuscript but she also gave valuable and thoughtful comments to both contents and lay-out. Without her skillful input this book would never have become what it is now.

Copenhagen, June 2010   Per Kragh Andersen, Lene Theil Skovgaard

Contents

1

Introduction

Suppose we are studying blood pressure in humans based on a random sample from a specific population, say, inhabitants of some larger city. The very first step in such a study may be to get a summary of the level and variation of blood pressure, subject to criteria such as ethnicity, gender or age. The purpose of studying blood pressure may be to establish normal references to serve as future guidelines for when to start treatment for either too high or too low a blood pressure.

In order to illustrate the distribution of the blood pressure measurements from this sample, we usually calculate average and standard deviation and possibly produce a histogram or some other graphical illustration. These quantities are examples of *descriptive statistics*.

A small part of the variation in the blood pressure measurements can probably be ascribed to measurement error, however, a larger part of the variation is more likely due to individual fluctuations over time and to *population variation*, the true differences between subjects. Part of this population variation may be due to characteristics of the subjects that are easily recognized. For instance, men frequently have a somewhat higher blood pressure than women, and older people tend to have a higher blood pressure than younger people.

The example illustrates that, in many fields of research, information may be collected on various *features* in a number of *experimental units*. Other examples may be the serum bilirubin level in male and female patients with liver cirrhosis, whether persons in different job categories working in a given company have suffered from severe headaches in some specified period, the survival time from diagnosis of cancer patients in different stages of disease, the rise in blood glucose in experimental animals after feeding with different diets, the number of claims in a year for insurance policies of different types, the yield of some crop in differently treated field plots in an agricultural experiment, or the annual cancer rates in successive years in some country.

In the last three examples the experimental units are the insurance policy, the field plot, and the country. However, in this book we are mainly using examples from medical and public health research and we denote the experimental units by *individuals* and the features that are observed in the individuals as *variables*. Frequently, the aim of research is to study the *distribution* of one of the variables and to *compare* this distribution among subgroups of the individuals or, more generally, to *relate* this distribution to other features of the individuals. Thus, in the blood pressure example, we may wish to compare the blood pressure distributions between the groups of men and women and/or to relate the blood pressure distribution to the age of the individuals.

This illustrates the situation that we focus on in this book. We denote the variable whose distribution is under study as the *response* or *outcome variable* and that or those variables giving rise to the subgroups as *explanatory variables* or *covariates*. Alternative names for the response variable include *dependent variable* or *y-variable* and alternative names for the explanatory variables include *independent variables* or *x-variables*. However, we do not use the latter names in this book. In the blood pressure example the response variable is blood pressure whereas gender and age are explanatory variables.

Statistical techniques for studying the distribution of the response variable in relation to one or more explanatory variables are known as *regression methods* and if we manage to specify the dependence of blood pressure on gender, age, or other characteristics, we have performed a *regression analysis* and explained some of the population variation. (We later (Section 1.4.2) explain why the name "regression", meaning "decline", has been attached to this situation.) The unknown quantities involved in the description of the relation between outcome and covariates are denoted *parameters* . We aim at providing *estimates*, that is, "informed guesses" of these parameter values when analyzing the data.

A regression model may result in better diagnostics regarding too high or too low blood pressure and, as a consequence, we have better results in the overall treatment of abnormal blood pressure because the correct patients may be identified for treatment.

The specification of a useful regression model must rely on two components: theoretical knowledge of the problem at hand and graphical representations of the data. It cannot be emphasized too much that graphics are an extremely important part of regression analysis and, whenever possible, data and results from analyses should be illustrated graphically. Therefore, graphical displays of various sorts are used throughout the text.

Following a regression analysis for the problem just described, we can give sex- and age-specific reference values for normal blood pressure. In the former case, we have two sets of references, whereas in the latter case we get a reference curve covering an appropriate age range reflecting the age distribution in our sample.

When performing a regression analysis and thereby studying the distribution of a (response) variable, the relevant techniques to use depend on the *type* of this variable. Thus, methods for studying the distribution of a *quantitative* or *numerical* variable (i.e., a variable that may take (several) numerical values) are different from methods for studying the distribution of a *categorical* variable which may take few, and not necessarily numerical, values. However, it is one of the main purposes of this book to highlight *similarities* among a number of different regression methods, all of which are frequently applied in medical and public health research, as well as in several other scientific branches.

The rest of Chapter 1 is organized as follows. In Section 1.1 we introduce three examples from medical research with different types of outcome variables. Both these examples and those introduced in Section 1.5 are based on our own experience and are used as illustrations throughout the book. Having introduced these examples we next summarize the characteristics of the distribution of the outcome variable which is the focus for regression modeling when, as in these examples, the outcome is either quantitative, binary, or a survival time. These characteristics are the mean value, the failure risk, and the survival function, respectively. In Section 1.2 we discuss models with a single covariate and in Section 1.3 we explain how this covariate is related to the relevant outcome characteristic via the *link function*. In Section 1.4 we demonstrate how, for all types of outcome, covariates are combined into a *linear predictor* when building a regression model for the outcome. In these sections we illustrate the basic ideas in regression analysis using these three examples. As part of the illustration, some parameter estimates in simple regression models are presented without specifying details about how the estimates are obtained. Such details are given later in the book. Thus, the general ideas of estimation are presented in Chapter 2 (Section 2.3.1) and specific methods are discussed systematically in subsequent chapters. Section 1.5 presents other examples to be used for illustration and the final Section 1.6 summarizes how the rest of the chapters of the book are organized.

1.1 Introductory examples and types of outcome

The following examples are used for illustration throughout the book.

1. A substudy of a European investigation of vitamin D status where the outcome variable is quantitative
2. A substudy of the Danish National Birth Cohort Study where the outcome variable is binary
3. The PBC-3 trial in liver cirrhosis where the outcome variable is a survival time

1.1.1 Introductory examples

Example 1.1. Body mass index and vitamin D status

The data presented here come from a larger study on vitamin D status in four European countries (Ireland, Poland, Finland, and Denmark) conducted by Andersen et al. (2005). The data provide age, body mass index, and vitamin

D status for 420 females (girls and elderly women). Body mass index (BMI) is a height-corrected weight measure defined as weight (in kg) divided by height (in m) squared. BMI is considered normal when between 18.5 and 25 (kg/m^2), underweight when below 18.5 and overweight when above 25. The group of overweight individuals may be further subdivided into slight overweight and obese (> 30 kg/m^2). Vitamin D status is given via a measurement of 25-hydroxy-vitamin D (25OHD) in serum (nmol/l). Among the questions to be addressed using these data is whether the 25OHD-level depends on BMI and on age and how these levels vary between countries. There were 41 adult Irish women who were not underweight and where both BMI and 25OHD were available. Table 1.1.1 presents average 25OHD values for these women. There are 16 normal weight women and 25 overweight women. For the latter group the averages are also given separately for the 16 slight overweight and the 9 obese women. It seems as if the vitamin D measurements decrease with increasing body mass index.

Table 1.1.1. Average 25OHD vitamin D values for 41 adult Irish women in subgroups given by body mass index.

BMI Group	n	Vitamin D
Normal	16	56.138
Overweight	25	42.804
Slight overweight	16	45.831
Obese	9	37.422

This example is used as an illustration in Sections 1.2, 1.4, 2.2.2, 2.3.2, 3.1.1, 3.2.1, 4.1.1, 5.1.1, 5.1.2, 5.2.1, 5.2.2, 5.3.1, 6.2.1, 7.3, and 8.2.

Example 1.2. Fever in early pregnancy and risk of fetal death — A substudy of The Danish National Birth Cohort Study

The Danish National Birth Cohort Study was a nationwide study of pregnant women and their offspring (Olsen et al., 2001) . Between 1997 and 2002 more than 100,000 women were recruited to the study at their first antenatal visit to the general practitioner. When an informed consent form was received by the study secretariat, the women were invited to complete a computer-assisted telephone interview, scheduled to take place in pregnancy weeks 12–16 (although, for a number of women, the interview took place a little later). The interview provided information on a number of "exposures" suspected to be related to subsequent health outcomes in the child. Andersen et al. (2002a) analyzed a subsample of the cohort, consisting of women recruited before March 31, 1999, with the aim of studying the relation between fever in early pregnancy and fetal death. Here we present data on women interviewed before pregnancy week 17, who were still pregnant at week 17, and for whom information on episodes of fever in pregnancy was obtained. The average number of pregnancy weeks at interview was 14. These women were then followed from week 17, with the response variable of interest being fetal death.

Table 1.1.2. Distribution of fetal death by number of fever episodes before pregnancy week 17 in 11,778 women recruited to the Danish National Birth Cohort Study.

| Fetal Death | Number of Fever Episodes | | | | |
	0	1	2	3+	Total
No	9595	1852	182	30	11659
Yes	98	20	1	0	119
Total	9693	1872	183	30	11778

Table 1.1.2 shows the distribution of the response variable, fetal death, in subgroups given by the explanatory variable, number of fever episodes, for the 11,778 women included in our substudy. Thus, among women without fever episodes before the 17th week of pregnancy, $98/9693 = 1.0\%$ experienced a fetal death after week 17; among women with one or more fever episodes the corresponding number was roughly the same: $(20 + 1 + 0)/(1872 + 183 + 30) = 1.0\%$. However, a number of other explanatory variables may confound this simple comparison between the groups. We study the influence of smoking, alcohol consumption, coffee consumption, age, number of previous pregnancies, and number of previous spontaneous abortions.

Even though the main question addressed using these data deals with the risk of fetal death following fever in early pregnancy, it is also of interest to study predictors for the number of fever episodes.

This example is used as illustration in Sections 1.3, 2.2.1, 2.3.2, 3.1.2, 4.1.2, 5.1.1, 7.4, and 7.2.

Example 1.3. The PBC-3 trial in liver cirrhosis

PBC-3 was a multicenter randomized clinical trial conducted in six European hospitals (Lombard et al., 1993). Between January 1, 1983 and January 1, 1987, 349 patients with the liver disease primary biliary cirrhosis (PBC) were randomized to treatment either with Cyclosporin A (CyA, 176 patients) or placebo (173 patients). The purpose of the trial was to study the effect of treatment on the survival time. However, during the course of the trial an increased use of liver transplantation for patients with this disease made the investigators redefine the main response variable to be time to "failure of medical treatment" defined as either death or liver transplantation. Patients were then followed from randomization until treatment failure, drop-out or January 1, 1989; 61 patients died (CyA: 30, placebo: 31), another 29 were transplanted (CyA: 14, placebo: 15) and 4 patients were lost to follow-up before January 1, 1989. In this example, the response variable, time to failure of medical treatment, is not observed in all patients. For patients lost to follow-up and for those alive without having had a liver transplantation on January 1, 1989, only a lower limit of the response variable is observed, namely time from randomization to end of follow-up. These incomplete observations of the response are denoted *right-censored* observations. The presence of such observations in the dataset prevents the use of simple means (as in Example 1.1) or simple percentages (as in Example 1.2) when describing the data. The simple descriptive method that is used instead for right-censored data is the empirical Kaplan–Meier survival curve where the probability of staying event-free is estimated as a function of follow-up time. This is introduced in Section 2.2.3 with details deferred to Section 3.1.3. Figure 1.1.1 shows the estimated survival curves in the two treatment groups. It is seen that the two curves are nearly identical; for example at three years the fraction of event-free patients in both groups is estimated to be slightly below 80%. However, a number of other explanatory variables, including serum bilirubin, serum albumin, sex, and age are strong *prognostic factors*. Imbalances with respect to these factors among the treatment groups, which may exist in spite of the randomization, may affect the simple treatment comparison between the survival curves.

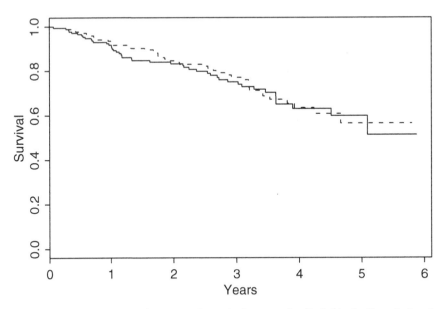

Fig. 1.1.1. Comparison of estimated survival curves for CyA (dashed) and placebo (solid) treated patients with PBC.

This example is used as an illustration in Sections 1.3, 3.1.3, 3.2.3, 4.1.3, 4.2, 5.1.1, 5.1.2, 5.2.2, and 6.2.3.

1.1.2 Types of outcome

We now revisit the examples from the previous section with the purpose of emphasizing the three main types of outcome variable. The mathematical symbol for the response variable is y, and the value observed in individual i is y_i. The explanatory variable is denoted x and the value for subject i is x_i.

Quantitative outcome

In Example 1.1 the outcome y is the *quantitative* variable vitamin D status measured by the concentration of 25OHD. When we talk about quantitative responses we often think of the situation where y is in fact *continuous*, (i.e., the outcome may take on any value in some interval). For such an outcome variable, the object for regression modeling is the *level of* y, typically taken to be the *mean* (or *expected*) value which we formally introduce in Section 2.1. It is denoted $E(y)$ where $E(\cdots)$ stands for "expectation". The mean values of 25OHD in subgroups given by categorization (grouping) of the explanatory variable body mass index (BMI) x are estimated by the averages shown in Table 1.1.1. For the level of the outcome to be described adequately by the mean, the distribution of y should be reasonably symmetric. If the distribution of y is skewed, the mean may provide a poor description of the level and it may be advantageous to transform y prior to regression modeling. For instance, if a logarithmic transformation of y gives rise to a distribution closer to symmetry then the object for regression modeling may be taken to be instead the mean value $E(\log(y))$ of the transformed variable. In such situations, a suitable back-transformation is crucial for interpreting the results as we do in later chapters.

The grouping of BMI in Table 1.1.1 provides an example of a categorical covariate. Another categorical covariate from Example 1.1 is country. Comparing the 25OHD mean values in two BMI groups (overweight versus normal weight) typically leads to the t-test (Section 3.1.1) whereas comparison among several groups is carried out using "one-way analysis of variance" (Section 3.2.1). We show in these sections how these simple methods are special cases of linear regression. However, avoiding categorization of BMI and treating it instead as a quantitative covariate x may often be advantageous. This leads to simple linear regression (Section 4.1.1) where $E(y_i)$ is related directly to x_i assuming a linear relationship. Modeling $E(y_i)$ by means of several covariates (e.g., both BMI and country) is done using multiple linear regression (the general linear model)(Chapter 5).

Binary outcome

In Example 1.2 the response variable, fetal death, is *binary* (i.e., with two levels: fetal death versus no fetal death) and we may code it as $y_i = 1$ if woman i experiences fetal death and $y_i = 0$ otherwise . For this binary outcome the object of regression analysis will typically be the *risk* of fetal death: $\text{pr}(y_i = 1)$ where $\text{pr}(\cdots)$ stands for "probability" (cf. Section 2.1). The probabilities of fetal death in subgroups given by the covariate x, number of fever episodes in early pregnancy, are estimated by the relative frequencies shown in Table 1.1.2. Comparison of the risk of fetal death between two groups (e.g., no fever episodes versus some) is often carried out using the chi-square test for a two by two table (Section 3.1.2) and a comparison among several groups (e.g., the four categories of number of fever episodes from Table 1.1.2 is done via the chi-square test for a two by four table (Section 3.2.2). The small numbers of fetal deaths in the categories 2 and 3+ fever episodes may prevent one from doing that comparison in a meaningful way, however. We show in these sections that both chi-square tests are closely connected to logistic regression analysis including the categorical covariate number of fever episodes .

Relating the risk of fetal death to the quantitative covariate alcohol consumption is performed using simple logistic regression (Section 4.1.2). As mentioned in Example 1.2 adjusting for other covariates, such as alcohol consumption, may be needed to obtain an unconfounded comparison between women with or without fever episodes. Relating the risk of fetal death to both of these covariates is carried out using multiple logistic regression (Chapter 5) .

Survival time outcome

In Example 1.3 the response variable y is a *survival time*; time to failure of medical treatment (death or liver transplantation) . Recall that for patients dropping out of the PBC-3 trial as well as for patients still alive without a transplantation on January 1, 1989, the exact value of y is not observed and only a lower limit (the time of right-censoring) is known. This has important consequences for the way in which the distribution of y may be described and related to explanatory variables. For example, the mean time to failure of medical treatment $\text{E}(y)$ may *not* be estimated as a simple average as used in Example 1.1 due to the censored observations. Also, for any fixed value t of time since randomization the probability $\text{pr}(y > t)$ of surviving time t may *not* be estimated as a simple relative frequency (as used in Example 1.2) if there are censored observations less than t. We extend the discussion of this problem in later sections (Sections 2.2.3 and 3.1.3) and here just briefly mention that the characteristic of the distribution of a survival time response variable y that is most frequently used for relating y to covariates is the whole *survival function*, that is, the survival probability $\text{pr}(y > t)$ studied as a function of time, t.

Note that, although $\text{pr}(y > t)$ may not be estimated as a simple relative frequency when there are censored observations, it may be estimated using the so-called Kaplan–Meier estimator (Section 2.2.3 and 3.1.3). Figure 1.1.1 shows Kaplan–Meier estimates of the survival function for PBC-3 patients in the groups given by the binary covariate treatment (CyA versus placebo). Comparison of the survival function between the two treatment groups may be carried out by the two-sample logrank test or using a Cox regression model (Section 3.1.3). Also quantitative covariates such as bilirubin may be relevant to study in the PBC-3 trial for which purpose the "simple" Cox regression model may be used (Section 4.1.3). Treatment comparisons after adjustment for prognostic variables such as bilirubin are carried out using the multiple Cox regression model (Chapter 5).

1.2 Covariates

In Section 1.1 we showed how different types of response variables (quantitative, binary, survival time) appeared in different studies and how the characteristics used both to describe the distributions and to relate them to explanatory variables differed among them. However, we also saw how the structure of the covariates (any combination of categorical and quantitative explanatory variables) was the same, no matter the type of the outcome variable and we exemplified how regression techniques were relevant in Examples 1.1 to 1.3. In this section focus is on the two types of *explanatory variables*, categorical (Section 1.2.1) and quantitative (Section 1.2.2), and we exemplify simple regression models with a single covariate. For a quantitative outcome variable we show that such models may be obtained in a rather direct way whereas, for binary and survival time outcomes, it is advantageous to introduce *link functions* (Section 1.3).

For notation, index i always refers to individuals, y is always the outcome variable, and the explanatory variable is x. Sometimes a basic explanatory variable is used directly in the regression models, however, frequently categorized, or otherwise transformed, versions of x are also used. Other mathematical symbols are model parameters or indices for groupings other than individuals. The notation used in the book is summarized in Appendix A.

1.2.1 Categorical covariates

To describe the distribution of y in the x-subgroups, certain summary measures were used depending on the type of response variable. Thus, for the quantitative outcome in Example 1.1 the average was used as an estimate of the mean (or expected) value $E(y_i)$ of the vitamin D status measured as the concentration of 25OHD. For the binary outcome variable in Example 1.2 the relative frequency was used as an estimate of the probability $pr(y_i = 1)$ of fetal death. For the survival time outcome in Example 1.3 the empirical survival curve (the Kaplan–Meier estimator) was used as an estimate of survival probabilities $pr(y_i > t)$ for relevant values of time t.

To be more specific, we assumed in Example 1.1 that there were separate mean values, say m_0 and m_1, in the two groups defined from BMI; that is

$$E(y_i) = \begin{cases} m_0 \text{ if } x_i = 0 \\ m_1 \text{ if } x_i = 1, \end{cases} \tag{1.2.1}$$

where $x_i = 1$ if woman no. i is overweight and $x_i = 0$ if she is normal weight. The similar assumption in Example 1.2, defining the explanatory variable x_i as 1 if woman i had fever before week 17 and $x_i = 0$ if not, was that there were separate risks of fetal death, say p_0 and p_1, in the two groups; that is

$$\text{pr}(y_i = 1) = \begin{cases} p_0 \text{ if } x_i = 0 \\ p_1 \text{ if } x_i = 1. \end{cases} \tag{1.2.2}$$

Finally, in Example 1.3, defining the explanatory x_i as 1 if patient i was treated with CyA and $x_i = 0$ if not, we assumed that there were separate survival functions, say $S_0(t)$ and $S_1(t)$, in the two groups, i.e.

$$\text{pr}(y_i > t) = \begin{cases} S_0(t) \text{ if } x_i = 0 \\ S_1(t) \text{ if } x_i = 1. \end{cases} \tag{1.2.3}$$

Focusing on Example 1.1, Equation (1.2.1) may be rewritten as

$$\text{E}(y_i) = m_0 + (m_1 - m_0)x_i, \tag{1.2.4}$$

or

$$\text{E}(y_i) = a + bx_i. \tag{1.2.5}$$

In the linear regression model (1.2.5) we have introduced the standard regression parametrization where $a = m_0$, the *intercept* or *constant term*, is the mean response in the *reference group* corresponding to $x = 0$, and $b = m_1 - m_0$ is the *effect* of the explanatory variable or the *regression coefficient* for the explanatory variable, x, that is, the difference between the mean responses for individuals with $x_i = 1$ and individuals with $x_i = 0$. The effect b of x is sometimes denoted the "slope" (for reasons that should become apparent when quantitative explanatory variables are introduced below). Note that when $b = 0$ the mean of y does not depend on x. (In Section 1.4.2 we give some cautionary remarks concerning the use of the word "effect".) In Example 1.1 we find from Table 1.1.1, denoting the estimate of a parameter by a "hat", that the estimate of b is $\hat{b} = -13.334$ and $\hat{a} = 56.138$; both estimates are measured in the same units as the outcome variable.

For the other types of outcome variables, binary in Example 1.2 and survival time in Example 1.3, Equations (1.2.2) and (1.2.3) may be rewritten in a similar fashion. However, it turns out that the convenient way of doing this is after having introduced *link functions* which we do in Section 1.3.

In Equations (1.2.1)–(1.2.3) the basic covariate x_i was defined to take values 0 or 1 whereby x_i could be used directly as the explanatory variable in Equations (1.2.4) and (1.2.5). If a binary covariate x_i more generally takes values g_0 and g_1, say, then (1.2.4) and (1.2.5) are applicable when replacing x_i by the *indicator* or *dummy* variable defined by

$$I(x_i = g_1) = \begin{cases} 1 \text{ if } x_i = g_1 \\ 0 \text{ if } x_i = g_0. \end{cases} \tag{1.2.6}$$

This approach is also used for a general categorical explanatory variable, that is, with possibly more than two categories. Here, the model formulation (1.2.1) is directly applicable: if x_i takes the $k + 1$ values $g_0, g_1, \ldots, g_k$, say, we may write

$$\mathrm{E}(y_i) = \begin{cases} m_0 & \text{if } x_i = g_0 \\ m_1 & \text{if } x_i = g_1 \\ \cdots \; \cdots \\ m_k & \text{if } x_i = g_k. \end{cases} \tag{1.2.7}$$

To rewrite equation (1.2.7) like (1.2.4) or (1.2.5) we then introduce the k indicator variables $I(x_i = g_j), j = 1, \ldots, k$ and Equations (1.2.4) and (1.2.5) become

$$\mathrm{E}(y_i) = m_0 + (m_1 - m_0)I(x_i = g_1) + (m_2 - m_0)I(x_i = g_2) \\ + \cdots + (m_k - m_0)I(x_i = g_k)$$

and

$$\mathrm{E}(y_i) = a + b_1 I(x_i = g_1) + b_2 I(x_i = g_2) + \cdots + b_k I(x_i = g_k), \tag{1.2.8}$$

respectively. Again, Equation (1.2.8) uses standard regression parametrization, where $a = m_0$, the intercept, is the mean response in the reference category corresponding to $x = g_0$, and the regression coefficients $b_j = m_j - m_0, j = 1, \ldots, k$, represent the effects of x with the interpretation that b_j is the difference between the means when $x = g_j$ and $x = g_0$, respectively. Note again that if $b_1 = b_2 = \cdots = b_k = 0$ then the mean of y does not depend on x.

In Example 1.1 we may study the body mass index divided into three groups: 0: normal, 1: slight overweight, and 2: obese, and from Table 1.1.1 we find the estimates $\hat{a} = 56.138$ and we get $\hat{b}_1 = -10.307$ for the comparison of slight overweight and normal weight and $\hat{b}_2 = -18.716$ for the comparison of obese and normal weight.

1.2.2 Quantitative covariates

Frequently, the groups are *ordered* (e.g., the categories may be obtained by grouping a *quantitative* explanatory variable x into certain intervals). Thus, in Example 1.1 we were studying the subgroups: "normal," "slight overweight," and "obese" given by the BMI cutpoints 25 and 30 kg/m^2. In Example 1.2, the risk of fetal death may be related to alcohol consumption whereas in Example 1.3 the distribution of time to treatment failure is likely to depend on the patients' serum bilirubin levels.

In such examples it is often a plausible a priori assumption that the level of the response variable varies in a *monotonic* way among the groups: the response level either increases or decreases through the ordered groups. Often a natural *score* $s(x_i)$ can be attached to each group. Thus, if the groups correspond to intervals of a quantitative explanatory variable x, the score attached to interval j could be a typical x-value (like the midpoint) from that interval. Otherwise one may simply use the group numbers $0, 1, \ldots, k$ as scores.

In Figure 1.2.1 the averages of the response variable y (25OHD) in Example 1.1 are plotted against the BMI scores defined as the midpoints 21.75 and 27.5 for the first two intervals and 32.5 for the last.

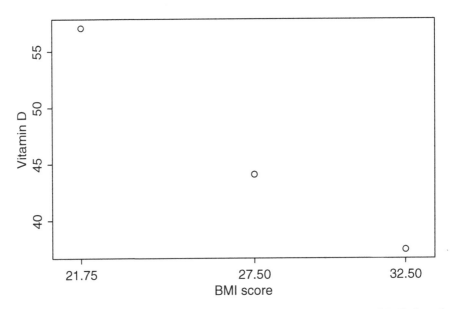

Fig. 1.2.1. Average 25OHD-values plotted against the BMI scores 21.75, 27.5, and 32.5 in Example 1.1.

A graphical representation such as Figure 1.2.1 may (as we show below) be well suited for illustration for other types of outcome variables. However, for a quantitative outcome it is more natural to use a *scatterplot* where the individual response y_i is plotted against the explanatory variable x_i, in particular if x_i is "truly quantitative" or *continuous* (i.e., if it takes many different values). In Figure 1.2.2 this is done for the data from Example 1.1.

A simple way of describing a relation like the one we see in Figure 1.2.2 is to assume a *linear* relation between x and the expected value, $E(y)$ of y, that is,

$$E(y_i) = a + bx_i. \tag{1.2.9}$$

Equation (1.2.9) expresses that the scatterplot, on average, is a straight line with *slope* b (hence the name "slope" for this parameter introduced above) and *intercept* a (which is the mean value when $x_i = 0$). The interpretation of

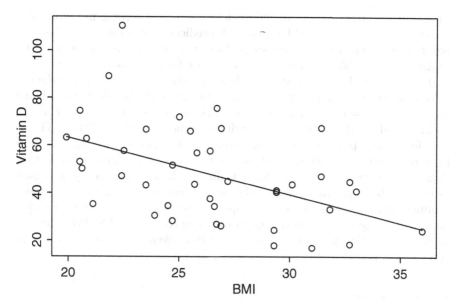

Fig. 1.2.2. Scatterplot: values of the quantitative outcome y (25OHD) plotted against the quantitative covariate x (BMI) in Example 1.1.

b is the difference in mean response between subjects whose difference in x is one unit. That is, if $b = 0$ then the line is horizontal and the mean of y does not depend on x.

The straight line in Figure 1.2.2 has slope $\widehat{b} = -2.388$ and intercept $\widehat{a} = 110.941$. Note that the interpretation of a as the mean 25OHD value for women with a BMI of zero is not very useful and a *reparametrization* of the model (1.2.9) is advantageous for presentation purposes. One solution could be to use the explanatory variable $x_i - 25$ instead of x_i in (1.2.9). Thereby, the intercept in the reparametrized model would be the expected 25OHD value for women with a BMI value of 25 kg/m^2 and the estimate of this new intercept would be $\widehat{a} + 25 \cdot \widehat{b} = 110.941 - 25 \cdot 2.388 \doteq 51.241$ which is certainly a more typical value for observed 25OHD values. The model as such and the slope are not affected by the reparametrization as is further illustrated in Section 4.1.1.

1.3 Link functions

In (1.2.9) the line will (if $b > 0$) take arbitrarily large (positive) values for large positive values of x and arbitrarily small (i.e., large negative) values for large negative values of x (vice versa if $b < 0$). For this to be a sensible model for $E(y_i)$ it is implicitly assumed that the quantitative outcome variable y may take both positive and negative values with no strict limitations. If, however, the range of y is restricted to positive values, for example, then extreme predictions from the model (1.2.9) may become meaningless if the covariate is unrestricted because such predictions eventually may become negative. Whether this is a serious problem will depend on the range of the explanatory variable x and the range of $a + bx$ for reasonable values of x.

For binary and lifetime outcomes, however, the range restriction of the parameter is a serious challenge. This is because, for both the failure probability for a binary y, $p = \text{pr}(y = 1)$, and for the survival probability, $S(t) = \text{pr}(y > t)$ for lifetime data, the parameter is restricted to the interval from 0 to 1. Therefore, for these types of outcome, one typically does not assume that it is the basic parameter (p or $S(t)$) which is, itself, a linear function of x but rather that some function of p or $S(t)$ depends linearly on x. This function is known as the *link function*. In the remainder of this section we introduce the most common link functions for binary responses and for survival times. Finally, we return to the situation with a quantitative outcome variable. When studying the link function, material concerning *logarithmic* functions collected in Appendix B is useful.

Binary outcomes

Let us begin by considering the simple case of a binary outcome as in Example 1.2 (cf. Equation (1.2.2)). The link function most frequently used for binary outcomes is the *logit* link function which relates to the *odds* parameter. When p is the failure probability then $p/(1 - p)$ is the odds of failure, that is, the ratio between the failure probability and its complementary probability (the "success" probability, $1-p$). The odds is just another measure of the frequency of a failure. It is nonnegative; it is 0 if $p = 0$ and undefined or "plus infinity" if $p = 1$. This means that the log(odds)

$$\ell = \text{logit}(p) = \log\left(\frac{p}{1 - p}\right) \tag{1.3.10}$$

can be both negative and positive; it is undefined or "minus infinity" if $p = 0$ and undefined or "plus infinity" if $p = 1$. Equation (1.2.2), dealing with a binary covariate x, can then be rewritten as

$$\ell_i = \text{logit}(\text{pr}(y_i = 1)) = \begin{cases} \text{logit}(p_0) \text{ if } x_i = 0 \\ \text{logit}(p_1) \text{ if } x_i = 1 \end{cases} \tag{1.3.11}$$

and the equation equivalent to (1.2.5) becomes the logistic regression model

$$\ell_i = a + bI(x_i = 1) = a + bx_i. \tag{1.3.12}$$

The function $\text{logit}(p)$ is shown graphically in Figure 1.3.3 (left panel). In (1.3.12) the interpretation of the intercept parameter a is $\log(p_0/(1 - p_0))$, the log(odds) in the reference group of women without fever episodes, and the slope b is

$$b = \text{logit}(p_1) - \text{logit}(p_0) = \log\left(\frac{p_1/(1-p_1)}{p_0/(1-p_0)}\right)$$

the *log(odds ratio)* between women with and women without fever episodes. Thus $b = 0$ again corresponds to no dependence on x of the distribution of y. Note that, as a consequence of (1.3.10), the failure probability is given by the *logistic* function

$$p = \frac{\exp(\ell)}{1+\exp(\ell)} \qquad (1.3.13)$$

shown in Figure 1.3.3 (right panel).

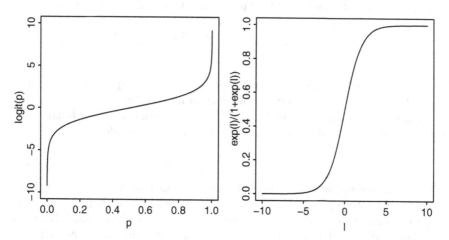

Fig. 1.3.3. Left: the logit function $\ell = \text{logit}(p) = \log(p/(1-p))$. Right: the logistic function $p = \exp(\ell)/(1+\exp(\ell))$.

In Example 1.2, the estimate for p_0 was $\widehat{p}_0 = 98/9693 = 0.01$; that is, the estimate for a becomes $\log(\widehat{p}_0/(1-\widehat{p}_0)) = -4.584$ whereas that for b is $\log(\widehat{p}_1/(1-\widehat{p}_1)) - \log(\widehat{p}_0/(1-\widehat{p}_0)) = -4.588 - (-4.584) = -0.004$. These estimates are in a scale that is hard to interpret and, instead, the estimated odds ratio $\exp(\widehat{b})$ is usually quoted. For this example the value is 0.996, close to the null value of 1 for an odds ratio, meaning that the odds of fetal death are practically the same for women with or without fever episodes.

For a categorical explanatory variable expressions like (1.2.7) and (1.2.8) may be set up for the log(odds) parameter leading to regression coefficients $b_1, \ldots, b_k$ which are log(odds ratios) for categories $1, \ldots, k$ in relation to the reference category 0.

As an illustration we study Example 1.2 and the reported weekly alcohol consumption during pregnancy. Table 1.3.1 presents the data. It is seen that the risk of fetal death is rather constant over alcohol categories. The table also

Table 1.3.1. Distribution of fetal death by reported number of drinks per week during pregnancy in 11,778 women recruited to the Danish National Birth Cohort Study. (One woman had missing value for the alcohol consumption.)

Fetal death	Number of drinks per week					
	0 (0)	0.5–1 (0.73)	1.5–2 (1.85)	2.5–3 (2.83)	3.5+ (4.89)	Total
No	6954	3241	962	308	193	11,658
Yes	68	34	12	3	2	119
Total	7022	3275	974	311	195	11,777
Risk ($\hat{p}$) (%)	0.97	1.04	1.23	0.96	1.03	1.01
log(odds) (log($\hat{p}/(1-\hat{p})$))	−4.63	−4.56	−4.38	−4.63	−4.57	−4.58
log(odds ratio)	0	0.07	0.24	0.00	0.06	
odds ratio	1	1.07	1.28	1.00	1.06	

gives the estimated log(odds) parameters and the corresponding odds ratio estimates relative to the reference category of nondrinkers.

Again, an analogue to Equation (1.2.9) may be considered for binary outcomes. Here the model is the simple logistic regression model

$$\ell_i = a + bx_i, \tag{1.3.14}$$

where x_i denotes the weekly alcohol consumption reported by woman i. In (1.3.14), the intercept a is the log(odds) for individuals with $x = 0$ and the slope or regression coefficient b is the difference in the log(odds) between subgroups whose difference in their values of x is one unit (i.e., the log(odds ratio) associated with one x-unit). This means that the most natural regression parameter to quote is $\exp(b)$, the odds ratio associated with one x-unit. Again $b = 0$ (or $\exp(b) = 1$) corresponds to the situation where the distribution of y is independent of x. In this model the estimates become $\hat{a} = -4.627, \hat{b} = 0.078$. Thereby, $\exp(\hat{b}) = 1.08$ meaning that the odds of fetal death are 8% higher for women who have one more drink per week.

To evaluate the model (1.3.14) we may define the score $s(x_i) = \bar{x}(j)$, the average number of weekly drinks for women in alcohol category j, if woman i belongs to that category. These averages are shown in brackets in Table 1.3.1 and in Figure 1.3.4 the log(odds) estimates are plotted against these averages. Note that this figure is analogous to Figure 1.2.1 for the example with a quantitative outcome variable (Example 1.1). Also note that, for a binary outcome, the scatterplot used in Figure 1.2.2 for a quantitative outcome is not very informative, although adding a *scatterplot smoother* (introduced more formally in Section 4.2) aids the interpretation. We do that in Section 4.1.2. For the model

$$\ell_i = a + bs(x_i)$$

we find $\widehat{b} = 0.0455$, not dramatically different from the slope estimated in model (1.3.14). The line in Figure 1.3.4 has this slope corresponding to an estimated odds ratio per weekly drink of $\exp(\widehat{b}) = 1.05$. The interpretation is that the odds of fetal death increase by 5% for each extra weekly drink in the sense that the estimated odds ratio for women differing by 1 drink per week is 1.05. The intercept is $\widehat{a} = -4.609$.

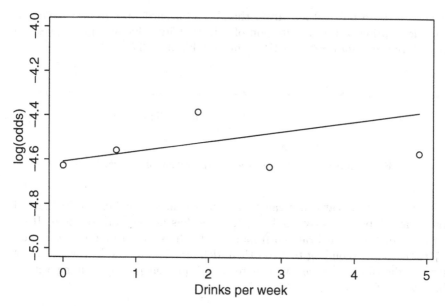

Fig. 1.3.4. Log(odds) of fetal death (and fitted regression line) for categories of weekly alcohol consumption in the Danish National Birth Cohort Study.

We later (Section 6.1.3) return to a general discussion concerning merits and drawbacks of the grouping of a quantitative explanatory variable.

Survival time outcomes

For the survival data in Example 1.3 we also have the restriction $0 \le S(t) \le 1$ similar to the restriction on p in Example 1.2. This means that one possible link function to use for survival data would be the logit transformation. However, because of its relation to the *log(hazard ratio)* parameter (defined shortly), a different link function has been used more frequently for survival data.

The hazard rate is defined, intuitively, in the following way. If y is a survival time outcome then the survival function, as explained above, is

$$S(t) = \mathrm{pr}(y > t),$$

the probability that the outcome exceeds time t. The hazard rate $h(t)$ (which is also a function of time t) is then given as follows. The *conditional probability* that the survival time y is between t and $t + dt$ *given that* y exceeds t is, approximately, for small $dt > 0$, equal to $h(t)dt$. This conditional probability, defined properly in Section 2.1, is written as

$$\text{pr}(t < y < t + dt \mid y > t)$$

where "|" is to be read as "given that." The hazard rate gives a "dynamical" description of the distribution of y in that its value at time t gives the *instantaneous failure rate* per time unit; see Figure 1.3.5.

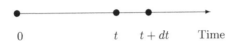

$$0 \qquad\qquad\qquad t \quad\; t + dt \qquad \text{Time}$$

Fig. 1.3.5. Illustration of the interpretation of a hazard rate.

Because the hazard rate can be any nonnegative number the log(hazard rate) can be both positive and negative and has no range restrictions. If we let $h_0(t)$ be the hazard rate corresponding to the survival function $S_0(t)$ and $h_1(t)$ that corresponding to $S_1(t)$ then, defining $l_i(t)$ as the log(hazard rate) for the distribution of y_i, we can rewrite Equation (1.2.3), dealing with a binary covariate, as

$$l_i(t) = \begin{cases} \log(h_0(t)) & \text{if } x_i = 0 \\ \log(h_1(t)) & \text{if } x_i = 1. \end{cases} \tag{1.3.15}$$

The equation analogous to (1.2.5) then becomes

$$l_i(t) = \log(h_0(t)) + bI(x_i = 1) = \log(h_0(t)) + bx_i; \tag{1.3.16}$$

that is, the hazard rate for individual i is given by the *Cox regression* model

$$h_0(t)\exp(bx_i). \tag{1.3.17}$$

In Equation (1.3.16) the crucial assumption that the difference $b = \log(h_1(t)) - \log(h_0(t))$ does not depend on t has been imposed. This is known as the *proportional hazards* assumption as it implies that the hazard ratio $h_1(t)/h_0(t) = \exp(b)$ is constant; see (1.3.17). This may be a severe restriction that may simply be inadequate in certain examples and, at any rate, it is a model assumption which must be checked carefully in actual data analyses. If the proportional hazards model fits the data then the hazard ratio $\exp(b)$ is the natural parameter to quote and $\exp(b) = 1$ (or log(hazard ratio), $b = 0$) corresponds to the situation where the distribution of y does not depend on x. Note that, as a consequence of the proportional hazards assumption, the intercept term in (1.3.16), that is, the log(baseline hazard rate) $\log(h_0(t))$, is not a single number (like a in (1.2.5) or (1.3.12)) but itself a function of time, t. The baseline hazard rate $h_0(t)$ is the hazard rate in the reference group, $x = 0$. For the PBC-3 data from Example 1.3 the estimated hazard ratio for treatment is 0.94 close to the null value of 1 indicating, as shown in Figure 1.1.1, that there is no substantial difference in time to treatment failure between the two treatment groups.

For a categorical explanatory variable, following the approach for quantitative and binary outcome variables, expressions like (1.2.7) and (1.2.8) may be set up for the log(hazard rate) $l(t)$ leading to regression coefficients $b_1, \ldots, b_k$ which are log(hazard ratios) for categories $1, \ldots, k$ in relation to the reference category 0. Under the assumption of proportional hazards between all $k + 1$ groups we then get the equation

$$l_i(t) = \log(h_0(t)) + b_1 I(x_i = 1) + b_2 I(x_i = 2) + \cdots + b_k I(x_i = k). \quad (1.3.18)$$

As an example we again study the PBC-3 trial and the explanatory variable serum bilirubin recorded at entry into the trial. This is a strong prognostic factor as indicated by Table 1.3.2 which presents the number of patients and observed number of treatment failures in bilirubin *quintile groups* (i.e., dividing patients into five (approximately) equal-size groups according to their value of bilirubin). The same tendency is seen in Figure 1.3.6 which shows the estimated survival curves in the same five groups.

Table 1.3.2. Number of patients and observed ("expected") number of treatment failures in serum bilirubin quintile groups in the PBC-3 trial in liver cirrhosis.

	Serum Bilirubin (μmol/L)					
Interval	$\leq$10.3	10.3–16	16–26.7	26.7–51.4	>51.4	Total
Average	(7.66)	(13.26)	(20.23)	(37.32)	(148.83)	
Patients	70	73	66	70	70	349
Treatment failures	6	3	13	23	45	90
("Expected")	(23.26)	(20.34)	(16.78)	(16.89)	(12.73)	90
Hazard rate ratio	1	0.57	3.00	5.28	13.70	

The numbers given in the last row of Table 1.3.2 estimate $\exp(b_1)$, $\exp(b_2)$, $\exp(b_3)$, $\exp(b_4)$, the hazard rate ratios for the last four bilirubin groups compared to the first (cf. Equation (1.3.18)). (These estimates may be based on the "expected" numbers of treatment failures; see Section 3.2.3.) A general increase of the hazard rate with bilirubin is seen and it may be advantageous to treat bilirubin as a quantitative explanatory variable, that is, to study a model like the *simple Cox regression* model

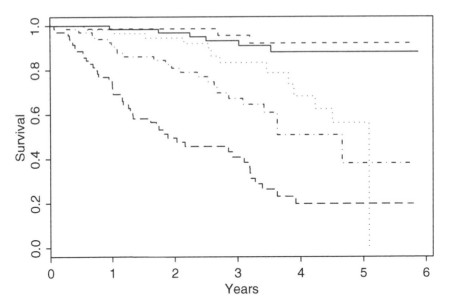

Fig. 1.3.6. Comparison of estimated survival curves for patients with PBC in quintile groups of serum bilirubin: first quintile (solid), second (upper dashed), third (dotted), fourth (dotted-dashed), fifth (lower long-dashed).

$$l_i(t) = \log(h_0(t)) + bx_i, \qquad (1.3.19)$$

where x_i is the bilirubin value at entry for patient i. To evaluate this model let us first define the score $s(x_i)$ to be the average bilirubin value for the quintile group to which individual i belongs:

$$s(x_i) = \begin{cases} 7.66 & \text{if } x_i \leq 10.3 \\ 13.26 & \text{if } x_i \in (10.3, 16] \\ 20.23 & \text{if } x_i \in (16, 26.7] \\ 37.32 & \text{if } x_i \in (26.7, 51.4] \\ 148.83 & \text{if } x_i > 51.4. \end{cases}$$

In Figure 1.3.7 the estimated log(hazard ratios) $b_0 = 0, \widehat{b}_1, \ldots, \widehat{b}_4$ are plotted against the scores $s(x_i)$. We may note that, also for survival time data, due to the presence of right-censored observations, scatterplots analogous to Figure 1.2.2 are not available. Instead in later chapters we introduce "scatter-type plots" based on so-called pseudo-observations for survival data (Section 3.1.3).

Although, according to Figure 1.3.7, linearity of the log(hazards) is questionable, we consider the model

$$l_i(t) = \log(h_0(t)) + bs(x_i), \qquad (1.3.20)$$

where $\exp(b)$ is the hazard rate ratio between groups differing by 1 μmol/L for their values of bilirubin. The estimate becomes $\exp(0.0150) = 1.02$. In this example it is more informative to quote the hazard rate ratio associated with a bilirubin difference of 10 μmol/L. This is $\exp(0.150) = 1.16$. Replacing $s(x_i)$ by each patient's individually recorded serum bilirubin value at entry x_i the estimate corresponding to 10 μmol/L is $\exp(0.093) = 1.10$, the discrepancy partly arising from the nonlinearity seen in Figure 1.3.7.

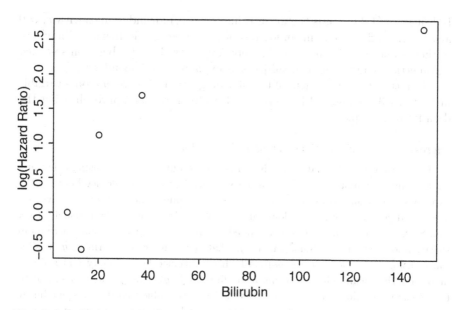

Fig. 1.3.7. Estimated log(hazard ratios) plotted against average bilirubin value $s(x)$ in quintile groups of serum bilirubin.

Quantitative outcomes. Transformations

We now return to a quantitative outcome variable y as discussed in the introduction to this section. For a positive y an obvious link function to use would be log, that is, to study a model like

$$\log(\mathrm{E}(y_i)) = a + bx_i. \tag{1.3.21}$$

In Equation (1.3.21) a is the log of the mean value of y_i for individuals with $x_i = 0$ and b is the difference in the log of the mean response between individuals with a difference in their value of x equal to one unit; that is, $b = 0$ corresponds to no dependence on x for the mean of y. For this model the parameter $\exp(b)$ is the one with the most obvious interpretation being the ratio between mean responses in subjects whose difference in their values of x is one unit.

However, for a positive quantitative outcome variable it is often simpler to log-transform y before the analysis than to apply a model such as (1.3.21) with the log link function. This transformation leads to considering a linear model for the log-transformed outcome $\log(y)$:

$$\mathrm{E}(\log(y_i)) = a + bx_i. \tag{1.3.22}$$

In Equation (1.3.22), a is the mean value of $\log(y_i)$ for individuals with $x_i = 0$ and b is the difference in mean log-response between subjects whose difference in their values of x is one unit. Thereby, $\exp(b)$ is the ratio between so-called "geometric means" for such subjects as explained in Appendix B.

We return to the problem of transforming a quantitative outcome variable in Sections 3.1.1 and 3.2.1 where we also illustrate this approach using the data from Example 1.1.

Digression. Transformations versus link functions

Using a log-transformation of the quantitative outcome y and using a log link for $\mathrm{E}(y)$ may, at first glance, look rather similar. The main difference between the two approaches has to do with an aspect of the linear model that we have not mentioned yet, namely the random variation of y. The linear model is usually (see, e.g., Sections 3.1.1 and 4.1.1) accompanied by an assumption of a constant random variation for y ("variance homogeneity"). That is, when log-transforming y, it is for the transformed scale that we assume to have variance homogeneity and a linear model for the mean, whereas, using a log link for $\mathrm{E}(y)$, it is y that is assumed to have constant random variation, but it is the log mean value that depends in a linear way on x. In Section 7.3 we contrast the use of a log link with a log-transformation. ◇

1.4 Building a regression model

In the previous sections we introduced ways in which the distribution of an outcome variable y may be related to a single explanatory variable x. We were dealing with outcome variables of different types: quantitative, binary, and survival times, and both situations where x was categorical and situations where x was quantitative were studied. Different statistical models were relevant for different types of outcomes. However, both for categorical explanatory variables and for quantitative explanatory variables, the ways in which a covariate was dealt with were quite similar for the three types of outcome. Thus, a categorical x with $k + 1$ different values $(g_0, g_1, \ldots, g_k)$ gave rise to adding terms of the form

$$b_1 I(x_i = g_1) + b_2 I(x_i = g_2) + \cdots + b_k I(x_i = g_k) \tag{1.4.1}$$

to the intercept a. In particular, for a binary x a single term

$$b_1 I(x_i = g_1) \tag{1.4.2}$$

was added to a. Furthermore, a quantitative x gave rise to adding a term of the form

$$bx_i \tag{1.4.3}$$

to a. Recall that, for survival data, the intercept a is to be understood as the log(baseline hazard rate), that is, the function that expresses how the log(hazard rate) depends on time t for covariates equal to 0.

In the three examples introduced in Section 1.1 focus was on a single explanatory variable at a time: body mass index in Example 1.1, fever or alcohol in early pregnancy in Example 1.2, and treatment or bilirubin in Example 1.3. Nevertheless, other explanatory variables may be of interest or adjustment for such variables may be warranted to obtain an accurate estimate of the effect of the explanatory variable of primary interest. This may, for instance, be the case in the second example where fever episodes may be more prevalent in women with a high alcohol consumption during pregnancy. A simple comparison of the risk of fetal death between women with or without fever episodes may, therefore, be confounded by the possibly different levels of alcohol consumption in the two groups. Thus, we can see that there is a need for studying *multiple regression models* , that is, models with several simultaneous explanatory variables.

In Section 1.4.1 we present the basic idea for doing this, namely simply to add terms of the form (1.4.1)–(1.4.3) to the model, thereby obtaining the *linear predictor*. We show what the corresponding consequences of doing this are in relation to the interpretation of the regression coefficients in the model. We do this in detail for the case of modeling the mean of a quantitative outcome as a function of two explanatory variables that are either both binary or one is binary and the other is quantitative. Other situations are just mentioned briefly with details deferred to later chapters. An important feature is that the linear predictor in all cases is linked to the distribution of the response variable via the link function as explained in Section 1.3.

In Section 1.4.2 we discuss a number of different purposes for undertaking a regression analysis and give some cautionary remarks about difficulties in attaching causal interpretations to the results from a regression analysis.

The notation when there are several, say n_c, explanatory variables is that, for individual i, the observed value of the first of these is denoted $x_{i,1}$, the second $x_{i,2}$, and so on; the last one is x_{i,n_c}. Recall that sometimes these basic explanatory variables are used directly in the regression models however, frequently categorized, or otherwise transformed, versions of the xs are also used.

1.4.1 The linear predictor and the link function

Our starting point for the discussion is the women from Ireland and Poland in Example 1.1 and the quantitative outcome variable y_i, 25OHD measurement of vitamin D status for woman no. i. For this study we have the two explanatory variables:

$$x_{i,1} = \text{BMI for woman } i.$$

and

$$x_{i,2} = \begin{cases} 1 \text{ if individual } i \text{ is from Ireland} \\ 0 \text{ if individual } i \text{ is from Poland.} \end{cases}$$

We first consider a model with the two binary explanatory variables $I(x_{i,1} \geq 25)$ (overweight versus normal weight) and $x_{i,2}$. Adding terms of the form (1.4.2) for these two variables leads to the model

$$E(y_i) = a + b_1 I(x_{i,1} \geq 25) + b_2 x_{i,2} \tag{1.4.4}$$

for the expected value of y_i. In tabular form, the model is presented in Table 1.4.1.

Table 1.4.1. Expected values in four groups according to model (1.4.4).

	Normal Weight	Overweight
Poland	a	$a + b_1$
Ireland	$a + b_2$	$a + b_1 + b_2$

From (1.4.4) and Table 1.4.1 we can compute the effect of the dichotomized body mass index, $I(x_1 \geq 25)$, for women from Ireland ($x_2 = 1$) and for women from Poland ($x_2 = 0$). The former is

$$(a + b_1 + b_2) - (a + b_2) = b_1$$

and the latter is

$$(a + b_1) - a = b_1.$$

Thus, the interpretation of the regression coefficient b_1 for the dichotomized body mass index in the model which also includes country x_2, is an *effect of body mass index for separate values of country*. Furthermore, it is seen that this effect is assumed to be the same for all values of x_2, that is, both for Ireland and for Poland. Similarly, we can compute the effect of country x_2, that is, a difference between countries for overweight women and for normal weight women. The former is

$$(a + b_1 + b_2) - (a + b_1) = b_2$$

and the latter is

$$(a + b_2) - a = b_2.$$

It is seen that the interpretation of the regression coefficient b_2 for country x_2 in the model which also includes body mass index x_1 is the *effect of country for separate values of body mass index* and, again, this effect is assumed to be the same for all values of x_1, that is, for normal weight and for overweight women. We say that the effects of body mass index and country are *mutually adjusted*.

In conclusion, a consequence of simply adding the terms for the explanatory variables is that the effect of one explanatory variable is assumed to be the same no matter the value of the other explanatory variable(s). We say that there is *no interaction* between the explanatory variables. This is a crucial assumption and it is often part of the regression analysis to examine whether such an assumption is reasonably fulfilled.

For the vitamin D study (cf. Example 1.1) we find $\widehat{a} = 42.298, \widehat{b}_1 = -11.942, \widehat{b}_2 = 12.990$. We can compare these estimates with the average 25OHD values computed in each of the four countries by BMI groups (cf. Table 1.4.2). The estimate $\widehat{b}_1 = -11.942$ is an average of the two differences between averages for overweight and normal weight: $30.613 - 41.167 = -10.554$ in Poland and $42.804 - 56.138 = -13.334$ in Ireland, *weighted according to group size*. Similarly, $\widehat{b}_2 = 12.990$ is a weighted average of the differences between averages for Ireland and Poland: $56.138 - 41.167 = 14.971$ among normal weight women and $42.804 - 30.613 = 12.191$ among overweight women. The fact that these differences in rows and columns, respectively, are not very different suggests that the *additive* model (1.4.4) provides a satisfactory fit to the data and, hence, there seems to be *no interaction* between country and BMI. We return to a more careful evaluation of this in Section 5.2.1.

We can also illustrate the concept of *confounding* by comparing these mutually adjusted effects of BMI ($\widehat{b}_1 = -11.942$) and country ($\widehat{b}_2 = 12.990$) with the corresponding unadjusted estimates. For BMI the latter is the difference between the "marginal averages": $34.520 - 49.722 = -15.201$ and for country it is the difference $48.005 - 32.561 = 15.444$. The difference between the adjusted and unadjusted estimates is due to confounding and we can say that the unadjusted effect of BMI "does not provide a fair comparison" between overweight and normal weight women because of the influence of country: the group of overweight women is dominated by the women from Poland (Polish women constitute $53/(53 + 25) = 68\%$ of the overweight women and only $12/(12 + 16) = 43\%$ of the normal weight women) and the Polish women tend to have lower 25OHD-values than the Irish. Therefore the adjusted BMI estimate is smaller in absolute terms than the unadjusted. We can interpret the change in the estimated effect of country similarly. However, the differences are not great so there is not much confounding in this example.

Table 1.4.2. Average 25OHD values (and number of women) in four groups defined acccording to country and BMI.

	Normal weight	Overweight	Total
Poland	41.167 (12)	30.613 (53)	32.561 (65)
Ireland	56.138 (16)	42.804 (25)	48.005 (41)
Total	49.722 (28)	34.520 (78)	38.536 (106)

If we replace the binary $I(x_{i,1} \geq 25)$ by the quantitative explanatory variable $x_{i,1}$ (BMI for woman i) and study a model including this variable and country $x_{i,2}$, we get the following expression for the expected value of vitamin D for woman i:

$$E(y_i) = a + b_1 x_{i,1} + b_2 x_{i,2}. \tag{1.4.5}$$

Considering two women with the same BMI $x_{i,1}$, one from Ireland (i.e., with $x_{i,2} = 1$), and one from Poland ($x_{i,2} = 0$) the difference between their expected y-values is

$$a + b_1 x_{i,1} + b_2 - (a + b_1 x_{i,1}) = b_2$$

no matter the value of $x_{i,1}$. That is, b_2 is again the effect of country (Ireland versus Poland) adjusted for BMI. Similarly, b_1 is the difference in expected vitamin D value for two women *from the same country* whose BMIs differ by 1 unit (kg/m^2). Note that this is true for women from Ireland as well as for women from Poland; also in model (1.4.5) there is *no interaction* between country and body mass index. The effect of country does not depend on the level of BMI and vice versa.

Fitting the model (1.4.5) to the data from Example 1.1 we find the estimates $\hat{a} = 70.156, \hat{b}_1 = -1.299, \hat{b}_2 = 12.084$. The expected y-values in this model can be displayed graphically as done in Figure 1.4.1. We see that the two lines are *parallel*, both with slope $\hat{b}_1 = -1.299$, and with (constant) vertical distance $\hat{b}_2 = 12.084$. The intercepts for the two lines are $\hat{a} = 70.156$ (for the line corresponding to women from Poland) and $\hat{a} + \hat{b}_2 = 82.240$ (for the line corresponding to Irish women), respectively. As in Section 1.2 it may be advantageous to reparametrize the model to obtain an intercept corresponding to the expected 25OHD value for a sensible BMI value, for example 25 kg/m^2 instead of 0. Such a reparametrization does not affect the estimates of b_1 and b_2 but the estimate of the intercept in the reparametrized model becomes $\hat{a} + 25\hat{b}_1 = 70.156 - 25 \cdot 1.299 = 37.681$ and has the interpretation as the expected 25OHD value among Polish women with a BMI of 25.

Again, we can illustrate the concept of confounding by comparing with unadjusted estimates. For country this is (again) 15.446 whereas for BMI it is -1.698, both numerically slightly larger than the unadjusted effects as explained when studying the model with two binary covariates.

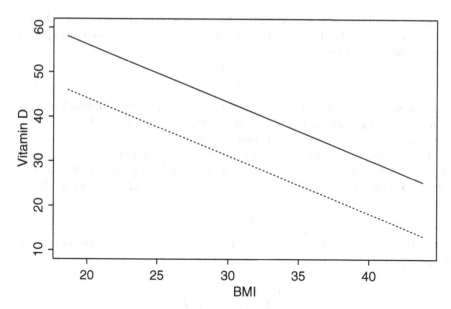

Fig. 1.4.1. Expected values from the model (1.4.5): two parallel lines with slope b_1 and vertical distance b_2. Dashed curve is for Ireland, solid for Poland.

The assumption of no interaction is crucial and in actual data analysis it is often important to examine the hypothesis more closely. In Section 5.2.2 we return to a closer discussion of the concept of interaction in multiple regression models.

We have presented linear regression models with two binary explanatory variables (1.4.4) and with one binary and one quantitative explanatory variable (1.4.5) and we have seen that a consequence of simply adding the terms for each variable is a model with no interaction between the two variables. We have also seen consequences of potential confounding by comparing adjusted and unadjusted estimates. In a similar vein we could study linear models for the log(odds) of a binary outcome and for the log(hazard rate) for a survival time outcome. In both cases, terms for the explanatory variables can be added leading to models where there is no interaction and where the effects of the variables are mutually adjusted. Also, for all types of outcome variables, other kinds of explanatory variables can be combined in multiple regression models by adding their corresponding terms. This includes general categorical and quantitative covariates.

This leads us to a way of building *regression models*. When we want to relate the distribution of a single outcome variable y_i to explanatory variables $x_{i,1}, \ldots, x_{i,n_c}$ for subject i, terms $b_j x_{i,j}$ (or $b_j f(x_{i,j})$ for some transformation, $f(\cdot)$ when x_j is used in a transformed fashion) are added to a common intercept, a. Each term then depends on a separate *regression parameter* (or *regression coefficient*) b_j. Common to the models obtained in this way is their *linear* structure because an expression that is linear in the parameters is obtained. This is the kind of model we study in the rest of this book and for all models the expression

$$LP_i = a + b_1 x_{i,1} + b_2 x_{i,2} + \cdots + b_{n_c} x_{i,n_c} \tag{1.4.6}$$

is denoted the *linear predictor* for individual i. The regression coefficient b_j is also denoted the *effect* of $x_{i,j}$ although, as we discuss in the next section, this terminology should be used with some caution.

Depending on the type of response the linear predictor (1.4.6) is then *linked* to the distribution of the outcome variable using the proper link function. Thus, for a quantitative outcome y (possibly transformed; see Section 1.3) we typically have

$$E(y_i) = LP_i,$$

(i.e., "the link is the *identity* function"), whereas for a binary y the link is the log(odds) ℓ_i; that is,

$$\ell_i = \log\left(\frac{\mathrm{pr}(y_i = 1)}{1 - \mathrm{pr}(y_i = 1)}\right) = LP_i.$$

For a survival time y the linear predictor will depend on time t, and $LP_i(t)$ is introduced via the log(hazard rate)

$$l_i(t) \approx \log(\frac{1}{dt}\mathrm{pr}(t < y_i < t + dt \mid y_i > t) = LP_i(t).$$

Here, the linear predictor is

$$LP_i(t) = \log(h_0(t)) + b_1 x_{i,1} + b_2 x_{i,2} + \cdots + b_{n_c} x_{i,n_c}$$

where "the intercept a" in (1.4.6) is now the log(baseline hazard rate) $\log(h_0(t))$ as explained in Section 1.3.

1.4.2 Regression models and their interpretation

The word "effect" introduced in the previous section should be used with some caution because the regression models under study do not necessarily allow us to make "causal" interpretations of the results. We can take gender as an example of a very common explanatory variable that is observable, but not controllable. This means that whenever we study sex differences for the distribution of a particular outcome variable, we must be aware that men and women differ in a lot of respects that may or may not account for the sex difference for this particular outcome. If we mean to quantify the sex difference as such, we should include no such "intermediate covariates" in the model. However, if we want to see whether, for example, height, is the true cause of the difference and gender only appears important because of its obvious relation to height then we are in a situation where both covariates should be taken into account simultaneously.

On the other hand, in a clinical trial where two or more treatments are compared we have an example of an explanatory variable, treatment, which can be controlled in the sense that the experimenter can decide which patients are to receive which treatment. Such a subjective choice is not advisable because it will almost inevitably lead to selection differences in the treatment groups (differences in stage of illness, age, etc.) causing possible bias in the treatment comparisons. Instead, it is common practice to *randomize* patients to the treatment groups in order to ensure that the groups become comparable. An example of such a situation is provided by the PBC-3 study in Example 1.3. Any differences (apart from the treatment itself) that may be present after (proper) randomization may be ascribed to chance and for large group sizes, such differences will therefore on average be small. This ensures that a simple comparison between treatment groups (i.e., with treatment group as the only covariate) will be valid and will even allow us to make causal interpretations. However, inclusion of other explanatory variables in the model may still often be advisable, for example, if a study is not sufficiently large to ensure identical covariate distributions among the treatment groups or, more important, at least for quantitative outcomes, to reduce the unexplained variation and thereby obtain increased precision for the estimation of treatment differences.

This leads us to a discussion of the different scientific purposes for performing a regression analysis. One such purpose could be a simple prediction: given a number of potential explanatory variables, how well are we then able to predict the outcome? In such a case the interpretation of a single "effect" is not crucial; it is merely the joint contribution of all predictors that matters. In our discussion of models in subsequent chapters, in particular in Chapter 6, prediction is *not* what we primarily have in mind. In fact, for the purpose of pure prediction, a number of other approaches (including neural nets and classification trees; see e.g. Hastie, Tibshirani, and Friedman, 2001, Ch. 9 and 11) may be superior to the kinds of linear models that are our focus, although models with a linear predictor have the advantage of providing a simple and explicit "prediction rule."

A second major purpose of a regression analysis is to *understand* a relationship between one or few explanatory variables and the outcome. However, to obtain an accurate estimate of such a relationship it is often necessary to account for a number of other covariates, the effects of which are not of primary interest. Such a point of view is the core of most observational studies in epidemiology. Here, interest frequently focuses on an *exposure* variable, such as fever in early pregnancy in the study introduced in Example 1.2. However, due to the observational design where, obviously, exposure groups are not randomized, a number of *confounding factors* must be taken into consideration in order to obtain a "fair" comparison between exposure categories. This is the kind of situation which we will often have in mind when discussing regression models in the following.

Digression. The word "regression"

Finally, a brief remark on the term "regression" itself; why is a word meaning "decline" attached to this extremely common analytical approach to statistics? The explanation seems to date back to Francis Galton (1822–1911) who noticed a tendency to "mediocrity" (i.e., "more like average") in the offspring compared to the parents. In particular he, and later Karl Pearson, observed that the height of sons whose fathers were very tall tended to be closer to the mean height and similarly for sons of fathers with small heights. This situation of "regression towards the mean" is still an important one in many studies, however, the word also seems to be stuck to the kind of models that we work with in this book; see for example, Farewell (2005). ◇

1.5 Further examples

In this section, more examples used for illustration in subsequent chapters are introduced.

Example 1.4. Surgery complications

The study conducted by Berg et al. (1997) was concerned with postsurgery pulmonary complications. The investigation included 691 patients undergoing either orthopedic, gynecological or abdominal surgery. The number of complications in the three groups (the actual counts as well as the percentage of the corresponding group) are shown in Table 1.5.1.

Table 1.5.1. Complications in relation to type of surgery.

Operation Type	Complications No	Yes	Total	%
Orthopedic	200	6	206	2.9
Gynecological	235	5	240	2.1
Abdominal	210	35	245	14.3
Total	645	46	691	6.7

This table suggests that abdominal surgery is more subject to complications than the other types of surgery. However, for each patient we have additional information about age and duration of anesthesia, and these may account for some of the discrepancy, inasmuch as abdominal patients may be older and the surgery may last longer.

The main purpose of the study, however, was to determine whether some types of neuromuscular blocking agents (NBA) were more prone to complications than others. Furthermore, it was of interest to know whether residual neuromuscular block (RNB, here quantified by the "TOF-ratio", a measure of neuromuscular function) was a mediating risk factor in this connection.

This example is used as an illustration in Sections 3.1.2, 3.2.2, and 6.2.2.

Example 1.5. Fatty acids

An experiment studying lymphatic absorption of fatty acids was conducted (Fruekilde and Høy, 2004) by feeding 40 rats with different dairy products. The rats were subdivided into five groups and each group was fed one specific dairy product (I: cream cheese, II: sour cream, III: cream, IV: mixed butter, V: butter). The rats were fed at time 0 and, after 8 hours, the accumulated lymphatic absorption of fatty acids (in mg) was measured.

The aim of the experiment was to study the effect of diet on uptake of fatty acids. We may get a first idea about the possible differences by simply looking at a scatterplot of accumulated lymphatic absorption versus diet type, as seen in Figure 1.5.1. The absorption of mixed butter and butter (products 4 and 5) seems to be at a lower level than the other three types of fatty acids.

This example is used as illustration in Section 3.2.1.

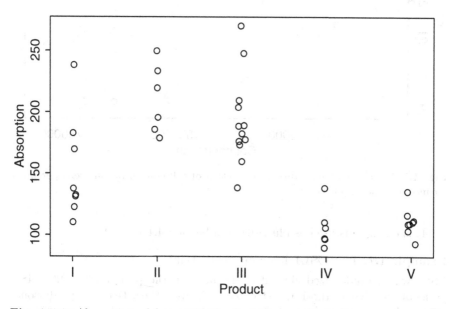

Fig. 1.5.1. Absorption of fatty acids for five dairy products, I: cream cheese, II: sour cream, III: cream, IV: mixed butter, V: butter.

Example 1.6. Cell concentration of tetrahymena

In an experiment with the unicellar organism tetrahymena (Hellung-Larsen et al., 1990), we are interested in determining how cell concentration (number of cells in 1 mL of the growth media) may affect the cell size (average cell diameter, measured in μm).

Moreover, the effect of adding glucose to the growth media is investigated, by studying 19 cell cultures with no glucose added and comparing to 32 cell cultures grown with glucose added. The relation between cell size and cell concentration for the group without glucose is seen in Figure 1.5.2. We note that the effect of an increased concentration is to decrease cell size and that this effect diminishes for large concentrations leading to an apparent nonlinear relationship between cell concentration and cell size.

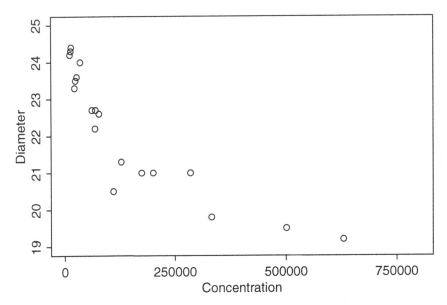

Fig. 1.5.2. Cell diameter (μm) as a function of cell concentration (cells per mL) for media without glucose.

This example is used as illustration in Section 4.1.1.

Example 1.7. The CSL1 liver cirrhosis trial

CSL1 was a randomized clinical trial where, in the period 1962–1969, 488 patients with liver cirrhosis were treated with either the active drug prednisone (251 patients) or placebo (237 patients) (Copenhagen Study Group for liver diseases, 1969; Schlichting et al., 1983). After randomization patients were followed to either death, drop-out, or end of study (September, 1974): 142 prednisone patients and 150 placebo patients died. The survival times for the remaining patients are right-censored. An important prognostic factor for these patients is ascites, that is, excess fluid in the abdomen. The presence of ascites at entry was recorded as absent, slight, or moderate/marked. The numbers of patients and deaths are given in Table 1.5.2. The fraction of deaths is seen to increase with the amount of ascites whereas the treatment seems to have a minor influence on mortality.

Table 1.5.2. CSL1 trial: number of patients (% deaths) in six treatment by ascites groups.

		Ascites		
Treatment	No	Slight	Moderate/Marked	Total
Prednisone	191 (49%)	34 (71%)	26 (92%)	251 (57%)
Placebo	195 (60%)	20 (75%)	22 (82%)	237 (63%)
Total	386 (55%)	54 (72%)	48 (88%)	488 (60%)

This example is used as illustration in Sections 5.2.1, 5.2.4, and 5.3.2.

Example 1.8. Birthweight and ultrasound measurements

The birth weight (BW) in grams for 107 babies was ascertained. For all babies, both the abdominal (AD) and biparietal (BPD) diameters (in mm) were measured shortly before birth using ultrasound (Secher et al., 1987). The purpose of this study was to describe the relationship between birthweight and these two ultrasound measurements in order to establish a way to predict birthweight (or fetus weight). For a preliminary examination, Figures 1.5.3 and 1.5.4 show the scatterplots of birthweight versus AD and BPD, respectively. It is seen that birthweight, as expected, increases with both of the measured diameters.

This example is used as an illustration in Sections 5.1.3 and 5.2.3.

Example 1.9. Identifying markers for liver fibrosis

For patients with liver diseases, an important part of the diagnostic procedure can be to quantify the degree of liver fibrosis. However, this requires a liver biopsy which is an invasive and time-demanding procedure with potentially serious side effects. It would therefore be advantageous to replace such a biopsy with something simpler, preferably some markers that may be quantified from blood samples.

An investigation was carried out by Nøjgaard et al. (2003) among 127 patients with liver problems. Based on a liver biopsy, the degree of fibrosis was determined on a four-point scale (0: "no," 1: "slight," 2: "modest," 3: "severe" occurrence of granulation tissue) and from blood samples, three different markers: "hyaluronan" (ha), "type III procollagen peptide" (p3np), and "human cartilage glycoprotein 39" (ykl40) were measured. The task is to use

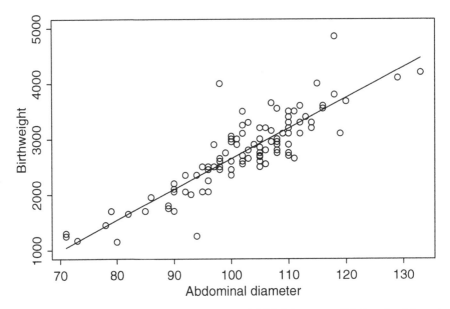

Fig. 1.5.3. Birthweight study: scatterplot of BW (g) versus AD (mm) with estimated regression line.

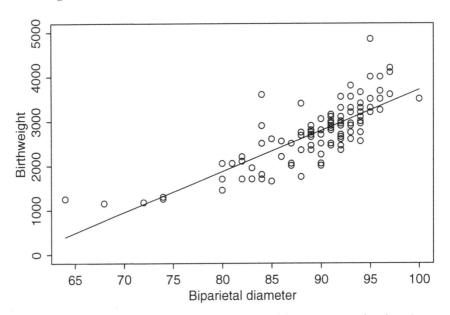

Fig. 1.5.4. Birthweight study: scatterplot of BW (g) versus BPD (mm) with estimated regression line.

one or more of these markers to predict the degree of fibrosis, so that in the future, a liver biopsy may be replaced by a simple blood test. A preliminary look at the data is presented in Table 1.5.3 as medians and ranges, subdivided according to the degree of fibrosis. The levels of all three markers seem to increase with the degree of fibrosis.

Table 1.5.3. Median of blood markers in the four fibrosis groups.

Degree of Fibrosis	Count	ha	Median (Range) p3np	ykl40
0	27	27.5 (21.0–126.0)	5.00 (1.7–25.0)	174.0 (50.0–408.0)
1	40	42.0 (25.0–2920.0)	5.90 (2.6–27.0)	270.0 (111.0–967.0)
2	42	211.5 (25.0–3060.0)	15.85 (3.8–62.0)	466.0 (82.0–2430.0)
3	20	242.5 (105.0–4730.0)	14.55 (8.2–70.0)	676.0 (180.0–4850.0)

This example is used as an illustration in Section 7.1.

Example 1.10. Survival with malignant melanoma

In the period 1962–1977, 205 patients with malignant melanoma (cancer of the skin) had a radical operation performed at Odense University Hospital, Denmark (Drzewiecki and Andersen, 1982). All patients were followed until the end of 1977 by which time 134 were still alive and 71 had died (out of whom 57 had died from cancer and 14 from other causes).

The object of the study was to assess the effect of risk factors on survival. Among such risk factors were the sex and age of the patients and the histological variables tumor thickness and ulceration (absent versus present). For a preliminary presentation of the data, Table 1.5.4 shows the number of patients and the number of deaths according to thickness and ulceration. It is seen that the fraction of deaths seems to increase with thickness and with presence of ulceration.

Table 1.5.4. Number of deaths/number of patients (%) by thickness and ulceration for the malignant melanoma survival data.

Thickness	0–2 mm	2–5 mm	5+ mm
Ulceration absent	14/87 (16%)	7/21 (33%)	2/7 (29%)
Ulceration present	6/22 (27%)	26/43 (60%)	16/25 (64%)

This example is used as an illustration in Sections 7.5 and 8.1.3.

Example 1.11. Cardiac output

Measuring cardiac output requires an invasive procedure and to minimize discomfort for the patients, the time involved in the measuring process should be minimized. However, the precision of the measurement is important and several consecutive measurements are needed in order to limit the estimation uncertainty.

An investigation was carried out by Nilsson et al. (2004) in order to study the number of measurements required, and to determine possible explanatory variables for the standard deviation of the measurements. The study involved 80 patients, who each had eight consecutive measurements of cardiac output (in L/min) taken (except for a single patient where one observation is missing for technical reasons). One additional measurement was deleted because of an obvious error in measurement.

A within-patient standard deviation based on the eight consequtive measurements was calculated for each patient and in Figure 1.5.5 these are plotted against the corresponding average value of cardiac output.

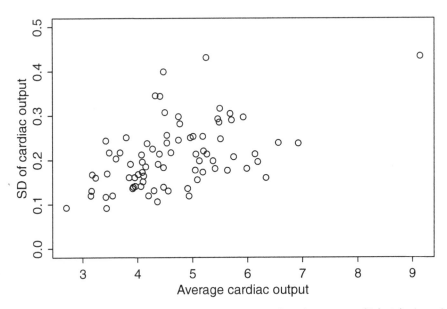

Fig. 1.5.5. SD of eight consecutive measurements of cardiac output (L/min) plotted against the mean.

This example is used as an illustration in Section 7.3.

Example 1.12. Tryptase and allergic reactions

Tryptase is found in mast cells in the human body and all individuals have a baseline level of tryptase in the blood (serum tryptase). The tryptase level can increase in connection with severe allergic reactions and is used to confirm these reactions.

Garvey et al. (2010a,b) conducted investigations of serum tryptase with the following purposes.

- To determine possible predictors for the baseline level of serum tryptase
- To determine the effect of general anesthesia and surgery on serum tryptase
- To investigate possible increases in serum tryptase in patients with suspected allergic reactions during anesthesia

In one study (study 1) serum tryptase was measured in 120 patients immediately before and after orthopedic surgery in general anesthesia. None of these patients experienced any signs of allergy during anesthesia. For these patients, age, sex, and physical status (according to the ASA classification) is known. Figure 1.5.6 shows the tryptase values after surgery plotted against those before.

A second study (study 2) concerns patients with a suspected allergic reaction during anesthesia. For these patients, a blood sample for serum tryptase is measured 1–4 hours after the reaction and a baseline level is taken after more than 24 hours when the suspected allergic reaction has disappeared. For these patients, we have additional information regarding the severity of the reaction (1: mild, 2: more serious, 3: severe life-threatening reaction (anaphylactic shock), 4: cardiac arrest) and information on the result of subsequent allergy testing (0: negative, 1: positive).

The "before surgery" values from study 1 and the after 24-hour values for the suspected allergy patients in study 2 can be treated as baseline tryptase measurements. The values measured after surgery in study 1 can be used for studying the effect of surgery and anesthesia (an expected decrease due to dilution), whereas the values measured after the suspected allergic reaction in study 2 can be thought of as a combined effect of dilution and a possible allergic reaction.

These data are mostly used for exercises in the book and to ease data handling, they have been organized as three datasets as follows.

1. Before and after tryptase values for 120 orthopedic patients with no suspected allergic reaction (study 1).
2. Tryptase values taken in connection with a suspected allergic reaction for 318 patients undergoing various kinds of surgery. This dataset also includes subsequent baseline values (study 2).
3. Baseline tryptase values for 438 patients (study 1 and 2 combined).

This example is used as an illustration in Section 5.4.

1.6 The scope of this book and how to read it

This section summarizes how the rest of the book is organized and at the same time it provides some guidance on how to read it. Some sections are more

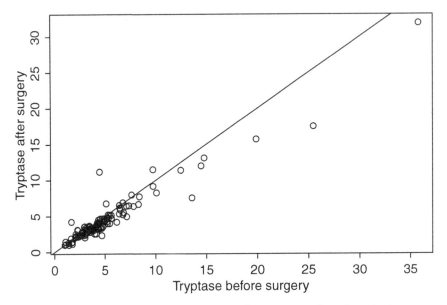

Fig. 1.5.6. Tryptase data: measurements after surgery plotted against measurements before; the line is the identity line.

difficult to read than others, simply because they deal with more complicated topics. Recall from the preface that our main readership is intended to be researchers from scientific areas where statistics are being used as a tool. However, it is our hope that also people with a more mathematical background who wish to enter into the field of biostatistics will benefit from using the book, for example, for self-study.

Chapter 2 first presents a review of background material on the principles of probability and distributions. Some of the material covered may be familiar to some readers but we have chosen to present it for completeness. Next follow sections on descriptive statistics and on statistical inference. The latter has separate subsections presenting the main ideas for the three steps of inference: estimation, model checking, and hypothesis tests. This section concludes with a subsection on the most important principle for inference, the likelihood principle. That subsection is more difficult to read than the rest of Chapter 2 as it contains more mathematical details. It may be skipped without missing the main flow of the book.

In Chapter 3 the simple building blocks for categorical explanatory variables are introduced for the three main types of outcome variable. We first deal with the simplest such covariate with only two levels and, subsequently, we discuss the general case with any number of levels. The chapter explains how simple, perhaps well-known, statistical techniques such as the t-test, the chi-square test for frequency tables, the logrank test for survival data, and others can be considered special cases of regression analysis.

Chapter 4 deals with one quantitative explanatory variable, first when a linear effect can be assumed. As is the previous chapter, Section 4.1 is subdivided according to the three types of outcome variables and the special cases of simple linear, logistic, and Cox proportional hazards regression, respectively, are presented. In Section 4.2 certain models with a quite flexible, nonlinear effect of the covariate (still described by a linear predictor) are introduced. A very common example of such a nonlinear effect is a polynomial but models using "splines" are also discussed. This section is more difficult to read because the models discussed are more complicated than those presented in previous sections.

Having presented the building blocks, Chapter 5 discusses multiple regression models, that is, models with several explanatory variables. For ease of presentation and interpretation we focus on models with two covariates and introduce the concepts of confounding and interaction. We emphasize that, although both of these concepts become relevant when studying multiple covariates, they have absolutely nothing in common. If we study the effect of an explanatory variable x_1 on an outcome y, then confounding by another covariate x_2 means that the effect of x_1 on y differs with or without adjustment for x_2. On the other hand, interaction means that the effect of x_1 on y depends on the value of x_2; that is, the effect varies between x_2-subgroups. We study models with and without interactions for combinations of the two covariates: two categorical, one categorical and one quantitative, and two quantitative. The chapter continues with a brief section discussing models with any number of covariates, introducing the rather technical concept of "higher-order interactions," and concludes with a brief section dealing with the situation where observations are paired or matched.

In Section 6.1 we discuss model-building strategies, in particular selection of explanatory variables for answering a given research question, and principles for model checking. We illustrate these principles in Section 6.2 via three worked examples (Examples 1.1, 1.4, and 1.3), and Chapter 6 concludes with a brief section dealing with sample size determination useful in the planning stage of a study.

Whereas Chapters 3 – 6 primarily deal with examples of linear models for quantitative outcomes, logistic models for binary data, and Cox models for lifetimes, Chapter 7 presents a number of other regression models with a linear predictor. These include the logistic models for ordinal and multinomial data and Poisson-type models for counts. Also models for quantitative, binary, or survival time data with *other link functions* than those studied in Chapters 3–6 are discussed. Sections 7.3 – 7.5 are more technical than most previous sections. Chapter 8 briefly mentions a number of extended models all involving a linear predictor. These include models with more than one response variable per individual, including repeated measurements and other types of correlated outcomes, for example random effect models and models with covariate measurement errors. The treatment of these topics is by no means meant to be exhaustive but serve mainly as a warning that models more complicated than the ones treated in this book occur quite frequently and will produce erroneous conclusions if not analyzed properly.

We conclude with four appendices summarizing: the notation used in the book (Appendix A), the use of logarithms (Appendix B), a number of recommendations otherwise "hidden" in the text (Appendix C), and very simple commands in R, SAS, and STATA for performing analyses like those reviewed in Tables 1.6.1–1.6.2 below (Appendix D).

Examples 1.1 – 1.3 from Section 1.1.1 and Examples 1.4 – 1.12 from Section 1.5 are referred to throughout all chapters. However, only in Section 6.2 are the examples meant to be exhaustive and to cover all aspects of the data analysis whereas, in other sections, the examples are merely meant to illustrate the methods under current discussion. Most chapters end with a section containing exercises dealing with additional analyses of the data from the examples.

We mentioned in Section 1.4.2 that our main motivation for doing regression analysis is to *understand* a relationship between one or a few explanatory variables and the outcome, rather than to make an accurate prediction of the outcome based on a set of explanatory variables. However, this point of view is most important for the discussion of model selection in Chapter 6 and we believe that the methods discussed in other chapters are relevant no matter the purpose of the regression analysis. In that respect, Chapters 3 – 5 constitute the core of the book, introducing the building blocks of a regression model, and Tables 1.6.1 and 1.6.2 summarize those three chapters. Thus, Table 1.6.1 presents, perhaps well-known, names of methods for *simple* regression (i.e., including only one covariate) with references to the relevant sections of Chapters 3 and 4. Table 1.6.2 does the same for *multiple* regression (Chapter 5). As mentioned above, Appendix D presents very simple commands (in R, SAS, and STATA) for doing most of the analyses reviewed in these tables.

A main feature of this book is that Chapters 3 to 5 correspond to *rows* of Tables 1.6.1 and 1.6.2, that is, taking *types of covariates* as a starting point and discussing analyses with various outcome types subsequently. Other books on regression models highlight the *columns* of Tables 1.6.1 and 1.6.2. Thus Hosmer and Lemeshow (2000) and Kleinbaum and Klein (2002) concentrate on logistic regression, Kleinbaum and Klein (2005), Collett (2003), and Kalbfleisch and Prentice (2002) on survival analysis, and Draper and Smith (1998) and Panik (2009) on linear regression. Also more general books, treating more than one class of regression model, tend to divide chapters according to outcome type rather than covariate type. This includes both the more technical books on "generalized linear models" by McCullagh and Nelder (1989) and Dobson (2002) and the more applied book by Vittinghoff et al. (2005). Among the books listed, the latter is probably the one that comes closest in aim and scope to this book.

Table 1.6.1. Overview of methods for simple regression (i.e., including only a single covariate): Chapters 3 and 4.

Explanatory Variable (or Covariate)	Outcome Type		
	Quantitative (e.g., blood pressure)	**Binary** (e.g., complication)	**Survival data** (e.g., time to treatment failure)
Binary (2 categories, e.g., gender)	*Comparison of*		
	two means: t-test	two probabilities: 2×2-table: χ^2-test	two survival curves: logrank test
	(Section 3.1.1)	(Section 3.1.2)	(Section 3.1.3)
Categorical ($k+1$ categories, e.g., treatment groups)	*Comparison of*		
	$k+1$ means: one-way ANOVA	$k+1$ probabilities: $2 \times (k+1)$-table, χ^2-test	$k+1$ survival curves: $k+1$-sample logrank test
	(Section 3.2.1)	(Section 3.2.2)	(Section 3.2.3)
Quantitative (e.g., age)	*Effect of a one-unit increase*		
	on the mean value: linear regression	on the log(odds): logistic regression	on the log(hazard rate): Cox regression
	(Section 4.1.1)	(Section 4.1.2)	(Section 4.1.3)
	Nonlinear terms		
	Categorization, polynomials, splines (Section 4.2)		

Table 1.6.2. Overview of methods for multiple regression (i.e., including several covariates): Chapter 5.

Explanatory Variables or (Covariates)	Outcome Type — Quantitative (e.g., blood pressure)	Binary (e.g., complication)	Survival data (e.g., time to treatment failure)
Generally	multiple linear regression	multiple logistic regression	multiple Cox regression

Specific terminology

Explanatory Variables or (Covariates)	Quantitative	Binary	Survival data
Two (or more) binary or categorical (e.g., gender and treatment)	two-way ANOVA	Mantel–Haenszel test (Section 5.1.1)	stratified logrank test

Comparison of groups, adjusted for a quantitative covariate

Effect of a one-unit increase in a quantitative covariate common to several groups

One quantitative and one binary or categorical (e.g., treatment and age)	analysis of covariance	(Section 5.1.2)	

Effect of one covariate, adjusted for all others

Two quantitative or generally **any number and type** (e.g., age and body mass index)	general linear model (Sections 5.1.3 and 5.3.1)		

With interaction

Comparison of effect of quantitative covariate in different groups

One quantitative and one binary or categorical	analysis of covariance	multiple logistic regression (Sections 5.2.1 and 5.2.2)	

Effect of one covariate, possibly depending on the value of others

Any number and type	Multiple linear regression	multiple logistic regression (Sections 5.2.3, 5.2.4, and 5.3.2)	multiple Cox regression

2

Statistical models

Research begins with theories and hypotheses. For instance, it may have been noted that many people experiencing a stroke tend to have high blood pressure. You get the idea that medication aimed at lowering blood pressure may therefore also reduce the risk of a stroke. However plausible this sounds, it requires an investigation (a study) to confirm or reject this suspicion. For instance, the apparent connection between high blood pressure and stroke may be simply due to the fact that people experience stroke at an older age where blood pressure is also increased and hence that lowering of blood pressure has no effect on the risk of a stroke because it does not change the age of the individual. Thus, empirical studies are needed in order to show which hypotheses are reasonable and which ones have to be abandoned. Studies create observations that show variation (people at identical ages differ in blood pressure, and people with identical blood pressure may or may not experience a stroke). Statistics is the discipline dealing with the interpretation of such observations in the search for overall patterns, for example, a description of the risk of a stroke as a function of age and blood pressure.

In this chapter, we describe the most fundamental mathematical concepts used in this process. We abstain from a thorough treatment that would require a solid mathematical training. We believe that this is not necessary in order to appreciate the ideas and logic behind the most commonly used statistical procedures.

Statistics uses *probabilities* and *probability distributions* to describe variation between the observations and to build models that enable us draw conclusions about the scientific problem in the presence of this variation. These concepts are introduced in Section 2.1.

Having obtained data, the next step is to make relevant summaries (frequencies, averages, etc.) and produce informative plots. Even though the type of data analysis may already have been more or less decided upon before data collection, it is very important not to skip this initial step of getting acquainted with your collected data. This process may reveal data errors or unexpected values that may lead to slight changes in the perspective of the analysis, for example, introducing a safety aspect. These topics are treated in Section 2.2 under the heading *descriptive statistics*.

The models specified for the data will typically contain one or more unknown quantities of interest, called *parameters*, for example, describing the relation (if any) between blood pressure and risk of experiencing a stroke. Analysis of the collected data will aim at deriving informative statements about these, as well as about other parts of the specified model, for example, the distribution. The principles behind data analysis (called *statistical inference*) are the focus of Section 2.3. That section is again subdivided according to the main steps of statistical inference, namely

1. *Model checking*; evaluation of the adequacy of the model to describe the data reasonably
2. *Parameter estimation*; finding the values of the parameters that provide the best model fit, according to some criteria
3. *Hypothesis testing*; to assess whether the data are compatible with simplified models with fewer unknown parameters

Several general principles for parameter estimation and testing exist, by far the most important one being *the likelihood principle*. This principle lies behind most of the procedures used in the remaining chapters and is therefore important to understand. It is described briefly in the introduction to Section 2.3 and this should be sufficient for appreciation of the ideas. Readers interested in a more detailed description of the idea and use of the likelihood function may find this in the separate Section 2.3.4, but material in this section may be skipped with no consequences for understanding the rest of the book.

2.1 Random variables and probability

Few things are certain or identical in all situations or units (a couple of exceptions being that all life must die or that the number of legs in humans or hearts in octopuses is rather constant).

The concept of *probability* expresses uncertainty, using numbers between 0 and 1. These two extremes denote certainty, either that an event will not occur (0) or that it will occur (1). Values between 0 and 1 denote varying degrees of uncertainty, the uncertainty being largest in the case of probabilities around 0.5 (the fifty–fifty situation; we have no idea whatsoever whether the event will occur). For instance, we could be interested in the probability of a pregnant woman experiencing fetal loss in pregnancy, the probability of a woman in Poland having an adequate level of vitamin D (above some fixed threshold) or the probability of surviving ten years or more following treatment of liver cirrhosis. We denote such probabilities as $\text{pr}(\cdots)$, for example, $\text{pr}(\text{fetal loss})$.

Uncertainty and variation are two closely related concepts. The presence of uncertainty implies that units (subjects, animals, etc.) may behave differently even if the circumstances are identical (same country, identical treatments, etc.). When variation is present, we may look for an explanation (a "cause") for the differences. Some characteristics (good health, low blood pressure) are more desirable than others and we may search for predictors of such character- istics with the aim of understanding the relationship and eventually perhaps to be able to perform an intervention to change things to the better.

In statistical terminology, we consider the observations or data as a *sam- ple* from a large (in fact, infinite) population . Hypothetical repetitions of the experiment would lead to similar, but not identical observations. We refer to the uncertain events about to occur (or about to be observed) as *random vari- ables* (random because we cannot predict the outcome before we observe it and variable because the outcomes will in general be different between units). Random variables are typically denoted by y. The collection of possible val- ues for a random variable y is denoted the *sample space.* For instance, in the fetal death Example 1.2, the sample space may be seen as the "values" {no, yes} or converted to *numerical* values, for example, {0,1}. If we instead count the number of fever episodes for each woman, we have the sample space {0, 1, 2, . . .}, because in principle there is no upper limit to the number of possible fever episodes (although we would probably demand a fever episode to have a certain extent so that in practice there *will* be an upper limit). In the vitamin D Example 1.1, as well as in Example 1.3 concerning survival for patients with liver cirrhosis, the sample space is an interval of nonnega- tive numbers (vitamin D level, respectively, years of survival). For remaining lifetime, the obvious lower endpoint is zero (patients dying immediately fol- lowing treatment) whereas the upper endpoint is more uncertain (although most certainly no more than a hundred years). For the vitamin D example, the endpoints are not known, although experts in the field may be able to set some limits. At the very least, we know that vitamin D concentration can- not be negative, so the sample space is restricted to the positive axis. This fact should lead to a consideration as to whether it is necessary to adjust the analyses accordingly, typically by using a logarithmic transformation as mentioned in Section 1.3 and further explained in Appendix B.

Each possible outcome u in the sample space has a certain probability $pr(y = u)$ of occurring. Some will be more probable than others. For instance, in the fetal death Example 1.2, it is most likely to experience no fetal death and in the vitamin D example, it is most likely to have a value in the neighborhood of 30–60 nmol/l. A distribution or a *probability distribution* is a description of the way in which the total probability (which is always 1) is distributed over the sample space (the collection of possible outcome values). This means that to each possible outcome we specify the associated probability. We introduce this concept through a couple of common examples in the subsections that follow.

The expected value of a numerical random variable is defined to be the weighted mean of all possible outcomes, weighted according to the probability of occurrence. We denote the expectation of a random variable y as $E(y)$, that is,

$$m = E(y) = \sum u \operatorname{pr}(y = u), \qquad (2.1.1)$$

where we have used the symbol $\sum$ as representing a sum over all possible values of y (i.e.. all us in the sample space). We also refer to this expectation as the *mean value of y*. Note that the mean has the same units as the variable itself.

The expected value tells us about the general level of the possible outcome values, but it tells us nothing about the amount of variation (variance or standard deviation, defined below). There are several reasons why it is important to have a measure of variation. First of all, it may be of scientific interest in its own right to know whether the phenomenon under study is stable or variable in the population. If it is very stable (number of legs in humans), it may be futile to study group differences, age effects, and so on, whereas a highly variable phenomenon such as vitamin D status suggests the presence of predictors associated with it. Moreover, we need a measure of variation to use for stating the precision of the conclusions that will follow from statistical analyses. For instance, if we claim that alcohol consumption has an impact on the probability of fetal death, we need to quantify this, for example, as a risk ratio, equipped with a measure of precision or uncertainty.

In mathematical terms, the *variance* of a random variable y is defined as the expected squared distance from its mean:

$$s^2 = \operatorname{Var}(y) = E(y - m)^2. \qquad (2.1.2)$$

Because this is a quadratic expression, it has (inexplicable) quadratic units, so for practical use this variance is most often quoted as a *standard deviation* instead. This is simply the square root s of s^2 with units identical to the variable itself; that is,

$$s = \operatorname{SD}(y) = \sqrt{\operatorname{Var}(y)} = \sqrt{E(y - m)^2}. \qquad (2.1.3)$$

The interpretation of variance or equivalently of standard deviation is not as intuitive as for the mean. Whereas the mean is often used and understood as a sort of theoretical average (that we would get as an actual average if we had an unlimited number of observations), the corresponding interpretation of the variance as a theoretical average of squared distance does not help us very much. Also, the practical use of the standard deviation (or variance) will in general depend on the specific distribution for the observations.

In the subsections that follow, we introduce the most common types of distributions, namely the Bernoulli, Binomial, Poisson, and Normal distributions. Other distributions are only briefly mentioned.

2.1.1 The Bernoulli distribution

The simplest situation for illustration of a probability distribution is Example 1.2 concerning fetal death. For each single woman (or, rather, pregnancy), the random variable y can take on only two different values, 0 (no fetal death) and 1 (fetal death). We denote this a *binary variable* or *Bernoulli variable*. The probability distribution in this case simply consists of specifying, for example, the probability p of a 1-outcome, because then the probability of a 0-outcome must be $1 - p$. In this simple case, the parameter p is also the mean value (the expected value) of y so that $E(y) = m = p$. This very simple distribution on the numbers 0 and 1 is known as the *Bernoulli distribution*. The number p is an unknown *parameter*. We can think of it as the fraction of all pregnancies (in the past, now and in the future) resulting in fetal death.

The standard deviation of a Bernoulli variable is $SD(y) = \sqrt{p(1-p)}$, a quantity which as a function of the unknown p looks like an extremely steep hill (in fact, it is the upper part of a circle), as seen in Figure 2.1.1. This reflects the fact that if p is very close to either 0 or 1, we are pretty sure about the outcome previous to observing it (small standard deviation, i.e., low uncertainty), whereas a p close to 0.5 reflects a lot of uncertainty (large standard deviation).

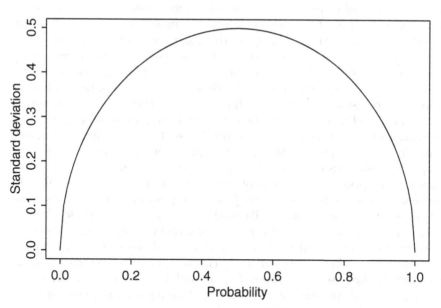

Fig. 2.1.1. The Bernoulli standard deviation $\sqrt{p(1-p)}$ as a function of the unknown p.

2.1.2 The Binomial distribution

In the fetal loss example, a possible predictor for fetal death is the number of fever episodes during early pregnancy (before pregnancy week 17). We might take an interest in this predictor in its own right (i.e., consider it as the response variable of interest) and study the distribution of the number of fever episodes. As long as we limit ourselves to considering only whether such episodes occur at all, we are conceptually in the exact same situation as in Section 2.1.1 concerned with the occurrence of fetal death. However, if we count the number of fever episodes rather than just noting whether any occurred, the probability distribution becomes more complex, because we now have to prescribe the probabilities for all nonnegative integer numbers: $0, 1, 2, \ldots$. In principle, we could introduce parameters $p_0, p_1, p_2, \ldots$ (with the restriction that these should sum to 1) but this would lead to many parameters (in principle infinitely many, if no upper bound to the number of fever episodes is specified) and in practice be untractable and uninformative. Instead, we show below how to use probabilistic (logical) arguments to derive a prescription for these probabilities, involving only a single parameter.

Suppose first that we have an upper limit on the number of fever episodes. To achieve this, let us assume that we count the weeks in which the woman experiences fever. As mentioned in Section 1.1, the average number of pregnancy weeks (before week 17) for the women was close to 14, so we assume here a maximum of 14 fever episodes for each single woman. In practice, this upper limit varies among women, so this fixed value serves only as an approximation. We denote this maximum by c for count, so that here, $c = 14$. Now, for each of the 14 weeks, the probability of a fever episode is denoted p. We assume these probabilities to be identical for all weeks, that is, fever is unrelated to gestational age. If we further assume that fever episodes occur *independently* of each other in different weeks (a disputable assumption that needs investigation in practice), we may calculate the probability of any given number u of fever episodes during a whole pregnancy. If we are talking about u *specific* weeks, this is simply $p^u(1-p)^{c-u}$, because of the assumed independence, because we have u weeks of fever (each with probability p) and the remaining $c - u$ weeks without fever (each with probability $1 - p$). This quantity does not depend on the specific weeks involving a fever episode, thus the only thing left is to figure out the number of ways in which we may choose the u weeks with fever out of the total $c = 14$ weeks of pregnancy. This number is called the *binomial coefficient* (or "c choose u") and is denoted $\binom{c}{u}$. If we let y denote the observed number of weeks with fever episodes during $c = 14$ pregnancy weeks then the total probability of having fever in exactly u weeks therefore becomes

$$P(u) = \operatorname{pr}(y = u) = \binom{c}{u} p^u (1 - p)^{c-u}. \tag{2.1.4}$$

The binomial coefficient $\binom{c}{u}$ may be calculated as $\binom{c}{u} = c!/(u!(c-u)!)$, where $c! = 14!$ denotes the factorial of c, that is, the product $14 \cdot 13 \cdot 12 \cdots 1$.

The distribution (2.1.4) is called the *Binomial distribution* with probability parameter p and count parameter $c = 14$ and is denoted $\text{Bin}(c,p)$. The point probabilities for a Binomial distribution with count parameter 14 and probability $p = 0.015$ (a hypothetical value, indicating a probability of 1.5% for a fever episode in any given week of pregnancy) are illustrated graphically in Figure 2.1.2.

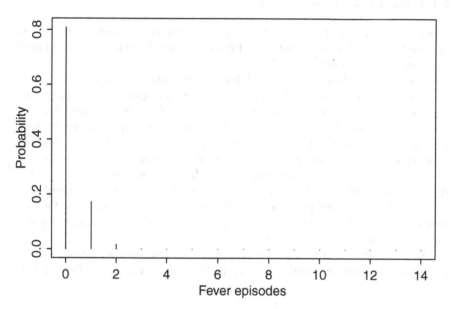

Fig. 2.1.2. The Binomial distribution Bin(14,0.015).

We see that most outcomes have very low probability and that the model predicts the number of fever episodes to be less than three for all practical purposes. This corresponds well with the observed data where only a tiny fraction ($30/11778 = 0.0025$) of the women experienced three or more episodes (cf. Table 1.1.2). Hence, $p = 0.015$ seems to be a plausible value for the unknown parameter.

In the Binomial distribution, the mean and standard deviation are given by

$$E(y) = cp, \text{ SD}(y) = \sqrt{cp(1-p)}.$$

The above specification (2.1.4) of a Binomial distribution constitues a *model* for the number of fever episodes. It may or may not fit the data, but if it fits, it may serve as a mathematical/probabilistic description that is tractable and useful for stating conclusions. Naturally, though, it should be checked in the light of data and rejected if it fails to describe the patterns of data that we see in practice. We deal with principles for model checking later in this chapter, in Section 2.3.2, where we return to this example.

In practice, the binomial coefficent (2.1.4) is cumbersome to calculate especially when the count parameter c gets large. Fortunately, in such situations, approximations to the Binomial distribution exist, namely the *Poisson* distribution (when p is close to either 0 or 1; see Section 2.1.3) and the *Normal* distribution (when p is not close to either 0 or 1; see Section 2.1.4).

2.1.3 The Poisson distribution

When counting the number of fever episodes for each pregnant woman in Section 2.1.2, we had an upper limit for each count, defined as the number of pregnancy weeks before week 17; $c = 14$.

In other situations we may be interested in counts with no well-defined upper limit, such as the number of cancer cases in a specific community during a specific year or the number of metastases following an experimentally induced cancer in laboratory rats. In order to describe such situations we have to specify point probabilities for all nonnegative numbers $(0, 1, \ldots)$. We can do so by thinking of these counts as binomially distributed with an unknown, large count parameter c (corresponding to the number of inhabitants in the specific community or the number of places in the mouse where cancer may occur) and a very small probability p (the probability that a single individual develops cancer during a specific year or the probability of a metastasis in a precisely defined spot on the mouse).

As the count parameter c in a Binomial distribution gets larger and the parameter p gets close to either 0 or 1, the Binomial probabilities from (2.1.4) approximate

$$P(u) = \text{pr}(y = u) = \frac{m^u}{u!} \exp(-m), \tag{2.1.5}$$

where the parameter m is given by the product $m = cp$. The distribution described by the point probabilities 2.1.5 is denoted the *Poisson* distribution. The parameter m is the *mean value*, interpreted as the expected count, and the standard deviation equals $\sqrt{m}$. This approximation to the Binomial distribution is sometimes referred to as the *law of rare events*, referring to p being close to 0. Note that in the case of an abundant event, we might simply shift the definition of an "event" to denote the opposite of before. The approximation will work quite well for combinations like $(p < 0.05, c > 20)$ and $(p < 0.1, c > 100)$. The larger the p, the larger c also has to be for the approximation to be reasonable.

For the number of fever episodes during pregnancy, the count parameter $c = 14$ was somewhat arbitrarily chosen, by defining the number of fever episodes to be the number of weeks in which the woman experienced fever. If we instead regard a fever episode to last only one or two days, c would be larger and the associated probability p of a fever episode in any one of these periods would be smaller. If we can still trust our assumptions regarding independence between fever episodes, we may therefore also describe the number of fever episodes as being Poisson distributed.

Figure 2.1.3 shows the Poisson distribution with mean value $m = 0.21$, chosen to match the mean value in the Binomial distribution from Figure 2.1.2 $(0.21 = 14 \cdot 0.015)$. We see a close resemblance between the two distributions; in fact, we can hardly see a difference at all.

We return to modeling of fever episodes as a Poisson variable in Section 7.2.

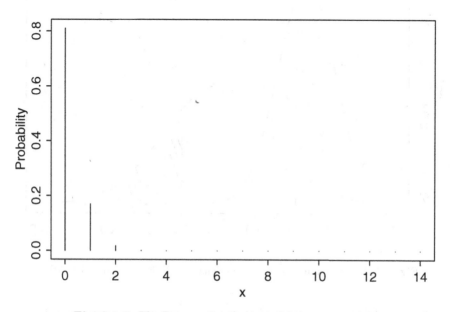

Fig. 2.1.3. The Poisson distribution with mean $m = 0.21$.

2.1.4 The Normal distribution

In the vitamin D Example 1.1 we were interested in the vitamin D levels for women in four European countries. Vitamin D concentration is an example of a quantitative and *continuous* variable, in the sense that any value (in some interval on the positive axis, not needed be specified further) is a possible value for a vitamin D concentration. This means that the sample space for vitamin D concentration is an interval on the positive axis and the distribution of vitamin D therefore in principle has to describe the probability for each single value in this interval. This would involve uncountably many values, therefore we instead specify a *probability density* (or just a *density*) as a function on the sample space, that expresses the expected denseness of observations around each value.

By far the most common distribution for continuous quantitative variables is the *Normal distribution* (also often called the *Gaussian distribution*). The sample space of the Normal distribution is not limited to the nonnegative integers but rather covers all numbers, nonintegers as well as integers, negative values as well as positive values.

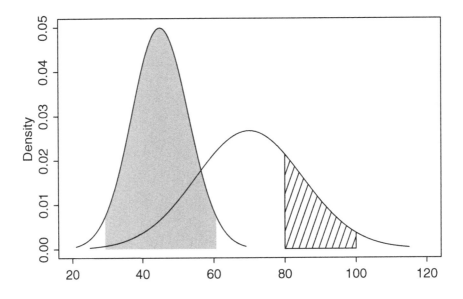

Fig. 2.1.4. Two examples of normal densities, $N(45, 8^2)$ and $N(70, 15^2)$.

Figure 2.1.4 shows examples of densities corresponding to Normal distributions with various means and standard deviations (e.g., densities corresponding to vitamin D concentrations for women in two hypothetical countries). The densities determine the probability of any given interval (e.g., values between 80 and 100) as the area below the curve in this interval (the hatched area for the rightmost density in Figure 2.1.4). The Normal distribution is seen to have a symmetrical, bell-shaped appearance, with its mean m (the expectation) in the center and with tails that approach 0 at a rate determined by the standard deviation SD, often denoted by s. The density is denoted $N(m, s^2)$. The larger the standard deviation, the heavier the tails are, that is, the wider is the distribution. In fact, we can give a precise definition of standard deviation in relation to the density, inasmuch as the interval

$$(E(y) - 1.96\,SD(y), E(y) + 1.96\,SD(y)) \tag{2.1.6}$$

covers approximately 95% of the probability mass, that is, an area of 0.95, shown as the shaded area in the leftmost density of Figure 2.1.4.

The Normal distribution may serve as an approximation to the Binomial distribution in situations where the probability p of a particular event is not too close to either 0 or 1. For instance, assume that we perform a study among subjects with asthma and ask them about the number of days in a specific month that they have had to take asthma medicine. If we fix the probability (for having a need for asthma medicine on a particular day) arbitrarily to 0.3, we would get a distribution like the one in Figure 2.1.5.

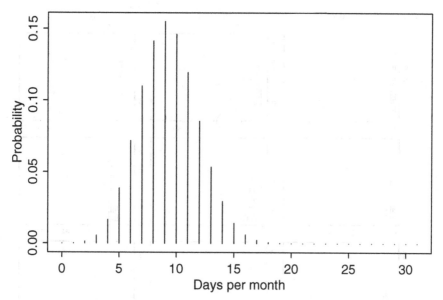

Fig. 2.1.5. Hypothetical distribution for frequency of asthma medication, Bin(31,$p = 0.3$).

Comparing Figures 2.1.4 and 2.1.5, we see that the number of asthma episodes may well be approximated by a Normal distribution. This approximation is based on a probabilistic result referred to as the *Central Limit Theorem* . In brief, this theorem says that a sum (or average) of many "well-behaved" independent quantities will have a distribution resembling the Normal. Because the Binomial variable as introduced above was exactly of the form "a sum of many independent, identically distributed quantities" (a sum of binary variables indicating fever episodes in each specific week of pregnancy, or the need to take asthma medicine on each day in a given period), it follows from this theorem that the Normal distribution may in "well-behaved" cases be used as an approximation to a Binomial distribution. The term "well-behaved" refers to a demand that the products cp as well as $c(1 - p)$ (the

expected counts of zeroes and ones, respectively) are both sufficiently large
(at least 5–10, according to the desired closeness of approximation). Figure
2.1.6 shows examples of Binomial distributions that illustrate the approximation of the Normal distribution. Each row of pictures corresponds to identical
count parameters, but varying probabilities $p = (0.2, 0.5, 0.8)$. The count parameters are chosen as $c = (5, 10, 20, 50)$. Note that a Normal approximation
for modeling the number of fever episodes during pregnancy is *not* warranted,
because the expected number of episodes is only around 0.21, that is, far below
the required threshold of 5–10.

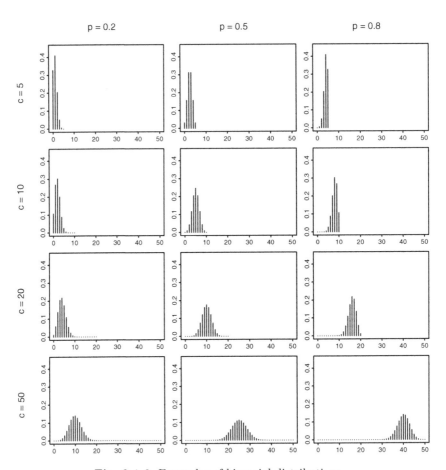

Fig. 2.1.6. Examples of binomial distributions.

2.1.5 Other common distributions

indexdistribution!MultinomialIn the above Subsections 2.1.1 – 2.1.4, we described three discrete distributions (Bernoulli, Binomial, and Poisson) and one continuous (Normal). These are the distributions most often used to describe response variables. In this subsection, we introduce a few more that are also used in subsequent chapters. The *Multinomial* distribution is a discrete distribution used for classifications into more than two categories, (e.g., degree of pain on four levels: no pain, moderate pain, heavy pain, and unbearable pain) or choice of health plan among three different possibilities (A, B, and C, say). The former is an example of an *ordinal* variable (an ordered categorical variable, inasmuch as pain has a natural ordering by severity) whereas the latter is an example of a *nominal* (unordered) categorical variable. In both situations, in the case of $k+1$ categories, $0, 1, \ldots, k$, we specify the distribution through the probabilities $p_1, \ldots, p_k$ of categories $1, \ldots, k$ and the probability of category 0, p_0, is defined so that the sum is 1.

The Multinomial distribution may be seen as a generalization of the Binomial distribution, because focusing on any given category (i.e., considering the outcome to be the number of occurrences in this particular category) will lead to a Binomial distribution. We discuss models for Multinomial data in Section 7.1.

The only distribution for continuous data considered so far is the Normal distribution. As mentioned, this distribution has positive probability for all values, negative as well as positive. Therefore, in principle, it is theoretically unjustified to use it for random variables that can take only positive values and such positive (or at least nonnegative) variables are abundant in applied contexts such as medicine, economics, and even physics. For variables such as birthweight of babies or blood pressure among 40-year-old women, the Normal distribution may still serve as a very good description because for all practical purposes, the probability mass below zero will be negligible. For a variable such as blood concentration of some hormone, however, the Normal distribution may be a very poor description, inasmuch as most values will be very small (close to zero, perhaps even truly zero, but never negative), whereas a few will be rather large. The distribution used to describe such data should therefore not be symmetrical.

To describe nonsymmetrical *skewed* data, we briefly mention the following possibilities

- The log-Normal distribution:
  A logarithmic transformation of the data follows a Normal distribution. We use logarithmic transformations in several examples throughout the book, for example in Chapters 3, 4, and 7 (see also Appendix B).
- The Weibull distribution:
  Derived to describe the distribution of particle sizes, but most commonly used for survival data because of its flexibility to model increasing as well

as decreasing hazard rates over time. We deal with this distribution in Section 7.5.

- The Exponential distribution:
  A specific form of the Weibull distribution assuming constant failure rate and, therefore, some times used to model waiting times.
- The Gamma distribution:
  A family of distributions including the Exponential as well as the Chi-squared distributions that appear in connection with variances. We deal with models of this kind in Section 7.3.

2.1.6 Conditional probability

In all the above subsections, we have been concerned with probability distributions that may be used as theoretical models for the variation in the response variable under consideration, for example, the occurrence of fetal death (Bernoulli), the number of fever episodes during pregnancy (Binomial or Poisson), or the level of vitamin D (Normal).

However, most often, in fact nearly always, the observed quantities will appear to have distributions that are rather mixtures of such distributions, for example, a mixture of Binomial distributions with different ps (corresponding to, e.g., different alcohol groups) or a mixture of several Normal distributions (levels of vitamin D in different countries). We express this by saying that the *conditional probability* of a certain outcome y, *given* the value of a covariate x (or many such covariates) can be described by a certain probability distribution. We use the notation $pr(y \mid x)$ for such a conditional probability (e.g., pr(fetal loss | alcohol consumption)) or pr(vitamin D < 30 | overweight Irish woman).

The conditional probability of fetal loss given either none, moderate, or high alcohol consumption may be described as a Binomial distribution, in which the parameter p depends on the alcohol consumption, that is, varies between the three subgroups,

$$pr(\text{fetal loss} \mid \text{alcohol consumption group } j) = p_j.$$

In the vitamin D example, we may specify that the conditional distribution of the vitamin D level given the country is a Normal distribution, with parameters (mean and standard deviation) that depend on the specific country. If we condition also on the body mass index, we could even specify the mean to depend linearly on some function of body mass index.

Actually, this whole book can be said to be concerned with specification of conditional probability distributions and in particular how aspects of these distributions (e.g., mean value, the probability of a specific event, or the hazard rate) relate to various explanatory variables through a link function and a linear predictor.

2.2 Descriptive statistics

Even before data collection we may have certain ideas concerning the distribution of the response variable in question. At least we know what kind of response (categorical, counts, or continuous) we are dealing with and we have some ideas about relationships of interest between the response variable and possible explanatory variables.

Nevertheless, it is important to make informative plots and calculate key statistics before undertaking the actual data analysis, partly to become acquainted with the data and detect abnormalities of any kind and partly to get an initial idea of possible patterns in the data. This initial step in data analysis is known as *descriptive analysis* and although the basic principles for this are universal, the precise contents depend on the nature of the variables.

This section is therefore subdivided in three, according to the type of the outcome variable: categorical, quantitative, and survival time.

2.2.1 Binary outcome

So far, the categorical variable that we have mainly focused on is very simple, namely a Bernoulli variable taking only values 0 (no fetal loss) and 1 (fetal loss). The obvious way to summarize this variable is of course to sum up the number of 0s and 1s and possibly present these sums in a (very simple) table. We see this information as the margin of Table 2.2.1 which just tells us that 119 pregnancies resulted in fetal loss whereas 11,659 did not.

Table 2.2.1. Distribution of fetal death by number of fever episodes before pregnancy week 17 in 11,778 women recruited to the Danish National Birth Cohort Study.

Fetal Death	Number of Fever Episodes				
	0	1	2	3+	Total
No	9595	1852	182	30	11659
Yes	98	20	1	0	119
Total	9693	1872	183	30	11778
Yes, in %	1.01	1.07	0.55	0	1.01

If our only aim were to count the number of failed pregnancies, we would hardly present it as a table and descriptive statistics in this setting would simply consist of the numbers 11,659 and 119, or the proportion 111/11,778, often expressed as the percentage 1.01%. For research purposes, we are typically more interested in studying the conditional distribution of fetal loss (as introduced in Section 2.1.6), given some explanatory variable such as the number of fever episodes during pregnancy. The body of Table 2.2.1 illustrates this conditional distribution through observed counts of fetal deaths in each group separately (groups being defined by the number of fever episodes in early pregnancy). In the absence of any other relevant explanatory variables for the probability of fetal loss, this table summarizes all the relevant information available from our study. To facilitate interpretation, the table also contains percentages computed within the columns because we are interested in the conditional distribution of fetal loss, given the number of fever episodes.

Small tables such as Table 2.2.1 are clear in their message simply because of their small size. For larger tables and in situations where the explanatory variable is quantitative, it can be an advantage to present the information in graphical form. For instance, if we relate fetal loss to alcohol consumption instead, we could subdivide alcohol consumption into five groups as shown in Table 1.3.1 in Section 1.3 and presented in graphical form in Figure 1.3.4. Here, we present Figure 2.2.1, showing simply the observed percentages of fetal loss in the five alcohol groups.

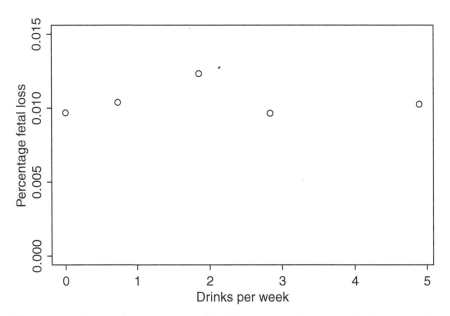

Fig. 2.2.1. Observed percentages of fetal loss, according to alcohol consumption during pregnancy.

If the covariate is subdivided into many (naturally ordered) groups, we saw in Section 1.3 that parsimonious models may be constructed by assuming linearity on the logit scale. In Section 4.1.2, we treat such models in detail.

2.2.2 Quantitative outcome

A quantitative variable takes on values for which it is meaningful to carry out arithmetic operations such as addition, subtraction, and so on. As such, the number of fever episodes also qualifies as a quantitative variable. However, unless specifically stated otherwise, we think of quantitative outcomes as variables that can take on any value in some interval, that is, variables such as the vitamin D concentration in blood, the birthweight of a newborn baby or the lung capacity, measured as forced expiratory flow rate. As mentioned in Section 2.1.4, we denote such variables as continuous.

Whereas for categorical outcomes, Section 2.2.1 described the natural form of presentation as tables of counts in various categories, perhaps converted into figures, for quantitative outcomes, figures are mandatory. Any table or summary statistic (such as an average) will necessarily throw away a lot of information whereas a plot will retain much more, if not even all. Moreover, the human eye is very efficient in detecting patterns and abnormalities in a graphical display.

As an example of a quantitative outcome, let us consider Example 1.1 concerned with vitamin D levels among Irish women. We may investigate the distribution of this variable by constructing a *histogram* (i.e., a picture of the *empirical* (the actually observed) distribution). This is constructed as follows. Observe that the range of the 41 observations is from 17.0 to 110.4. Subdividing into intervals of length 10, with midpoints ranging from 15 to 115 and counting the number of observations in each interval gives us the histogram as shown in Figure 2.2.2, with columns indicating the counts in each interval.

Because of the limited amount of information available from only 41 women, the histogram looks a bit rough and not at all like the nice curves from Figure 2.1.4, although the shape of the histogram bears some resemblance to these.

It can be quite difficult to judge the adequacy of an assumption of a Normal distribution from a histogram. Figure 2.2.3 shows three simulated data sets of size 25, 75, and 200, respectively, from a Normal distribution, with superimposed probability densities. We see that for small sample sizes, the histogram may well show signs of deviation from Normality, even though we know that this is not the case. An alternative way of judging Normality is to produce a *Normal quantile plot*. We introduce this kind of plot in Section 2.3.2 in connection with model checks in order to stress that a Normality assumption in general refers to the *residuals* (defined in Section 2.3.2) and not to the outcome variable as such.

Whether or not the distribution looks like a Normal density, we need to define descriptive statistics as a way of summarizing such a collection of quantitative observations. Typically, we want to specify a location (i.e., a center or a typical value) along with some sort of measure of the variation in the data.

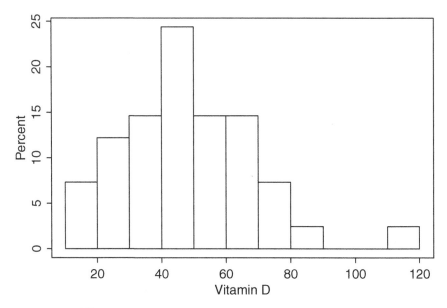

Fig. 2.2.2. Histogram of vitamin D for 41 Irish women.

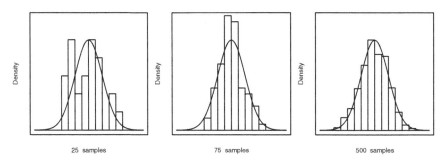

Fig. 2.2.3. Histograms for simulated observations from Normal distributions, with sample size 25, 75, and 200, respectively. Theoretical Normal probability densities are superimposed.

As a measure of location, there are two main alternatives, the *average* and the *median*. The average is the observed counterpart of the theoretical mean, and is simply defined as the sum of all observations, divided by the total number of observations. If y_i denotes the vitamin D level for the ith woman, we denote the average as $\bar{y}$ (called *y-bar*) so that

$$\bar{y} = \frac{1}{41}(y_1 + y_2 + \cdots + y_{41}) = \frac{1}{41}\sum_{i=1}^{41} y_i.$$

The average represents the center of gravity, which for symmetrical distributions is the intuitive center of the observations. For skewed distributions, however, the average may be pushed towards one of the tails, as a consequence of the fact that extreme observations have a pronounced influence on the center of gravity (a well-known fact that may be observed when children are playing on a seesaw).

For skewed distributions it is therefore often more meaningful to report instead the *empirical median*, defined as a "value" that cuts the observations in two halves, one containing smaller values and the other containing larger values. For odd-sized samples, this value is uniquely determined but for even-sized samples, various interpolation methods exist. For practical purposes, the choice of interpolation method will rarely give substantially different results; averaging the middle two values is typically appropriate.

The median is also denoted the *50% quantile* (or the *50th percentile*, due to the fact that 50% of the values fall below this value. In a similar way, we may define quantiles corresponding to any other fraction of the data, for example, the *lower and upper quartiles*, defined as the 25% and, respectively, the 75% quantile. Because 25% of the data fall below the lower quartile and 25% of the data fall above the upper quartile, we conclude that the interval between the lower and upper quartiles contains the central half of the data. This interval is known as the *inter-quartile range (IQR)*. In a similar way, we may construct an interval containing, for example, 95% of the observations by choosing the lower endpoint as the 2.5% quantile and the upper endpoint as the 97.5% quantile. Now, 2.5% of the observations will fall below this interval, and another 2.5% will fall above, that is, a total of 5% outside of the interval. The resulting interval is denoted a 95% *reference interval*, because by construction it contains the 95% most typical observations, that is, those that one would normally see (also in the future) and therefore use for reference when diagnosing abnormalities.

The quantiles tell us something about the distribution of the observations, location as well as variation, but they are cumbersome to report and compare between groups. For location, we have the average or the median, but we also need a single quantity describing variation. For this purpose, we have the empirical counterpart of the variance from Equation (2.1.2) or preferably the square root of this, the standard deviation from Equation (2.1.3). Traditionally, the standard deviation is estimated by

$$\widehat{s} = \sqrt{\frac{1}{n-1} \sum_{i=1}^{n} (y_i - \bar{y})^2} \tag{2.2.1}$$

a formula that is further explained in Section 2.3.1.

For the vitamin D observations on the 41 Irish women, *summary statistics* include the average (48.01), the standard deviation (20.22), and the quantiles given in Table 2.2.2.

Table 2.2.2. Quantiles for vitamin D observations, calculated from 41 Irish women.

Percentage point, p	0%	1%	2.5%	5%	25%	50%
	Minimum				Lower Quartile	Median
pth quantiles	17.0	17.0	18.0	18.5	34.4	44.8

Percentage point, p	100%	99%	97.5%	95%	75%	50%
	maximum				upper quartile	median
pth quantiles	62.7	75.7	89.1	110.4	110.4	44.8

As seen from Table 2.2.2, we have some difficulties with the outermost quantiles, because these are found to be identical to the absolute extremes: minimum and maximum. This is due to the small sample size in this example. Taking a fraction corresponding to 1% of 41 observations is not meaningful and hence this quantile should not be reported. We may say almost the same thing about the 2.5% and 97.5% quantiles, because the calculation of these involves an attempt to divide the sample into groups of 1 and 40, a division that is hardly very robust and trustworthy.

Digression. Precision of quantile estimation

A sufficient sample size for estimation of quantiles is hard to determine inasmuch as it depends, not only on the quantile itself (a 1% quantile demands a larger sample size than a 5% quantile) but also on the shape of the distribution (a skewed or heavy-tailed distribution may demand a larger sample size than does a distribution close to a Normal). We would recommend a minimum of 200 observations when estimating the 2.5% and 97.5% quantiles. ⋄

Hence, because of an insufficient sample size, we cannot sensibly report a 95% reference interval based on quantiles, unless we are willing to make some assumptions, for example, that the vitamin D level among Irish women follows a Normal distribution. In this case, a 95% reference interval may be constructed from the average and standard deviation, using the empirical counterpart of equation (2.1.6)

$$\bar{y} \pm 1.96\widehat{s} = 48.01 \pm 1.96 \cdot 20.22 = (8.38, 87.64).$$

We note that in this example, the upper endpoint is close to the 97.5% quantile, whereas the lower endpoint is somewhat smaller than the 2.5% quantile, reflecting the fact that the distribution as seen in Figure 2.2.2 is not entirely symmetric. In Section 2.3.2 we discuss methods for checking the adequacy of a Normal distribution. However, with a limited amount of information (such as in the present example), such methods are only rough guidelines. This is unfortunate because it is precisely in these situations with a limited number of observations that we may need this extra assumption in order to construct a 95% reference interval. The solution to this apparent dilemma is, however, quite simple. Do not construct reference intervals for clinical use based on so few observations!

In this discussion of Normality, it is to be stressed that in most situations involving quantitative outcomes, we do *not* assume the observations to follow the same Normal distribution *marginally* (i.e., that the observations as a whole come from the same Normal distribution), but only *conditionally* upon the relevant explanatory variables. In the case of vitamin D according to BMI groups, this means that we assume Normal distributions within each group, but quite possibly with different parameters in the two groups and thus marginally a more involved (possibly bimodal) distribution. In more complex situations, the assumption can be formulated as a Normal distribution for the *residuals* that we have not yet introduced but which are a part of all subsequent models for quantitative outcomes.

2.2.3 Survival time outcome

When the outcome variable y is a survival time or a time to treatment failure (indicated by a liver transplantation), as in the PBC3 study, Example 1.3, the data will almost certainly contain *censored* observations, either because subjects disappear or because we cannot wait for all events to occur before we start analyzing our data. Thus, in the PBC3 study, 4 patients were lost to follow-up before 1 January 1989 and 255 were alive without a liver transplantation at that date. For those 259 patients only a lower limit for the time to treatment failure was observed. This has the consequence that data cannot be described in a simple and meaningful way using averages. The averages for the patients with a treatment failure are likely to underestimate the true mean times to treatment failure (we are more likely to observe the short durations because the longer durations have not yet resulted in a failure). Also, the average of all observation times (observed treatment failures as well as censorings) will depend strongly on the fraction of censored observations and, at any rate, these averages will also underestimate the true mean values because the censored observation time for a specific subject by definition is smaller than the unobserved, true failure time.

Likewise, the presence of censored observations prevents us from making histograms and, in many situations, even medians cannot be calculated. We therefore have to look for a totally different approach for describing the distribution of survival times. This is achieved by looking at the process of deaths and censorings evolving dynamically over time. The risk of death at successive time points t is estimated and summarized by the empirical counterpart of the survival function $S(t) = \mathrm{pr}(y > t)$, called the *Kaplan–Meier curve*.

The Kaplan–Meier curve is a stepwise constant, nonincreasing curve, describing the fraction of individuals still alive at the current time. It has initial value 1 (all patients are alive) and has a downwards step at each observed failure time t_j. The relative height of such a step is given by a factor

$$1 - \frac{1}{R(t_j)},$$

where $R(t_j)$ is the number of subjects *at risk* or in the *risk set* at time t_j (i.e., the subjects that have not already died or been censored).

Note that a person with a censored time of observation t_0 is part of the risk set $R(t)$ for all times $t \leq t_0$ where, if that patient had experienced a treatment failure, this would have been observed. A censored observation does not give rise to a step in the Kaplan–Meier curve.

In Figure 1.1.1 in Section 1.1, we have already seen the Kaplan–Meier curves for the two treatment groups separately and we noted that these looked quite alike, suggesting no large discrepancy between the treatments. More details on Kaplan–Meier curves and their construction and use, including how the median survival time may (sometimes) be estimated, are given in Section 3.1.3.

2.3 Statistical inference

The purpose of statistical inference is to produce statements concerning the mechanisms generating the data, that is, to determine a plausible *statistical model* for our data.

In the previous sections, we have seen examples of such statistical models for various types of observed data. We have seen that the concept of a statistical model involves a specification of the *probability distribution* of the outcome referring to the population from which the sample was drawn, or at least some aspects of this, such as the effect of certain covariates on the mean value or the probability of surviving beyond some specific time.

We saw through examples that the interesting aspects of the models are given as certain *parameters*, such as a mean value of vitamin D concentration, the probability of fetal death, or more interestingly, parameters specifying the effects of certain covariates on these quantities. Examples include the number of fever episodes as a possible explanatory variable for the probability of fetal death, or the body mass index as an explanatory variable for the mean vitamin D concentration.

A particularly well-known scenario could be a model describing systolic blood pressure y for men of all ages, including age as an explanatory variable x. The mean value of systolic blood pressure might be specified as a linear function of age:

$$\mathrm{E}(y_i) = m_i = a + bx_i. \tag{2.3.1}$$

We call this model a *linear regression model* and models of this kind are treated in Section 4.1.1. Here we just note that the mean value is characterized through two parameters, the intercept a and the slope b of the line relating systolic blood pressure to age. We also use this kind of model to describe the relationship between vitamin D level and body mass index for the Irish women.

Typically, specific scientific questions have been formulated prior to data collection and the data serve as evidence for the answers to these questions. Through a model for the data, we reformulate our scientific questions in terms of model parameters and the statistical analysis of the data at hand. *Inference* will, as pointed out in the introduction to this chapter, consist of three steps: *parameter estimation*, *model checking* and *hypothesis testing*, each treated here in separate subsections.

The results of a statistical analysis can only be trustworthy if the model fits the data adequately. Therefore, it would seem that model checks should be the first issue to consider. However, for technical reasons (inasmuch as model checks often involve the *residuals*, discrepancies between observed and predicted outcomes), estimation has to be performed before such model checks can be made.

We therefore begin with Subsection 2.3.1 on estimation, in which we briefly mention various principles for estimation, referring details on the *likelihood principle* to a subsection of its own. The focus in Section 2.3.1 is instead the distribution of the estimates. This is a very important concept to understand because it provides the foundation for deriving statements of uncertainty, that is, judging the trust that we can have in a parameter estimate or the confidence with which we can state whether a hypothesis is true or false. We therefore advise the readers to go through this subsection in full.

Section 2.3.2 deals with general principles for model checking. Because the specific techniques depend on the type of outcome and model, the readers may want to read this section only cursorily and concentrate on the topic in later chapters dealing with specific models.

In Subsection 2.3.3 on testing statistical hypothesis, we focus on the general idea behind hypothesis testing and the errors that may result from judging a hypothesis to be true or false. Understanding these very general ideas is important whereas details of the derivation of test statistics are not.

At the end of this chapter, the separate Subsection 2.3.4 has been devoted to the most important inference principle, the likelihood principle. This section is rather technical and not necessary for understanding the subsequent chapters. It may therefore be skipped by readers not interested in theoretical details.

2.3.1 Estimation

Recall that statistical models involve *parameters* (i.e., unknown quantities that we want to learn about by conducting studies). Examples include a probability of fetal death or the increase in blood pressure for a one-year increase in age.

Obviously, we rarely get to actually *know* the true value of such parameters (inasmuch as this would have to involve observation of every single subject in the population), and we have to be satisfied with intelligent guesses based on observations for a sample of subjects. However, through lots of observations, our guesses will generally get close to the true value (provided of course that the model is sensible). We use the term *estimation* of the unknown parameter for this guessing process and obviously we want it to be as informative as possible.

Several objective estimation principles have been suggested, each leading to *estimating equation* that have to be solved to give the *parameter estimate*. In general, iterative methods (and thereby computers) will be necessary to solve such equations. Only in the simplest cases do the methods produce explicit solutions useful for illustrating the general logic behind the principles. Such simple situations include estimation of the mean in a Normal distribution and the estimation of a probability in a Bernoulli or Binomial distribution.

By far the most important general estimation principle is the *likelihood principle*. The likelihood principle builds upon the *likelihood function* which reflects the probability of the observed data as a function of the unknown parameters. Specifically, for each possible value of the parameters, we have an associated value of the likelihood function, namely the probability of observing what we actually did observe, under the assumption that this particular parameter value was the true one. The *law of likelihood* says that a parameter value (or in the case of more than one unknown parameter; a set of parameter values) is more credible than another if it has a larger value of the likelihood function. Hence, the *most* credible parameter value is the one that maximizes the likelihood function, the *maximum likelihood estimate* . If the parameter is called a, the estimate is commonly denoted by $\hat{a}$. The likelihood function and its use for estimation and testing is discussed in more detail and exemplified in Section 2.3.4.

No matter which principle lies behind the estimate of the unknown parameters, the result will be a function of the observations and therefore obviously subject to a certain degree of variability. The larger the sample size, the smaller this variability is and consequently the greater confidence in the stated estimate. In the remainder of this section, we are concerned with the interpretation of these statements.

Distribution of estimates

In a specific investigation, we only have one single estimate of a particular parameter, and therefore the concept of a distribution for this estimate leads to some confusion. *How can we talk about a distribution when we only have one single number?* The answer is that we mean the distribution of estimates obtained from *hypothetical repetitions* of the experiment. Such hypothetical repetitions would give similar but not identical values of the estimate, and from the model specifications we may infer properties of this (unobserved) distribution.

Consider once more the fetal death example, where among 11,778 women we observed 119 cases of fetal death, corresponding to an estimated probability of approximately 1%. Suppose we performed the investigation many more times (the following years, in other countries, etc.), taking every time a sample of 11,778 pregnant women. Which values of the estimated probability $\widehat{p}$ would we expect to see in such investigations? Provided that there are no changes over time or between countries, we would surely anticipate estimated probabilities in the vicinity of 1%, although they may vary somewhat due to natural variability between the women.

If we assume a *known* probability of fetal death (1.2%, say), we may *simulate* such a hypothetical investigation, or better yet, we may simulate a thousand such investigations in order to see what the distribution of $\widehat{p}$ would look like. In this way, we can picture the distribution of the estimate of a known value, see if it is centered around this true value, notice the variability, and so on, and we may then use this theoretical knowledge to make inference about the parameter, also in practical situations, where we of course do *not* know the true value.

In Figure 2.3.1 we show a histogram of estimated fetal death probabilities, based on a thousand simulated hypothetical replications corresponding to the fetal death example, each with a sample size of $n = 11,778$ and a true probability p, chosen to be $p = 0.012$. We note that the distribution of the estimate $\widehat{p}$ is quite symmetric and centered around the true value of 0.012 (which was chosen for simulation). Actually, the mean and standard deviation in the distribution of $\widehat{p}$ can be shown (theoretically) to be

$$\mathrm{E}(\widehat{p}) = p,$$
$$\mathrm{SD}(\widehat{p}) = \sqrt{\frac{p(1-p)}{n}}.$$

The *bias* of an estimate is defined as the difference between the mean value of the estimate and the true value of the parameter that we are trying to estimate: the discrepancy between our best guess and the truth. In this particular situation, the bias becomes 0, because the mean value of $\widehat{p}$ is seen to equal the true unknown value p. This property is called *unbiasedness* and we say that the estimate is *unbiased* (as opposed to *biased*). The uncertainty in the estimate $\widehat{p}$ is reflected in the standard deviation, and from the above formula, we see that this decreases with the square root of the sample size (n, the number of women in the study, here $n = 11,778$). This means that the more women we include in our study, the more certain we will be that the resulting estimate $\widehat{p}$ for the probability of fetal death is very close to the true value p. This property is called *consistency*, and the estimate is said to be *consistent* for the unknown parameter p.

We can illustrate this by performing simulations for sample sizes other than 11,778. In Figure 2.3.2 we have illustrated a thousand simulations for sample sizes of 100, 1000, 1000 repeated with a new scaling of the horizontal axis, and 10,000, all with an assumed true probability of 0.012. The figure illustrates

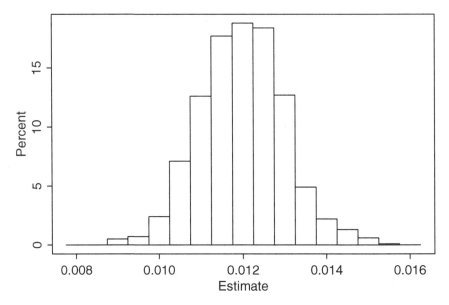

Fig. 2.3.1. Simulated distribution of estimated fetal death probability, assuming the true probability to be 1.2%.

the decrease in standard deviation (increase in precision) and the gradually centering around the true value, according to the increase in sample size. It also illustrates the *Central Limit Theorem* (CLT), which says that a sum of n ("many") single independent components with identical distributions will have a distribution that tends to look more and more like a Normal distribution, the bigger n is. We say that when n tends to infinity ($n \to \infty$, i.e., it becomes bigger and bigger), the distribution of the quantity will resemble a Normal distribution more and more closely. In the present case, we have a sum of many Bernoulli observations (i.e., a sum of either zeros or ones).

The distribution of an estimator is important because it can provide a *confidence interval* for the parameter. Confidence intervals are constructed to have a suitable probability, called the *coverage probability*, of containing the true, but unknown, parameter. Most often, this is chosen to be 95%, although other coverages may be reasonable in specific situations according to the nature of the problem (e.g., taking safety considerations into account). As the name suggests, we may be 95% confident that such a 95% confidence interval contains the true value.

A confidence interval can be thought of as a reference interval, only now for an estimate of some unknown parameter rather than for individual observations of some quantity. We are looking for a region covering the middle part of the distribution of the estimate. If the distribution of the estimate is close to Normal then a confidence interval may be constructed from the standard

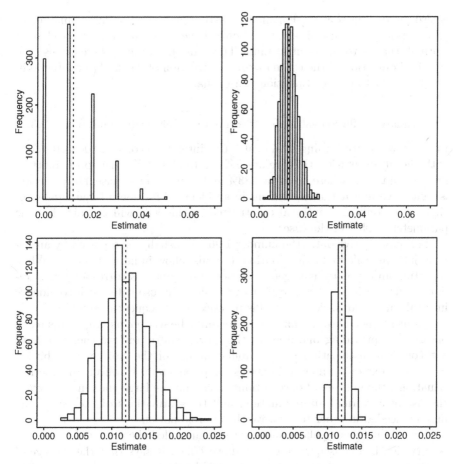

Fig. 2.3.2. Simulations of estimated fetal death probability, assuming $p = 0.012$, for sample sizes of 100 (upper left), 1000 (upper right), 1000 repeated with a new scaling of the x-axis (lower left), and 10,000 (lower right).

deviation in the distribution of the estimate. In a Binomial situation, such as the example concerning fetal death, we get the estimated standard deviation

$$\text{SD}(\widehat{p}) = \sqrt{\frac{\widehat{p}(1 - \widehat{p})}{n}} = 0.00092.$$

This quantity is often referred to as the *standard error of the estimate* (if the parameter to be estimated is a mean, the quantity is called the *standard error of the mean*). We, however, avoid these names altogether because they seem to introduce rather than eliminate confusion, and we simply use the term *standard deviation of the estimate*. As a standard deviation, it is only truly meaningful if the distribution is symmetric and only easily interpretable if it is also reasonably Normal. Fortunately, estimators based on large amounts of information (i.e., many observations) often have distributions that are close to Normal, thanks to the Central Limit Theorem and we may therefore use the standard deviation of the estimate for construction of a confidence interval in a way similar to that of Equation (2.1.6), namely

$$("estimate - 1.96 \ SD(estimate)", "estimate + 1.96 \ SD(estimate)"). \quad (2.3.2)$$

In the example concerning fetal death, this interval becomes $(0.0083, 0.0119)$, with the interpretation that we are 95% certain that the true probability of fetal death is somewhere between 0.83% and 1.19%. The precise interpretation is that if we repeat the experiment in an identical fashion a large number of times, the confidence interval constructed in this way will contain the true parameter in 95% of the cases.

For quantitative data, the number 1.96 will usually be replaced by an appropriate quantile in a t-distribution (details follow in later chapters). When reporting an estimate, it is general practice to quote its corresponding standard deviation in brackets, so that the reader may use it for such confidence interval calculations. We follow this practice in subsequent chapters.

As mentioned above, many estimators may be written as large sums (each observation providing one item to the overall sum), and we therefore have a theoretical justification for the abundant use of the Normal distribution in the context of confidence intervals for parameters. However, in practical situations, the number of observations n may not be large enough to warrant the use of a Normal approximation, and transformations of the estimators may be needed in order to improve the approximation.

Probability theory offers another theorem, called the *Law of Large Numbers* (which is a consequence of the above *CLT*). It says that the average of many such single independent items with identical means will be *consistent* for this mean, that is, get closer and closer to the true unknown parameter that we wish to estimate. This property was mentioned above for the estimate $\widehat{p}$ (the estimate of probability of fetal death).

Digression. Properties of estimators

We may ask whether such properties (unbiasedness, consistency, high precision, and so on) are important when choosing estimators. And what properties do we get by using the maximum likelihood principle described briefly above and in greater detail in Section 2.3.4? The answer to the last question is that the maximum likelihood estimate will in general be consistent and asymptotically Normal with a "high" precision, although it will not always be unbiased. This means that its mean value will not always be identical to the quantity that we aim at estimating, although the consistency implies that for large sample sizes, it will be approximately unbiased. In the fever example, the estimate $\widehat{p}$ is seen to be unbiased. On the other hand, the maximum likelihood estimate for the variance in the Normal distribution, as given in Section 2.3.4 later in this chapter, is *not* unbiased, only consistent, inasmuch as

$$E(\tilde{s}^2) = \frac{n-1}{n}s^2.$$

Because unbiasedness is intuitively considered to be a very attractive property, we may want to modify the above estimate to achieve the correct mean value. This is precisely why we use the estimate from Equation (2.2.1) instead of the maximum likelihood estimate. For practical purposes, this correction is unimportant, unless the sample size is very small. However, the very same problem appears for many other models considered in this book and the correction may not always be negligible. The general principle for correction involves using a slightly modified version of the likelihood function, the so-called residual (or restricted) maximum likelihood principle. A complete description of this principle is technical and beyond the scope of this book, but it has to do with accounting for the fact that whenever we estimate one parameter, we "use" one unit of information (called "a degree-of-freedom"). You could say, that we start out with n degrees-of-freedom (equal to the number of observations) but after estimation of the mean, we only have $n-1$ degrees-of-freedom left and hence we should divide by $n-1$ instead of n.

For small sample sizes, the asymptotic results do not apply and in general, simulations have to be performed in order to judge the appropriateness of a particular estimation method. If our sample in the fetal death example had consisted of only 100 pregnant women with a single incident of fetal death, we would still have had an estimated p of 0.01, although now with a much larger standard deviation, $SD(\hat{p}) = 0.0099$ and a corresponding confidence interval based on a Normal approximation would be calculated to be $(-0.0095, 0.0295)$. We immediately see that this is a ridiculous answer, because we cannot have a confidence interval including negative numbers when we are estimating a (nonnegative) probability! The problem is that a sample of only 100 women, in combination with such a small probability of the event under consideration (fetal death), does not warrant the use of a Normal approximation for the distribution of $\hat{p}$, as we could see from the simulation in the upper left panel of Figure 2.3.2. Therefore, the confidence interval constructed above is not valid and we have to use another method to construct an appropriate (asymmetric) interval.

An obvious way of constructing confidence intervals is to use the likelihood function. The maximum likelihood estimate is *the best*, in the sense that it gives maximum credibility to the observations that we actually got, therefore another value of the parameter with almost as high a likelihood value must be almost as likely as the best one. Therefore, we can construct a confidence interval consisting of all those parameter values that have a likelihood value above a certain value. The problem now changes to that of determining which threshold will result in a coverage of 95% and this is not always an easy task.

As mentioned above, small sample problems or problems involving very complicated models will often benefit from simulations. The idea is to fix the parameters and create a series of hypothetical datasets (as many as you like) of the same size as the original one and perform the estimation for each of these. By studying the resulting distribution of the estimates, we can get useful information regarding the shape (possible asymmetry) and size of confidence intervals. We have already used this approach above to illustrate the distribution of the estimate for the fetal death example. In this case, we assured ourselves that the distribution looked a lot like a Normal distribution so that we might use the simple way of constructing a confidence interval. If we instead simulate a small sample version of the fetal death example, such as the above-mentioned scenario with only 100 pregnancies, we get the simulated distribution of estimates as seen in Figure 2.3.3, which is seen to be far from Normal.

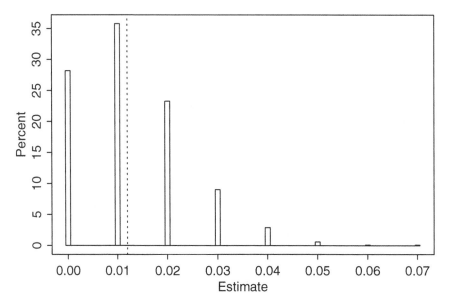

Fig. 2.3.3. Simulated distribution of estimated fetal death probability, based on 100 pregnancies, assuming the true probability to be 1.2%.

Simulations require full specification of the model and therefore cannot be used if the probabilistic mechanism is unknown, or partially unknown, and we are not willing to make assumptions. In such a case, we may instead use a *resampling method*. The idea is to create new (hypothetical) samples by taking a sample of the original data, in a sense as if we were simulating from the empirical distribution. These new samples are handled in exactly the same way as described above for simulations.

Two resampling methods are often used: *Jackknife* and *Bootstrap*. In the Jackknife method, we create new samples simply by deleting one observation at a time, so that all the new samples will contain one less observation compared to the original. On the other hand, the Bootstrap method may create samples of any size by randomly picking from the data at hand, with replacement (i.e., the chosen observation is re-entered into the pool from which we pick new observations). This means that a Bootstrap sample will (for all practical purposes) contain some observations multiple times, whereas others do not appear at all (e.g., Efron and Tibshirani, 1998, Ch. 6).

A very precise and slightly biased estimator may be preferable to an unbiased and imprecise estimate; see Figure 2.3.4 illustrating theoretical distributions of two possible estimators of the same unknown quantity, indicated by the vertical dashed line.

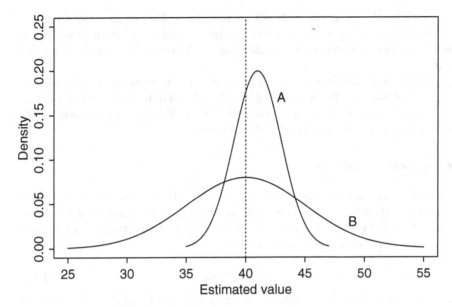

Fig. 2.3.4. Bias versus precision of estimates; see text.

In this fictive example, we want to estimate the unknown true value $a = 40$. One estimate (A) is rather precise (SD= 2) but has a small bias (1), whereas the other one (B) is unbiased, although with a larger SD(5). In most situations, estimate A will be closer to the true value, which may be seen by calculating the *mean squared error*, that is, the mean squared deviation from observation to true value

$$E(y - a)^2 = (\mathrm{SD}(y))^2 + (\mathrm{E}(y) - a)^2 = \begin{cases} 2^2 + 1^2 = 5 & \text{for estimate A} \\ 5^2 + 0^2 = 25 & \text{for estimate B} \end{cases} \qquad (2.3.3)$$

$\diamond$

2.3.2 Model checking

Statistical inference is based on a model for the data from our scientific investigation. Such a model can involve assumptions concerning type of distribution, specification of dependence upon covariates, and so on. In a particular study, model assumptions may be based on previous knowledge of the scientific substance, justified by previous data, but may also be based on the data gathered at present.

Conclusions derived from the model of course rely (at least to some extent) on these assumptions, and if they are not met to a reasonable degree, the conclusions may be imprecise or even erroneous and misleading.

Therefore, models should be checked before making conclusions and ideally even before we estimate in the model because otherwise this may not be worthwhile. However, the methods for model checking require calculation of quantities involving estimates from the model, and therefore in practice, the model checking cannot be performed before the estimation has been carried out.

Methods for model checking depend on the nature of the model, so only a flavor of the principles can be given in this introductory section whereas details are given in subsequent chapters. The techniques may be divided into two main categories: graphical and numerical.

Graphical model checking

Graphical methods of model checking involve the *residuals*, constructed to reflect the discrepancy between individual observations and their predicted (expected) values. For quantitative (continuous) observations y_i with mean value m_i, the residual is simply the difference

$$r_i = y_i - \widehat{m}_i \qquad (2.3.4)$$

or a *normalized* verison of this obtained by dividing by SD(y). For Bernoulli (binary) or Binomial data $y_i \sim \text{Bin}(c, p_i)$ the residuals (also denoted the *Pearson residuals*) are defined as

$$r_i = \frac{y_i - c\widehat{p}_i}{\sqrt{c\widehat{p}_i(1 - \widehat{p}_i)}}, \qquad (2.3.5)$$

whereas for a Poisson distributed variable the definition is $(y_i - \widehat{m}_i)/\sqrt{\widehat{m}_i}$. That is, Pearson residuals are also normalized by dividing by SD(y_i). For survival time outcomes, definition of residuals pose some nontrivial problems because of the presence of censored observations. Instead we use the so-called *pseudo-residuals*, defined from *pseudo-observations*, introduced in Section 3.1.3.

Digression. Other types of residuals

For quantitative observations, the residuals are defined as simple differences between observations and predicted values, and therefore measured in the same units as the observations themselves. This is convenient for interpretation when these units are intuitively interpretable. However, for identifying unusual observations, it is advisable to use instead *studentized* residuals, constructed from the ordinary residuals by dividing by their standard deviation (which need not be the same for all residuals).

In the search for outliers and influential observations, it may be even more revealing to use instead the *leave-one-out* residuals, in which the residual for an observation is calculated using a predicted value from an estimation in which this particular observation has not been included. This means that the predicted values are all based on different samples, using one observation less in the estimation. These leave-one-out residuals may also be standardized, so that we have a total of four different types of residuals (see, e.g., Cook and Weisberg, 1982). ⋄

No matter which kind of outcome we are dealing with (and which particular kind of residuals we have chosen), the use of residuals for model checking
is based on identical principles, although the specific appearance will depend
on the nature of the outcome. We illustrate the idea behind residuals and
their graphical use in the model relating vitamin D levels (y) for the 41 Irish
women (from Example 1.1) to their body mass index x through the linear
regression model (2.3.1); that is, $E(y_i) = m_i = a + bx_i$.

Figure 2.3.5 shows the observations and the fitted regression line, representing the *expected values* for any given body mass index. The residuals (i.e.,
the difference between observed and expected values), are therefore the vertical distances from observation to line, as also shown in Figure 2.3.5. This
vertical distance is unexplained by the linear regression model. The model
says that people with a high body mass index will generally have a low vitamin D level but it does not explain the discrepancies from this general line of
trend. This discrepancy is interpreted as the biological variation, that is, the
variation present among women with identical body mass indices.

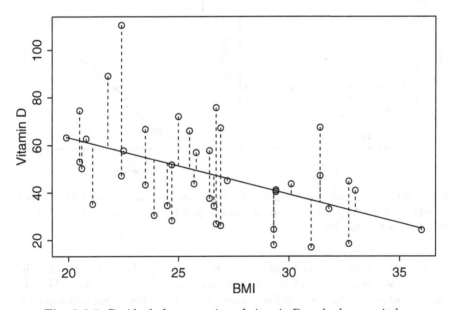

Fig. 2.3.5. Residuals for regression of vitamin D on body mass index.

Having calculated residuals, we proceed by looking for patterns in them.
For instance, we may produce plots of residuals against predicted values (to
see whether the variation is homogeneous), against body mass index (to see,
whether the specified linearity was reasonable), against various other charac-

teristics of the women in the study, such as age (to see whether this variable can account for some of the unexplained variation), or we may make histograms of the residuals to check their distribution.

If we, for instance, find that residuals vary with age of the individual, we should take this as an indication that an age dependence should be included in the model. If it has already been included, the form of the dependence has to be changed.

The left-hand side of Figure 2.3.6 shows a plot of residuals of vitamin D plotted against body mass index, which was the only covariate in the model. If any clear systematic pattern seems to be present, we should consider abandoning the assumption of a linear relation between vitamin D and body mass index. The definition of the residuals ensures that they will have an average of zero, and a reference line at zero has been added to the plot. In this example, there does not seem to be any systematic pattern, so we may conclude that the linearity is reasonable.

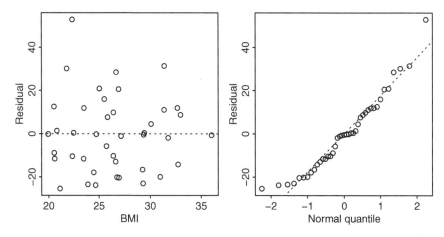

Fig. 2.3.6. Left panel shows residuals for regression of vitamin D on BMI, plotted against BMI. Right panel is a normal quantile plot for investigation of the Normal distribution assumption.

The right-hand side of Figure 2.3.6 shows a *Normal quantile plot* for the residuals for vitamin D, after regression on body mass index (i.e., the very same residuals as in the left-hand side plot). The idea behind this plot is to compare the observed distribution of the residuals with the best fitting Normal distribution (i.e., a Normal distribution with mean 0 and a standard deviation equal to that of the residuals themselves). For a specific residual, the vertical axis on this plot shows the value of the actual residual, whereas the horizontal axis shows the corresponding predicted residual in the best fitting Normal distribution scaled to a SD of 1. A systematic deviation from a straight line indicates that the Normality assumption is unreasonable, and more so if the sample is large.

This figure suggests a reasonable resemblance to a Normal distribution, although not perfect. A small systematic departure from the straight line is obvious, because points fall above the line in both ends (and tend to fall below the line in the middle). This is a very typical finding for positive data due to the fact that the range of possible values is limited by 0 to the left but with no fixed upper limit. In later chapters, we look into remedies for such discrepancies, such as a transformation of the original outcome variable, typically with a logarithm.

Numerical model checking

Even if graphs are most useful for spotting deviations from the stated model, it will sometimes be useful to add an objective decision as to whether deviating patterns are signs of real discrepancies between data and model or whether they may merely be a result of randomness.

A general idea for such a numerical model check is to build a larger (i.e., more general) model, for instance, by including an extra covariate or specifying a quadratic relationship instead of a linear and then making a formal hypothesis test (see Section 2.3.3 below) for reduction to the simpler model. The simpler model is then said to be *nested* in the larger model. For instance, the above-mentioned possible dependence between residuals and age may be too weak to be convincing and should therefore not be relied upon before additional evidence has been collected. We may investigate the strength of the observed pattern by including age in the model and perform a numerical test for significance of its effect.

A word of warning is that hypothesis tests driven by ideas arising in the analysis phase (i.e., generated by looking at the data) are to be regarded as fishing expeditions and possible findings should be regarded as spurious until they have been confirmed in future investigations.

To supplement the quantile plot in the right-hand side of Figure 2.3.6, a numerical test for Normality is sometimes carried out. We believe such tests to be of limited value because small samples will rarely reject Normality (we have too little information) whereas large samples will reject even small and unimportant deviations from Normality.

In situations involving categorical data, the information available may be too limited to warrant the use of graphical methods altogether. In such situations, a comparison of observed and expected values may be performed using simple tables. In Example 1.2 concerning fetal death, we discussed in Section 2.1.2 the distribution of the number of fever episodes and based on theoretical arguments, we found it to be Binomially distributed, $\text{Bin}(c, p)$, with $c = 14$. We now investigate the appropriateness of this assumption.

First of all, we realize that Table 2.2.1 falls short of detailed information concerning the number of fever episodes, because it only states that 30 women experienced three or more such episodes. Table 2.3.1 gives the full information on fever episodes, from which we can calculate the total number of fever episodes to be 2358, corresponding to an average number of fever episodes (per woman) to be

$$\frac{2358}{11,778} = 0.200$$

Equating this to the expected mean $cp = 14p$ in the Binomial distribution, we get an estimate of p to be

$$\widehat{p} = \frac{0.200}{14} = 0.0143$$

If we calculate the expected number of subjects in each category (number of fever episodes) according to this estimate, we get the results stated in the last row of Table 2.3.1.

Table 2.3.1. Comparison of observed and expected numbers of fever episodes before pregnancy week 17 in 11,778 women recruited to the Danish National Birth Cohort Study.

	Number of Fever Episodes										
	0	1	2	3	4	5	6	7	8	9	10
Observed	9693	1872	183	20	3	3	1	1	0	0	2
Expected	9627.2	1955.3	184.4	10.7	0.43	0.01	~ 0	~ 0	~ 0	~ 0	~ 0

The comparison of observed and expected counts constitutes a numerical model check. We note that there is a large discrepancy between observed and expected counts for both 0 and 1 fever episode, because we observe far too many women with zero episodes and far too few with a single fever episode. We cannot directly compare the discrepancies, however, because the expected counts are very different across fever episode classes. Instead, we must compare the normalized discrepancies

$$\frac{(\text{observed-expected})^2}{\text{expected}}$$

but in order to calculate these in a meaningful way (avoiding very small expected values, inasmuch as these appear in the denominator of the above ratio), we must again collapse the columns corresponding to three or more fever episodes. Doing this, we get Table 2.3.2. From this table, it is seen that the tail of the distribution is in fact where we see the most pronounced discrepancies between the observed and expected counts.

Table 2.3.2. Observed and expected numbers of fever episodes.

	Number of Fever Episodes				
	0	1	2	3+	Total
Observed (O)	9693	1872	183	30	11778
Expected (E)	9627.1	1955.3	184.4	11.1	11778
$O - E$		+65.9	-83.3	-1.4	+18.9	0
$\frac{(O-E)^2}{E}$		0.45	3.55	0.01	31.92	0

The discrepancies seen in Table 2.3.2 may be summed up to 35.9, a number that can be used to assess the adequacy of the Binomial distribution in the present context.

Digression. Test for goodness of fit

The sum of the $(O - E)^2/E$s in the above example is known as a test statistic for *goodness-of-fit* , and it should be compared to a Chi-squared distribution with two degrees-of-freedom. This will result in an extreme low P-value, indicating a very bad description. The theory behind tests and P-values is given in Section 2.3.3. ◇

When (as is the case here) there is a large discrepancy between the observed and expected findings, we must conclude that one or more assumptions regarding the Binomial distribution must be flawed. Two assumptions were made: (1) equal probability for fever episodes for all subjects and in all weeks of pregnancy, and (2) independence between the occurrence of fever episodes (i.e., the occurrence of fever in one specific week does not affect the probability of fever in any other week). Intuitively, both of these may be wrong: some individuals are more fragile than others, violating the first assumption (we look into this possibility by introducing covariates in Section 7.2) and, moreover, having had one fever episode may very well increase the vulnerability and make the individual more susceptible of getting another episode.

2.3.3 Hypothesis testing

When a suitable model for the data has been established and estimates with corresponding confidence intervals have been derived for the unknown parameters, we may consider one or more hypotheses of interest. *Hypotheses* are statements regarding the nature of the model, making it simpler, typically by fixing one or more parameters at specific values (often zero).

To illustrate the ideas, consider a simple example with a cross-over study comparing two pain killers, A and B. All subjects are randomized to receive one of the drugs in the first period and the other drug in the second period. A simple outcome could be the preferred drug, as stated by each individual in the study, so that our data would result in a list A,B,A,A,A,B,B, and so on. If we focus on a drug A preference as the *event*, we could represent this outcome as a 1 and a drug B preference as a 0. In this way, the situation can be seen to be totally equivalent to that of fetal death. The number of subjects preferring A to B is the number of 1s, and this sum will be Binomially distributed with some unknown probability parameter p and count parameter equal to the total number of subjects in the study. The parameter p will reflect the relative benefit of A (in relation to B), so that a large p (close to 1, or at least convincingly greater than 0.5) will make us conclude that A is the more effective painkiller of the two.

Suppose that we have 40 subjects in our study ($n = 40$), and that $y = 28$ of these prefer drug A. Then we know from Section 2.3.1 that p is to be estimated as $\widehat{p} = 28/40 = 0.7$. The standard deviation of this estimate is $SD(\widehat{p}) = \sqrt{0.7(1 - 0.7)/40} = 0.072$, yielding a 95% confidence interval of approximately (0.56, 0.84).

Because 0.5 is *not* included in this confidence interval, we can say that 0.5 is *not* a likely value for p and hence that there is in fact evidence that A is a better drug than B. The confidence interval provides further information about the likely discrepancy between the two drugs, indicating that there may be as many as 84% preferring drug A, but probably not more.

Even though the information contained in the confidence interval answers our scientific question, it is nevertheless very common also to perform a test of the *hypothesis* that the two drugs perform equally well (i.e., a hypothesis that $p = 0.5$). Such a hypothesis is often called the "null hypothesis" (for obscure mathematical reasons, probably because it often involves testing that "something" is equal to zero). We just use the word hypothesis, but we use the traditional notation

$$H_0 : p = 0.5.$$

The collected data may be used to assess the credibility of this hypothesis. If a vast majority of the subjects prefer drug A, it does not seem reasonable to think that $p = 0.5$, but rather that $p > 0.5$ and we therefore reject the hypothesis, whereas if there is more or less the same number of subjects preferring each of the two drugs, then we have to accept that $p = 0.5$ is a plausible value. For a hypothesis like this, involving only a single parameter, there can be a one-to-one correspondence between the test and the confidence interval: If the hypothesized value of the parameter is not enclosed in the confidence interval, the test should reject the hypothesis, and vice versa. Note that even though the simplification implied by H_0 is denoted "the hypothesis," it does not mean that we hypothesize this to be the truth. Actually, the scientific hypothesis that we believe to be true is more often the alternative hypothesis (here $p \neq 0.5$, often denoted H_A), and we carry out the investigation in order to gain support for this by rejecting H_0.

It is important to realize that a failure to reject the hypothesis does not mean that the two drugs are proven to be identical, only that we do not have enough evidence (at this stage at least) to conclude that they are different. Hence, also in the case of an acceptance of the hypothesis of no drug difference, we have to supplement with a confidence interval in order to be aware of the possible differences that *might be* between the drugs. This is very important because such a confidence interval tells us whether it is worthwhile continuing to investigate the problem and collect more data. If the confidence interval for the probability contains only values very close to 0.5 we may safely conclude that any difference between the two drugs is too small to be of any practical importance.

Similarly, in the hypothetical example concerned with systolic blood pressure as a function of age, we may be concerned with the hypothesis that there is no age dependency at all ($b = 0$ in Equation (2.3.1)). The idea is that if there is no actual dependence on age, it would be unnecessarily complicated to work with a model specifying such a dependency, whereas on the other hand, we want to be confident that we do not overlook any important dependence simply due to a small sample size.

Digression. Occam's razor

The underlying philosophy of hypothesis testing is that we are eager to find the most parsimonious model still consistent with our observed data, that is, the simplest mechanism that may possibly have generated our data. This philosophy, known as Occam's razor (e.g., Clayton and Hills, 1993, Ch. 24), has been applied to natural sciences through the centuries and may be formulated as a reluctance to assume more causes of the various phenomena than those that are necessary and sufficient to explain their appearances. The name comes from the fourteenth century English logician, William of Ockham, and has been frequently referred to later in history, for example by the twentieth century Austrian and British philosopher Karl Popper. ◇

We cannot trustworthily say that the simplest sufficient explanation is also necessarily the *right* one, or even the *best* one (whatever we mean by *best*) but it will often be the most robust and the one that gives the most precise estimates. Introducing unnecessary explanatory variables in a model will generally decrease precision in the individual estimates even though it gives a somewhat closer fit to our data. We discuss these issues to a greater extent in Section 6.1.

A model can be thought of as a collection of possible mechanisms that may have generated our data. All the mechanisms within the model will act more or less alike (they will have identical structures) but will correspond to different values of one or more parameters. For instance, the model for the hypothetical cross-over trial involving the drugs A and B consists of mechanisms specifying the subjects to behave independently of each other and having identical probabilities p of preferring drug A to B, in the sense that we have no knowledge of explanatory variables for this situation. However, the p will be different for the various mechanisms in the model. Identifying the mechanism most likely to have generated our data is another way of expressing the estimation of the unknown parameter p.

A hypothesis is simply a submodel, "nested" in the original model, that is, a specification that the true generating mechanism is to be found in a smaller subset than originally specified. For instance, in the cross-over example the hypothesis that the drugs perform equally well corresponds to the submodel consisting of a single mechanism, where $p = 0.5$.

The strategy for testing statistical hypotheses is to find a *test statistic* that reflects the discrepancy between the observations and the hypothesis to be investigated. There are several general principles for deriving reasonable test statistics, the most important one being the *likelihood ratio statistic*, which is defined as the ratio of the maxima of the likelihood function, taken in the submodel (defined by the hypothesis), respectively, in the original model. Other principles may also be derived from the likelihood function and more details can be found in Section 2.3.4. Having chosen a reasonable test statistic, we subsequently have to derive the distribution of this test statistic under the assumption that the hypothesis H_0 is true. For instance, the test statistic (T, say) could be large (numerically) when the hypothesis is not reasonable(H_0 false) and the distribution of the test statistic under H_0 (i.e., assuming that H_0 is true) tells us how large it may be due to randomness alone. If it is larger than what may typically be found due to randomness, we conclude that it reflects true discrepancy between data and hypothesis and hence that we have to reject the hypothesis.

Now the question remains to determine what we mean by *"larger than what may typically be found due to randomness."* A keyword in this connection is the *tail probability* which is defined as the probability that a test statistic (under H_0) reflects a larger discrepancy from the hypothesis than actually observed. More specifically, let T_{obs} denote the observed value of the test statistic T. If a large numerical value reflects discrepancy from the hypothesis, we calculate the tail probability

$$P = \mathrm{pr}_{H_0}(|T| > |T_{obs}|) \qquad (2.3.6)$$

and we denote this tail probability the *P-value* for the hypothesis. Note that we use a capital P in order to distinguish it from a possible parameter p. We have here used the notation $\mathrm{pr}_{H_0}(...)$ to indicate that the probability has to be calculated under the assumption that H_0 is true. In order to calculate the P-value (2.3.6) we, therefore, have to know the distribution of the test statistic T under the hypothesis H_0. It will often be a hard task to derive this distribution and we may have to rely on "asymptotic" results (i.e., an approximative result), appropriate only for large sample sizes. The idea is that if the P-value is low (e.g., 0.001), it is highly unlikely to observe such a large discrepancy between data and hypothesis just by coincidence (i.e., due to randomness alone). Hence we conclude that the hypothesis must be rejected. Now, precisely how small should the P-value be in order for us to reject the hypothesis? This question is hard to answer, because it really ought to depend on the circumstances: what kind of consequences a rejection versus a nonrejection might have. However, it has become common practice to consider 0.05 as a "small" value, so that we reject the hypothesis whenever the tail probability (the P-value) is less than 0.05. We denote this value the *significance level* and it is often written as 5% instead of 0.05.

Table 2.3.3. Classification of conclusions versus truth.

Truth	Statement/Conclusion	
	Accept H_0	Reject H_0
H_0 true	$1-\alpha$	α error of type I level of significance
H_0 false	β error of type II	$1-\beta$ power

Two desirable situations may occur in a testing situation: accepting a true hypothesis and rejecting a false hypothesis. On the other hand, there are also two types of error, namely rejecting a true hypothesis (error of type I, with a probability equal to the chosen level of significance) and accepting a false hypothesis (error of type II, typically not fixed). These possible scenarios have been arranged in the two by two Table 2.3.3. The rows correspond to the two possible truths: H_0 true or false, whereas the two columns correspond to the two possible conclusions: acceptance or rejection.

The risk of a type I error is often believed to be more serious and is therefore fixed at a low level (typically 5%). For instance, a comparison favoring a new expensive treatment to a traditional one (rejecting the hypothesis that they are equally good) may result in markedly increased expenses for the health care system and should therefore be based on very conclusive evidence (a low significance level). We may, however, also imagine a quite different situation in which a new and cheaper treatment is compared to the traditional one and found to be no worse than this. This is a very typical situation with small studies; they may fail to show anything significant simply because of a much too low power (insufficient ability to reject a false hypothesis).

With a fixed amount of information (the available data), we cannot have it both ways: an attempt to reduce the risk of a type I error is invariably associated with an increase in the risk of a type II error (a reduction of power), or vice versa. We may, however, at the planning stage of the investigation, perform a *power analysis*, that is, attempt to estimate the power to detect a certain difference of interest, as a function of the sample size. Better yet to do it the other way around and determine a sufficient sample size for avoiding an inconclusive study. We look into these matters in Section 6.3.

It is intuitively clear that for a fixed level of significance, power will increase with sample size. However, power is not a single number, but a function of the true discrepancy between model and submodel (the hypothesis). For instance, in the hypothetical drug preference example, the power will be high for rejecting the hypothesis $H_0 : p = 0.5$ if the true p is close to either 0 or 1, whereas it will be very low (close to the significance level of 5%) when the true p is close to 0.5. We may formulate this to say that the power depends on *the alternative*: "if p is *not* 0.5, what is it then?"

Some test statistics may have high power against some alternatives and low power for others, so it is not always easy to say which test statistic is the best. In general, however, testing a hypothesis regarding a submodel "close to" the original model (e.g., involving only one parameter less than the original model) will be more powerful than testing a much more restrictive submodel. We may formulate this as general advice about trying to avoid tests with too many degrees-of-freedom.

In the light of the possible erroneous conclusions that could arise from hypothesis testing, we once more stress the opinion that P-values should serve merely as a supplement to confidence intervals rather than the other way around. The P-value indicates only the strength of the evidence against a certain hypothesis, for example a difference between two groups (low P-values indicating strong evidence) and is *not* a measure of the difference itself. Therefore, a low P-value is not necessarily the same as a substantial difference and vice versa. In the same way, a high P-value does not ensure absence of differences, merely an absence of evidence of a difference and we need a confidence interval in order to see whether important differences might have gone undetected because of a bad study design or a small sample size (low power).

Recall the fact that for tests of simple one-degree-of-freedom hypotheses (i.e., for testing submodels that include just one parameter less than the original model), there is a close correspondence between P-value and confidence interval: If the hypothesized value of the parameter is enclosed in the confidence interval, the test statistic will not be significant, and vice versa. For testing more complicated hypotheses (such as the simultaneous equality of three means), no such correspondence exists.

2.3.4 The likelihood function

When data have been collected, we may calculate the probability (or probability density) for these particular data, based on the model for the situation. This probability will, of course, be a function of the unknown parameters, and we denote this function the *likelihood function*. The likelihood principle for estimation of the unknown parameter(s) is based on maximization of this function, that is, to find the values of the unknown parameters that maximize the probability of observing precisely what we actually did observe. In other words, we believe the parameters to have values that make the observed data the most plausible. We review some examples in order to explain the ideas.

In the fetal death example, we know that out of a total of 11,778 pregnancies, 119 resulted in fetal death. We wish to estimate the probability p of fetal death using the likelihood principle. If we let y_i denote the binary outcome for woman i (1 indicating fetal death), the probability of observing y_i may be written as

$$\text{pr}(y_i = u) = \begin{cases} p & \text{if } u = 1 \\ 1 - p & \text{if } u = 0 \end{cases} = p^u (1-p)^{1-u}. \quad (2.3.7)$$

All women must be assumed to behave independently of each other, thus the probability of observing exactly the sequence $y_1, y_2, \ldots, y_{11,778}$ becomes the product of $n = 11,778$ such terms. With the notation $\prod_{i=1}^{n}$ for such a product, we may write the probability of the observed data as

$$L(p) = \text{pr}(\text{observed } ys) = \prod_{i=1}^{n} \left(p^{y_i} (1-p)^{1-y_i} \right) = p^S \times (1-p)^{n-S}, \quad (2.3.8)$$

where S denotes the total number of fetal deaths; that is, $S = \sum_{i=1}^{11778} y_i = 119$, implying that $n - S = 11,778 - 119 = 11,659$.

This function $L(p)$ is the likelihood function and it describes the probability of observing the actually observed y_is if p is the true probability of fetal death, that is, a function of the unknown parameter p. For some values of p, it will be very small (it is highly unlikely to observe only 119 fetal deaths, if p were as large as, e.g., 10%, or 0.1), whereas for other values of p it will be larger. We wish to determine the value of p that makes this probability the largest possible, and we denote this value $\hat{p}$, the *maximum likelihood estimate of p*.

In Figure 2.3.7, the likelihood function is seen for values of p between 0 and 0.02. Beyond this value, the likelihood function is vanishing, and we see a maximum around 0.01. The maximum of the function $L(p)$ is to be looked for among values that have a horizontal tangent, that is, points where the derivative $L'(p)$ is zero. Because likelihood functions involve products and most often powers, it is analytically more tractable to find the maximum of the logarithmic transform of the likelihood function, the so-called *log-likelihood function*, $l(p) = \log L(p)$. Hence, we may find the maximum likelihood estimate by solving the *estimating equation*

$$l'(p) = 0, \quad (2.3.9)$$

where the derived function $l'(p)$ is also denoted the *score function*. In our problem, we have the log-likelihood function

$$l(p) = S \log(p) + (n-S) \log(1-p) \quad (2.3.10)$$

and therefore the score function

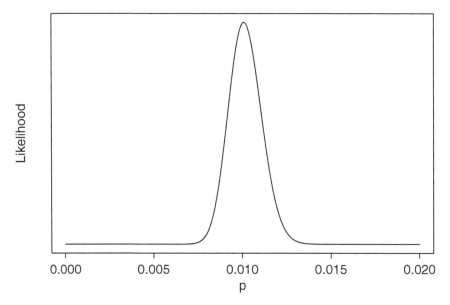

Fig. 2.3.7. Likelihood function for fetal death example.

$$l'(p) = \frac{S}{p} - \frac{n-S}{1-p}. \tag{2.3.11}$$

The log-likelihood function has a horizontal tangent at the maximum, thus we have by definition, that $l'(\hat{p}) = 0$, and the maximum likelihood estimate is therefore a solution to the equation

$$0 = \frac{S}{p} - \frac{n-S}{1-p} = \frac{S-np}{p(1-p)} \tag{2.3.12}$$

which is seen to give

$$\hat{p} = \frac{S}{n} = \frac{119}{11,778} \approx 0.010.$$

In Figure 2.3.8, the log-likelihood function as well as the score function is plotted as a function of the unknown parameter p. We see the horizontal tangent for the log-likelihood function at $\hat{p}$, corresponding to a score function value of zero.

The resulting estimate of p as the fraction of fetal deaths comes as no surprise in this context, because it is the natural way that one would proceed even in the absence of a principle. This is because the situation is so simple. It is, however, reassuring to see that in such a simple situation, the principle agrees with common sense.

When applying the maximum likelihood principle to models involving the Normal distribution, we need the mathematical description of the Normal

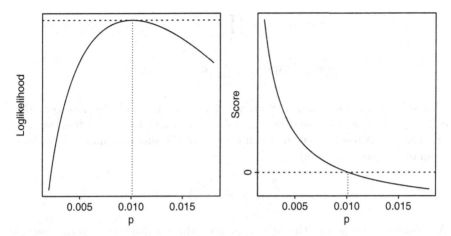

Fig. 2.3.8. Log-likelihood function and score function for fetal death example.

density for the distribution $N(m, s^2)$ with mean value m and standard deviation s, as a function of the observed u of y (cf. Figure 2.1.4). This is given by

$$\frac{1}{\sqrt{2\pi s^2}} \exp(-\frac{1}{2s^2}(u - m)^2).$$

When observing $y_1, \ldots, y_n$, assumed to come from this distribution, the likelihood function is therefore given by a product of such terms

$$
\begin{aligned}
L(m, s^2) &= \mathrm{pr}(\text{observed } ys) \\
&= \prod_{i=1}^{n} \frac{1}{\sqrt{2\pi s^2}} \exp(-\frac{1}{2s^2}(y_i - m)^2) \qquad (2.3.13) \\
&= (\frac{1}{\sqrt{2\pi s^2}})^n \exp(-\frac{1}{2s^2} \sum_{i=1}^{n}(y_i - m)^2).
\end{aligned}
$$

Mathematical theory tells us that the values of m and s^2 maximizing this function of two parameters (or equivalently, its logarithm) are $\bar{y}$ and $1/n \sum_{i=1}^{n}(y_i - \bar{y})^2$, respectively. Thus, the maximum likelihood estimate of the mean value, m is simply the average of the observed y_i-values, whereas the variance is estimated as the average squared distance from this average. Note that these estimates deviate somewhat from the usual estimate of standard deviation (2.2.1), a fact that we have already discussed in Section 2.3.1.

If we consider the more complicated situation of the linear regression model (blood pressure as a linear function of age, or vitamin D level as a linear function of body mass index), we find the likelihood function similarly to be

$$L(a, b, s^2) = \text{pr(observed } ys) = \prod_{i=1}^{n} \frac{1}{\sqrt{2\pi s^2}} \exp(-\frac{1}{2s^2}(y_i - a - bx_i)^2)$$

$$= (\frac{1}{\sqrt{2\pi s^2}})^n \exp(-\frac{1}{2s^2} \sum_{i=1}^{n}(y_i - a - bx_i)^2).$$

This situation is discussed in Section 4.1.1. It suffices here to note that the estimates for a and b based on maximization of this likelihood function are also those that result from the minimization of the sum of squared deviations (sum of squared residuals)

$$\sum_{i=1}^{n}(y_i - a - bx_i)^2.$$

As a consequence of this, the estimation procedure is also known as the *method of least squares* . This latter estimation method also works adequately in more general situations, that is, with no particular distributional assumptions.

The likelihood function may also be used for construction of test statistics for a hypothesis H_0. Most commonly, one considers the *likelihood ratio statistic*

$$Q = \frac{\text{max. Likelihood under } H_0}{\text{max. Likelihood under model}}. \tag{2.3.14}$$

Because the hypothesis is a submodel of the original model, it is obvious that the value in the denominator of Equation (2.3.14) will be greater than or equal to the value of the numerator and therefore the ratio Q will always be smaller than 1. For the likelihood ratio statistic, therefore, a small test statistic reflects an unreasonable hypothesis. Most often, it will not be possible to determine the exact distribution of Q. The logarithm of Q will usually be more tractable inasmuch as it is a sum instead of a product, and in particular, the quantity $-2 \log Q$ can be shown (under certain, not very restrictive, circumstances) to have an asymptotic *Chi-squared distribution*, with *degrees-of-freedom* equal to the difference in the number of parameters in model and hypothesis. A collection of distributions of this type, with varying degrees-of-freedom can be seen in Figure 2.3.9. These distributions arise quite commonly in connection with tests of hypotheses, but rarely as distributions for primary observations (see, however, Section 7.3). The Chi-squared distribution of $-2 \log Q$ is, as stated above, only *asymptotic*, meaning that the approximation gets better as the sample size increases. For hypotheses such as $H_0 : p = 0.5$, $H_0 : b = 0$ or $H_0 : m_1 = m_2$ (the identity of two means), it will have only one degree-of-freedom, corresponding to the upper-left panel of Figure 2.3.9.

In the hypothetical cross-over example with the two drugs, we test the hypothesis $H_0 : p = 0.5$ and letting again S be the number of preferences for drug A, we get the likelihood ratio

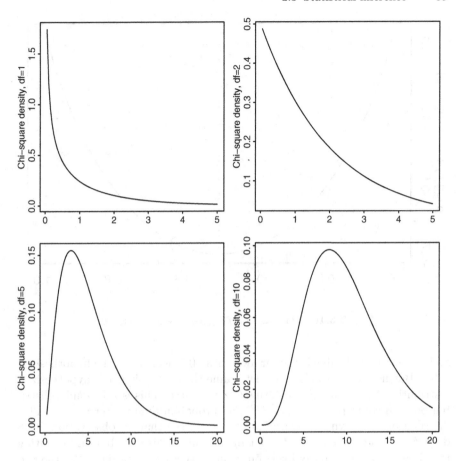

Fig. 2.3.9. Chi-squared distributions with 1, 2, 5, and 10 degrees-of-freedom.

$$Q = \frac{L(0.5)}{L(\widehat{p})} = \frac{0.5^S(1-0.5)^{n-S}}{\widehat{p}^S(1-\widehat{p})^{n-S}},$$ (2.3.15)

or rewritten as the quantity $-2\log Q$:

$$-2\log Q = 2n(\log 2 + \widehat{p}\log\widehat{p} + (1-\widehat{p})\log(1-\widehat{p})).$$ (2.3.16)

We reject the hypothesis if $-2\log Q$ is too large, that is, when the quantity

$$\widehat{p}\log\widehat{p} + (1-\widehat{p})\log(1-\widehat{p})$$

is too large. This function can be shown to be U-shaped and symmetric around $\widehat{p} = 0.5$ (see Figure 2.3.10) and hence, we simply reject the hypothesis, if $\widehat{p}$ is too far from 0.5, that is, when $|\widehat{p} - 0.5|$ or equivalently $|S - n/2|$ is too large.

In the hypothetical drug example, we get $\widehat{p} = 0.7$ and, thereby, $|\widehat{p} - 0.5| = 0.2$ and $|S - n/2| = |28 - 20| = 8$. It seems quite sensible to reject the hypothe-

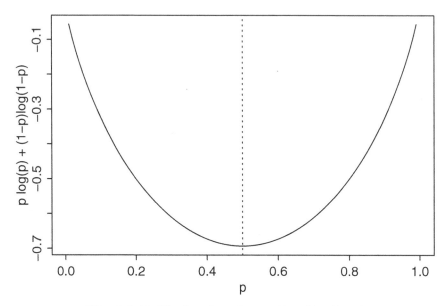

Fig. 2.3.10. The function $p \log p + (1 - p) \log(1 - p)$.

sis if the estimated value is too far away from 0.5, which was the hypothesized value. But how far is too far? To determine this, we look at the hypothesized distribution for the number of drug A preferences. This is a Binomial distribution with count parameter $n = 40$ and probability parameter $p = 0.5$. This distribution is shown in Figure 2.3.11 and we see that an observation of 28 drug A preferences is rather far out in the tail of this distribution indicating that it is not a particularly likely outcome if we are to postulate that the two drugs are equally effective. Rather, we are more inclined to believe that drug A is the more effective of the two drugs.

We can formalize this by calculating the tail probability (2.3.6) which in this case is the probability of observing a discrepancy of eight or more preferences either way if the drugs were truly equally effective. In Figure 2.3.11, such discrepancies are marked in bold, and their corresponding probabilities sum up to 0.0094, that is, less than 1% of the total probability. This means that the observed number of drug A preferences is too large to be a plausible observation if the hypothesis ($p = 0.5$) is true. Because we have actually observed this many drug A preferences, we choose to believe that the hypothesis is *not* true. We *reject* the hypothesis (with the P-value 0.0094) and declare A to be the more effective drug.

If we use the $-2 \log Q$ approach to the test, we get $-2 \log Q = 6.58$ which compared to a Chi-squared distribution with one degree-of-freedom gives a tail probability (P-value) of 0.0103, that is, very close to the above finding.

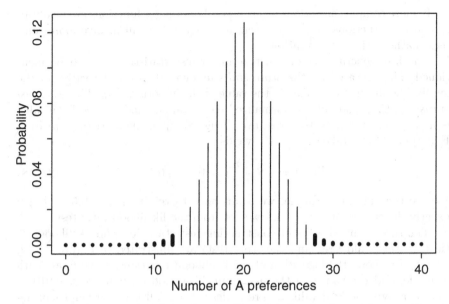

Fig. 2.3.11. Point probabilities for the Binomial distribution with $n = 40$ and $p = 0.5$.

Another quite general principle for deriving test statistics is to reformulate (if possible) the hypothesis to say that one (or more) parameter functions should be zero. In the examples considered thus far, this quantity could be $p - 0.5$, b itself, or $m_1 - m_0$. If comparing mean values of three groups, we would have a hypothesis of $m_0 = m_1 = m_2$ which may be reformulated as $m_1 - m_0 = m_2 - m_0 = 0$, that is, two parameter functions should be equal to zero.

In the case of a single parameter function which is hypothesized to be zero, the *Wald test statistic* is defined as the squared ratio between an estimate of this quantity (using the maximum likelihood estimate or any other sensible estimate) and its corresponding standard deviation

$$W = (\frac{\text{Estimate}}{\text{SD(Estimate)}})^2. \tag{2.3.17}$$

In situations where the Central Limit Theorem applies, the estimate will have an approximate Normal distribution. Therefore, the quantity W will be approximately distributed as a Chi-square with one degree-of-freedom and large values will lead to a rejection of the hypothesis. In the hypothetical drug example, we had $\hat{p} - 0.5 = 0.2$, and $\text{SD}(\hat{p} - 0.5) = 0.072$, which gives $W = (0.2/0.072)^2 = 7.72$. This is a little more than we got from the two approaches considered so far, and hence the P-value is a little lower, here 0.0055.

In more complex situations where several parameter functions are involved, similar constructions may be derived, although these will involve more complex mathematical computations.

One last general way of constructing a test statistic needs to be mentioned. This is based on the *score statistic*, defined as the derivative of the log-likelihood function, taken in the value of the hypothesis H_0. The *score test statistic* is the square of the normalized score statistic and rejects if the value is numerically large. In the cross-over drug example, the statistic $l'(p)$ from Equation (2.3.11) taken in $p = 0.5$ yields

$$l'(0.5) = 4(S - \frac{n}{2}) = 4n\left(\widehat{p} - 0.5\right). \tag{2.3.18}$$

We see that in this example, we again have to reject, if $|\widehat{p} - 0.5|$ is large: exactly the same conclusion that we got from the likelihood ratio test.

The three general ways of constructing test statistics (the likelihood ratio test, the Wald test, and the score test) are illustrated in Figure 2.3.12. This figure shows the logarithm of the likelihood function for the fetal death example, and the values of the maximum likelihood estimate, $\widehat{p} \approx 0.010$ as well as a hypothesized value p_0 are indicated. For all three principles of deriving test statistics, we look at the discrepancies between these two values, although in different respects: the likelihood ratio statistic looks at the vertical distance, that is, the difference between the values of the log-likelihood function itself, the Wald statistic looks at the horizontal distance, that is, the distance between the estimated and the hypothesized parameter values (squared and properly normalized), and the score test statistic looks at the slope of the curve in the hypothesized value (squared and properly normalized) and contrasts it to zero, which is the slope at the maximum likelihood estimate. Note that when calculating the score test we only need to estimate in the submodel given by the hypothesis and not in the original model. This may be a computational advantage in complicated situations. In the present example, this implies no estimation at all, because we have only the single parameter p, which under the hypothesis is fixed to 0.5.

No matter how we construct our test statistic, the idea behind the test will be the same: is it plausible that the simpler model may have generated our observed data, or can we reject this hypothesis? We do not know the truth but we use our observed data to make a statement about the perceived truth. Our statement may be correct or it may be wrong, and we can formulate the various possibilities in the two-way Table 2.3.3, which was discussed in Section 2.3.3.

2.4 Exercises

Exercise 2.1. Use the tryptase dataset 3 from Example 1.12 for investigating the distribution of baseline tryptase:

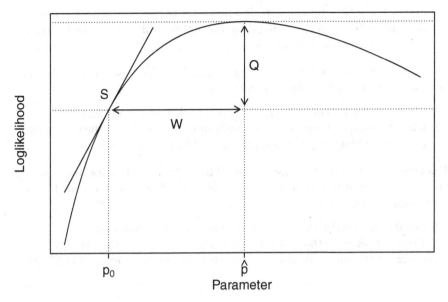

Fig. 2.3.12. Illustration of likelihood ratio test, Wald test, and score test. The notation Q, W, and S refers to the characteristics used for defining the likelihood ratio test, the Wald test, and the score test, respectively. For more information, see text.

1. Make a histogram and comment on the symmetry of the distribution. Calculate the average and the median and comment upon their discrepancy.
2. Try a logarithmic transformation of baseline tryptase and again make a histogram and calculate summary statistics.
3. How would we report a 95% reference interval for baseline tryptase values?
4. Based on the most appropriate scale as found from the above exercise, make a comparison between men and women, in terms of histograms as well as summary statistics and reference intervals.

Exercise 2.2. Use the vitamin D data for the girls from Example 1.1 and investigate the distribution of vitamin D levels, both graphically and by calculation of appropriate summary statistics.

Exercise 2.3. Use the PBC data from Example 1.3 to describe the distribution of bilirubin.

1. Calculate the average and the SD and use these to calculate a 95% reference region based on an assumption of Normality for bilirubin.
2. Compare this reference region to the empirical 2.5% and 97.5% quantiles and comment on the discrepancy.
3. Draw a histogram for bilirubin, as well as for a logarithmic transform of this. Is it reasonable to assume Normality for any of these two scales?

   4. Show that a 95% reference region based on the assumption of Normality on a logarithmic scale is given by the interval (3.3,182.1) and compare this to the empirical quantiles.

Exercise 2.4. Use the CSL data from Example 1.7 to describe the distribution of ascites in each of the two treatment groups:

1. Make a three by two table and calculate relevant percentages.
2. Does it look as if there is an even distribution of ascites in the two groups? (To answer this properly, see Exercise 3.14 in Chapter 3.)

Exercise 2.5. Use the tryptase dataset 2 from Example 1.12 for investigating the distribution of the reaction classes (the type of allergic reaction) for men and women separately:

1. Make a four by two table and calculate relevant percentages.
2. Does it look as if there is a genuine sex difference in the severity of the allergic reactions? (To answer this precisely, see Exercise 3.10 in Chapter 3.)

3

One categorical covariate

In this chapter, we discuss one of the two building blocks of regression models, namely models including only a single categorical covariate. This means that we compare groups, such as treatments, countries, stature groups based on body mass index, diet types, age groups, and so on.

Even if, in practice, it is often considered relevant or necessary to include the effect of other covariates as well, an initial comparison of groups is often called upon. This is particularly so in clinical trials, where a randomization secures an unbiased comparison between treatment groups.

We have divided the chapter into sections according to the nature of the covariate (binary or with more than two categories). For a binary covariate, the task is simply to compare two groups, and the challenge is to provide an interpretable measure of discrepancy between these, with a confidence interval. For covariates with more than two levels, a complicating feature is that we now have many possible group contrasts to look at, and we must take care to avoid spurious significances (if we ask too many questions, we will get too many wrong answers).

Each section is again divided into subsections according to the nature of the outcome. For quantitative outcomes, we look at differences in mean values, for binary outcomes, the focus is on odds ratios, whereas for survival data, the discrepancies are most naturally described as hazard ratios. However, as we show, the basic ideas are the same whatever the nature of the outcome, only the techniques differ according to the mathematics of the models. Along the way, simple and classical techniques are shown as special cases of regression. These include the t-test and one-way analysis of variance for quantitative outcomes, the Chi-square tests for 2×2- and $2 \times (k + 1)$-tables for binary outcomes, and the 2- and $(k + 1)$- sample logrank tests for survival data. It is important to notice that we do not assume that readers are familiar with these methods in advance.

For notation, let $y_1, \ldots, y_n$ denote the measured outcome values for the n subjects in the sample and let $x_1, \ldots, x_n$ denote the corresponding covariate values. We wish to specify how various aspects of the distribution of the ys may depend upon a single categorical covariate x in a way that is linear in the parameters, cf. Section 1.4.2.

3.1 Binary covariate

Categorical covariates with two levels are often called *dichotomous* or *binary*. Such variables are extremely common, an obvious example being gender. As mentioned in Section 1.4.2 gender is an example of a variable that is observable, but not controllable, and this means that whenever we study sex differences for a particular outcome variable, we must be aware that men and women differ in many respects and that some of these may account for the gender difference in this particular outcome. On the other hand, in a clinical trial the typical situation is a comparison of two treatments. The treatment is then another example of a dichotomous or binary variable, this time controllable, because we have the opportunity to choose, in particular by randomization, which patients receive which treatment.

For a categorical covariate with only two levels, the statistical problem becomes that of comparing two groups. For instance, we could be interested in estimation of the difference in mean blood pressure between men and women, the mean percentage of blood pressure reduction following an active drug compared to placebo, the odds ratio of fetal death for women experiencing fever during pregnancy in relation to those who do not, or the hazard ratio of treatment failure for cirrhosis patients receiving CyA compared to patients in the placebo group.

The precise way of summarizing the discrepancy between two groups will depend on the nature of the outcome but also on the particular problem at hand. Of primary importance is to derive a quantity that has a sensible and intuitive interpretation for the subject matter, and to provide a measure of uncertainty for this quantity, preferably in the form of a confidence interval.

Such a confidence interval summarizes our knowledge about the difference between the groups in an interpretable way, but may be supplemented (although not replaced) by a significance test, the hypothesis being that the groups are identical. It is important to note, however, that the result of a significance test is a P-value, indicating the strength of the evidence of a difference between the groups (low P-values indicating strong evidence) and not a measure of the difference itself. Thus, as mentioned in generality in Section 2.3.3, a low P-value is not necessarily the same as a substantial difference between the two groups but may simply reflect a large sample or a low variability, whereas the estimated difference itself may not be impressive nor of any practical importance. Likewise, a high P-value (indicating nonsignificance) does not necessarily imply that the two groups are identical but may instead merely indicate that we do not have enough evidence to conclude with any confidence.

3.1.1 Quantitative outcome: *t*-tests

In Chapter 1, we have mentioned examples of a quantitative outcome, for example, blood pressure measurements. If we combine this with a categorical covariate with two levels, we have the problem of comparing blood pressure in two groups. We look at data from a similar example, namely the vitamin D Example 1.1 concerned with body mass index (BMI) and vitamin D status.

You may recall that body mass index is a height-corrected measure of weight, defined as

$$\text{BMI} = \frac{\text{weight in } kg}{\text{height in } m, \text{ squared}}.$$

According to the predominant interpretation of this quantity, an individual is considered to be of normal weight if BMI is between 18.5 and 25, whereas we denote the individual as underweight (respectively, overweight), if BMI is below 18.5 (respectively, above 25). The group of older Irish women from the vitamin D example consists of 41 individuals, among whom we have 16 normal weight and 25 overweight women.

We are concerned here with the association (if any) between BMI and vitamin D status, as measured by 25-hydroxy vitamin D (25OHD) in serum (in nmol/L), and more specifically, we compare vitamin D status for normal weight and overweight women.

A graphical presentation of the S25OHD according to body stature group is given as a scatterplot in Figure 3.1.1.

From Figure 3.1.1 we note that in this particular example the distribution of S25OHD is quite symmetric, although perhaps with a slight tendency to right-skewness (tail of large values). The mean and standard deviation in each group are therefore meaningful quantities (Section 2.2.2).

We let y_i denote the outcome (S25OHD) for the ith woman, x_i the corresponding body mass index (BMI) for the ith woman and assume all the y_is to be independent with mean values given by

$$\text{E}(y_i) = \begin{cases} m_0 \text{ if subject } i \text{ is normal weight } (18.5 < \text{BMI} < 25), \\ m_1 \text{ if subject } i \text{ is overweight } (\text{BMI} \geq 25). \end{cases} \quad (3.1.1)$$

In terms of the covariate x_i, we may write the mean value structure in the regression form as

$$\text{E}(y_i) = m_0 + (m_1 - m_0)I(x_i \geq 25) = a + bI(x_i \geq 25), \quad (3.1.2)$$

where we have defined new parameters as

$$a = m_0, \ b = m_1 - m_0.$$

From Figure 3.1.1, we get the impression that overweight women have a slightly inferior vitamin D status compared to normal weight women: that

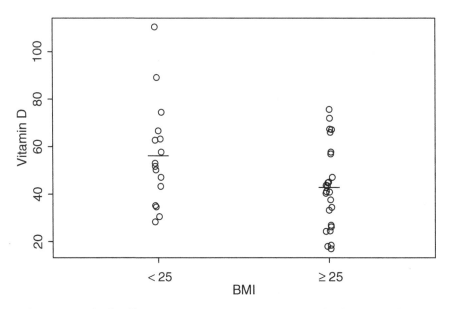

Fig. 3.1.1. The S25OHD in two stature groups, cutpoint body mass index= 25.

m_1 is slightly smaller than m_0, corresponding to a negative b-coefficient in the above notation (3.1.2). We quantify this difference in means between the two groups with a confidence interval and give a formal P-value for test of equality.

The estimates for the two means (simple averages for S25OHD in each group separately; cf. Section 2.3.1) are given in Table 3.1.1, together with the medians and the standard deviations, $\widehat{s}_0$ and $\widehat{s}_1$.

Table 3.1.1. Summary statistics for S25OHD according to BMI.

Group, j	Number, n_j	Average, $\widehat{m}_j$	Median, $\widehat{M}_j$	Standard Deviation, $\widehat{s}_j$
0: Normal weight	16	56.138	52.350	21.941
1: Overweight	25	42.804	41.100	17.562

The average and the median in each group look quite similar, indicating no large deviation from symmetrical distributions. The standard deviations in the two groups also look reasonably equal, with only a slightly larger variation in the normal weight group. When comparing mean values in two groups, it is common to assume such an equality between the population variations in the two groups as a prerequisite and initially, we follow this tradition. Later in this section, we return to a discussion on checks of the model assumptions as well as remedies for important violations of these.

Note that at this stage we have not made any assumptions of Normality or any other particular distributional form. The only distributional assumption so far lies in the demand that mean and standard deviation have to be meaningful quantities and this means that the distributions should be reasonably symmetric. As a consequence of this lack of distributional assumptions, the procedures derived are only approximate and may not be trustworthy for small samples. For large samples, however, the Central Limit Theorem as presented in Section 2.3.1 assures that the procedures will be valid.

Because the averages, $\bar{y}_0$ and $\bar{y}_1$ in the two stature groups are estimates of the two means, it follows that we may estimate the regression coefficient (the difference in means) $b = m_1 - m_0$ as

$$\hat{b} = \bar{y}_1 - \bar{y}_0$$

and that this quantity has mean value

$$E(\hat{b}) = E(\bar{y}_1 - \bar{y}_0) = m_1 - m_0 = b$$

and a standard deviation, estimated by

$$SD(\hat{b}) = SD(\bar{y}_1 - \bar{y}_0) = \hat{s}\sqrt{\frac{1}{n_0} + \frac{1}{n_1}}, \tag{3.1.3}$$

where n_0 and n_1 denote the two group sizes, and $\hat{s}$ denotes the pooled estimate of the common standard deviation in the two stature groups

$$\hat{s} = \sqrt{\frac{(n_0 - 1)\hat{s}_0^2 + (n_1 - 1)\hat{s}_1^2}{(n_0 - 1) + (n_1 - 1)}} = 19.296. \tag{3.1.4}$$

For large samples, the Central Limit Theorem ensures that $\hat{b} = \bar{y}_1 - \bar{y}_0$ will have an approximate Normal distribution, and an approximate 95% confidence interval for the difference $b = m_1 - m_0$ can therefore be calculated as

$$\hat{b} \pm 1.96 \cdot SD(\hat{b}) = \bar{y}_1 - \bar{y}_0 \pm 1.96 \cdot SD(\bar{y}_1 - \bar{y}_0) \tag{3.1.5}$$

where the term $SD(\hat{b}) = SD(\bar{y}_1 - \bar{y}_0)$ is taken from Equation (3.1.3).

Table 3.1.2. Summary statistics for the comparison of the two stature groups.

Parameter	Estimate	SD of Estimate	95% Confidence Interval
m_0	56.138	5.485	(45.387, 66.889)
m_1	42.804	3.512	(35.920, 49.688)
$b = m_1 - m_0$	-13.334	6.199	(-25.484, -1.184)

As mentioned, the above construction (3.1.5) of the confidence interval is based on an assumption of Normality of $\hat{b} = \bar{y}_1 - \bar{y}_0$ that will be reasonable for large datasets. However, even if this assumption is exactly fulfilled (i.e., if 25OHD is itself Normally distributed within each group), the construction is still only approximate, because the quantity $SD(\hat{b})$ is merely an estimate and not the true standard deviation. This means that for small samples, the interval above will have a slightly smaller coverage than the required 95%. In practice, this is most often of minor importance and need not lead to worries. For quantitative, Normally distributed observations it has, however, become tradition (in textbooks as well as in standard statistical software packages) to correct for this bias, and we therefore describe such a correction below, following the test for equal means.

Even though a confidence interval provides all necessary information to make conclusions about the discrepancy between the two groups, it is nevertheless common (and in connection with publications, often even mandatory) to assess the strength of the difference by performing an additional formal test of the hypothesis of identical means. We may formulate this as a test of the regression coefficient b being equal to zero:

$$H_0 : b = 0 \text{ or, equivalently } H_0 : m_0 = m_1.$$

In analogy with the above construction (3.1.5) of a confidence interval we get an intuitively interpretable test statistic (the signed square root of the Wald test statistic)

$$t = \frac{\hat{b}}{SD(\hat{b})} = \frac{\bar{y}_1 - \bar{y}_0}{SD(\bar{y}_1 - \bar{y}_0)}. \tag{3.1.6}$$

In the case of a Normal distribution assumption this also corresponds to the likelihood ratio test as well as the score test. For large samples, this quantity will have an approximate $N(0, 1)$ distribution and we therefore judge the test to be significant if its absolute value exceeds 1.96. This is in agreement with the confidence intervals constructed above, in the sense that a confidence interval excluding zero corresponds to a significant test statistic and vice versa.

Here, the test statistic becomes

$$t = \frac{-13.334}{6.199} = -2.15$$

which evaluated in a Normal distribution gives us a P-value of 0.032, that is, formally significant, corresponding to the confidence interval of $(-25.484, -1.184)$ found above in Table 3.1.2, not including zero. It is worth noticing that, in Table 3.1.2, the confidence intervals for m_0 and m_1 overlap: values betwen 45.387 and 49.688 belong to both intervals. It is a common mistake to conclude that two parameters do not differ at the 5% level if their 95% confidence intervals overlap but, as we can see from this example, this is, indeed, a mistake. However, arguing "the other way around," that is, concluding that two parameters differ at the 5% level if their 95% confidence intervals do not overlap is, in fact, correct. We show an example of that situation in Section 3.1.2.

In the construction of confidence limits and in the interpretation of the test statistic above, we have made use of a Normal approximation to the test statistic (3.1.6). However, due to the inherent uncertainty in the estimated standard deviation $\text{SD}(\widehat{b})$, this may be an inaccurate approximation for small samples, even if the estimate $\widehat{b}$ can be taken to be Normally distributed. Instead, we may base our inference on the so-called t-distribution (also known as the Student-distribution). If the observations are actually Normally distributed within each group, it can be shown that t from Equation (3.1.6) will follow such a t-distribution. This is slightly more heavy-tailed than the Normal distribution. Hence, the quantiles in the t-distribution are slightly (numerically) larger than the corresponding Normal quantiles, and more so the smaller the sample size. The t-distribution is characterized by a parameter called the degrees-of-freedom (df), reflecting the sample size (the degrees-of-freedom may be calculated as the number of observations minus the number of mean value parameters) .

In the case of comparison of two groups, the degrees-of-freedom become

$$df = (n_0 - 1) + (n_1 - 1) = (16 - 1) + (25 - 1) = 39$$

and the upper 2.5% quantile in the t-distribution with 39 degrees-of-freedom (i.e., the 97.5% quantile) is given by 2.023. Hence, the test statistic should only be judged significant, if the absolute value exceeds 2.023, rather than 1.96, and the confidence limit for $b = m_1 - m_0$ should correspondingly be calculated as

$$\bar{y}_1 - \bar{y}_0 \pm 2.023 \cdot \widehat{s}\sqrt{\frac{1}{n_0} + \frac{1}{n_1}}. \tag{3.1.7}$$

We have summarized the results in Table 3.1.3.

Table 3.1.3. Comparison of S25OHD in two BMI groups.

$b = m_1 - m_0$	Estimate	SD	95% Confidence Interval	Test Statistic	P-Value
Normal	−13.334	6.199	(−25.484, −1.184)	2.15	0.032
t	−13.334	6.199	(−25.875, −0.793)	2.15	0.038

We again note the correspondence between confidence limits and tests in the sense that confidence intervals, which almost include zero, correspond to P-values close to 5%. We also note that evaluation of the test statistic in a t-distribution instead of a Normal distribution gives rise to a slightly larger P-value and a slightly wider confidence interval. This is a consequence of the t-distribution being more dispersed than the Normal distribution. Intuitively speaking, we do not have quite as much precision as we think, inasmuch as $\widehat{s}$ is only an estimate, not the true value.

The confidence interval for the difference in means lies just below zero, indicating that formally, we have a significant difference between the two stature groups on a 5% level. On the other hand, compared to the range of values for S25OHD, the confidence interval is rather wide, so that our knowledge about the actual difference between the two groups is weak. There may be almost no difference, or there may be a difference as large as 25 units.

The assumption of Normality

The calculation of confidence intervals and the interpretation of the test statistic are often believed to rely heavily on the assumption of Normality in the original sample. It is true that the formula for the confidence intervals (3.1.5) and the test statistic (3.1.6) can be derived from the general likelihood theory presented in Section 2.3.1 when the original observations are Normally distributed within each group. A closer look at the calculations, however, shows that in order to obtain reasonable confidence limits and validity of the t-test, the Normality assumption needs only be fulfilled for the averages, $\bar{y}_0$ and $\bar{y}_1$, or rather, for the difference between these, $\bar{y}_1 - \bar{y}_0$. If the group sizes n_0 and n_1 are not too small, this will in most cases be a reasonable assumption due to the Central Limit Theorem, as described in Section 2.3.1, even if the distributions within groups deviate somewhat from Normality. We conclude that for large investigations, the procedures are quite robust to deviations from Normality, as long as the distributions are still reasonably symmetric.

On the other hand, as was also pointed out in Section 2.1, the interpretation of averages and standard deviations for descriptive purposes becomes doubtful if the distributions deviate systematically from Normality (e.g., if they are not reasonably symmetric). In such situations, confidence intervals for differences between means may also be hard to interpret. It is therefore of some value to have procedures for checking the closeness to Normality or at least for checking that Normality is not systematically wrong, for example in the form of a highly asymmetrical distribution.

Several procedures could be considered:

- Visual inspection of observations in each group separately
- Numerical tests of observations in each group
- Visual inspection of all residuals simultaneously
- Numerical tests of all residuals simultaneously

Recall from Section 2.3.2 that a residual is defined as an observation (y_i) minus its expected value ($\widehat{m}_i$); that is,

$$r_i = y_i - \widehat{m}_{j(i)},$$

the original observation minus the group average. We have here used the notation $j(i)$ to denote the number of the group containing subject i.

Investigating the Normality assumption for each group separately requires larger sample sizes than looking at pooled residuals and is not generally recommended because it may lead to conflicting results for the two groups and hence to an unclear conclusion.

Visual inspection of residuals follows the same lines as described for the one-sample situation in Section 2.3.2. In Figure 3.1.2, we show a sample of possible plots. We may or may not supplement these graphical displays with a formal test for Normality, but as mentioned in Section 2.3.2 we believe such tests to be of limited value, because small samples will often fail to reject Normality (even if it is far from fulfilled) whereas large samples will often reject Normality (even if deviations from this are small and unimportant).

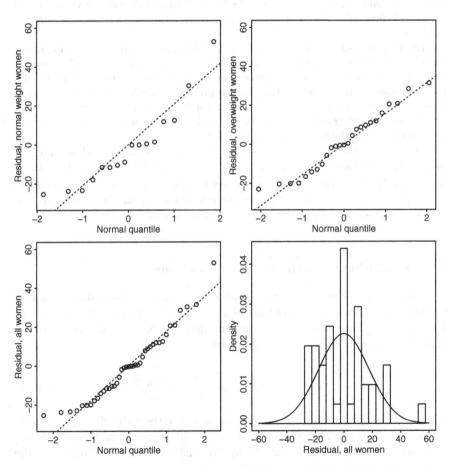

Fig. 3.1.2. Residual plots for model check.

The graphical displays show a slight tendency towards a heavy tail to the right, indicating a possible profit from a logarithmic transformation (Appendix B). We look into this possibility later in this section.

Digression. Nonparametric comparison

If the assumption of Normality is far from fulfilled, or if the sample size is very small, so that a justification of Normality is impossible, we may instead perform a nonparametric test of identity of the distribution of S25OHD for the two BMI groups. The term "nonparametric" may be slightly misleading, because it is often interpreted as free from assumptions of any kind. This is not the case, inasmuch as formally, the only assumption that is abandoned is the Normality assumption. We still assume the distributions to have the same shape in the two groups. The most traditional nonparametric test is the Mann–Whitney U-test, also known as the unpaired Wilcoxon test (e.g., Altman, 1991, Ch. 9; Armitage, Berry, and Matthews, 2002, Ch. 10).

The result of such a test is merely a P-value and no parameter estimates or confidence intervals are provided. Furthermore, the test cannot be used in general regression situations and it is therefore beyond the scope of this book to discuss the derivation or properties of this. In the present example, the test results in a P-value of 0.058, or with a continuity correction, 0.059. This is slightly higher than for the corresponding t-test due to the fact that a nonparametric test is generally less powerful than the parametric counterpart.

Due to the absence of a relevant estimate with an associated confidence interval, we are often reluctant to use the nonparametric approach. If the Normality assumption is clearly inadequate, another possibility may be to transform the outcome. In case of heavy right tails, the proper transformation will usually be the logarithm. As mentioned above, we return to this possibility later in this section. ◇

The assumption of equal standard deviations

The derivation of confidence limits and test statistic outlined above relies on the traditional assumption of identical standard deviations in the two groups. If this assumption is not reasonably fulfilled, we have to modify the 95% confidence interval for $b = m_1 - m_0$ to be

$$\bar{y}_1 - \bar{y}_0 \pm t_{97.5\%}(df) \sqrt{\frac{\hat{s}_1^2}{n_1} + \frac{\hat{s}_0^2}{n_0}}, \tag{3.1.8}$$

where $t_{97.5\%}(df)$ denotes the 97.5% quantile for the t-distribution with df degrees-of-freedom. This df will most often not be an integer, and the corresponding t-distribution is only an approximation to the distribution of the corresponding test statistic, given by

$$t = \frac{\hat{b}}{\text{SD}(\hat{b})} = \frac{\bar{y}_1 - \bar{y}_0}{\text{SD}(\bar{y}_1 - \bar{y}_0)} = \frac{\bar{y}_1 - \bar{y}_0}{\sqrt{\frac{\hat{s}_1^2}{n_1} + \frac{\hat{s}_0^2}{n_0}}}. \tag{3.1.9}$$

This version of the t-test is also denoted *the Welch test* (Armitage, Berry, and Matthews, 2002, Ch. 4), and the formula for the degrees-of-freedom is

$$df = \frac{(\frac{\hat{s}_0^2}{n_0} + \frac{\hat{s}_1^2}{n_1})^2}{\frac{\hat{s}_0^4}{n_0^2(n_0-1)} + \frac{\hat{s}_1^4}{n_1^2(n_1-1)}}.$$

In this particular example, the approximating number of degrees-of-freedom is 27.0, and the corresponding 97.5% quantile is 2.052, so that the confidence limit for the difference between means ($b = m_1 - m_0$) would become $(-26.700, 0.032)$, to be compared with the former result of $(-25.875, -0.793)$, that is, slightly wider. This is due to the fact that the largest standard deviation corresponds to the group with smallest size.

The test statistic changes similarly:

$$t = \frac{-13.334}{6.513} = -2.05 \sim t(27.0), \; P = 0.051$$

and formally, no significance is obtained.

Of course, the fact that the two approaches (standard deviations either equal or different) lead to different formal conclusions should not be regarded too seriously, because this is mainly due to the fact that we have made an arbitrary cutoff value (the significance level) of 5%. The standard deviations for the estimates differ by only 5% ($(6.513 - 6.199)/6.199 = 0.05$; cf. Table 3.1.4), and the actual P-values do not differ substantially ($P = 0.038$, respectively, $P = 0.051$).

The results based on the t-distribution are summarized in Table 3.1.4.

Table 3.1.4. Estimated differences in S25OHD in two BMI groups, according to whether the SDs are assumed equal.

$b = m_1 - m_0$	Estimate	SD	95% Confidence Interval	Test Statistic	P-Value
SDs equal	-13.334	6.199	(-25.875, -0.793)	2.15	0.038
SDs different	-13.334	6.513	(-26.700, 0.032)	2.05	0.051

In a practical situation, one would be reluctant to strongly emphasize a real difference between the groups based on this evidence alone. However, we would not be able to rule out a difference of the order of magnitude 25 units, a fact that at the same time prevents us from concluding that the two groups have identical means.

In the above presentation, we have looked at confidence intervals and test statistics both with and without assuming equal standard deviations in the two groups. We have noted that often it will be harder to obtain a significant result without an assumption of equal standard deviations and the corresponding confidence interval will be wider, in the spirit of "fewer assumptions lead to more vague conclusions."

It is very common to see conclusions based solely on the results relying on the assumption of equal standard deviations. This is especially true for the more complex situations where alternatives either do not exist or require specific programming. As we noted from Figure 3.1.1, the assumption of equal standard deviations seems reasonable in the present example, but we may consult a formal test in order to more safely conclude whether we may base our conclusion on this assumption. The traditional test for comparing two standard deviations is given by the squared ratio between the two:

$$F = \frac{\widehat{s}_1^2}{\widehat{s}_0^2} = \frac{21.941^2}{17.562^2} = 1.56. \tag{3.1.10}$$

If the two standard deviations were actually identical, and if the S25OHD values could be assumed to be Normally distributed within each group, then this F-quantity would be distributed as an F-distribution, with 15 degrees-of-freedom for the numerator and 24 degrees-of-freedom for the denominator. We write this as $F \sim F(15, 24)$. In the present example, the test statistic 1.56 corresponds to a P-value of 0.32, indicating that there is no real reason to doubt the hypothesis of equal standard deviations. On the other hand, with the limited amount of information available in these data, we cannot rule out quite large differences. Actually, a 95% confidence interval for the ratio s_1^2/s_0^2 is from $1.56/2.11 = 0.74$ to $1.56 \cdot 2.11 = 3.29$, where 2.11 is the 95%-quantile in the $F(15, 24)$-distribution. This wide confidence interval suggests that there is quite large uncertainty as to whether the two variances differ. It is, therefore, advisable to examine how much the conclusion concerning equality or not between the two mean values relies on the assumption of variance homogeneity.

Digression. The case of more than two groups

The above F-test for identical standard deviations does not generalize to more complex models (e.g., involving more than two possibly different standard deviations). Instead, such situations offer approximate solutions, valid for large samples that are not too non-Normally distributed. The most commonly used tests are *Levene's test* which here gives $0.87 \sim F(1, 39), P = 0.36$ and *Bartlett's test* , which gives $0.91 \sim \chi^2(1), P = 0.34$ (e.g., Draper and Smith, 1998, Ch. 2). We present more on this topic in Section 3.2.1. ◇

Transformation

As promised, we now return to the possibility of transformation. As we noted from the residual plots in Figure 3.1.2, there is a tendency to a skewness in the distribution of S25OHD within each group. A logarithmic transformation (cf. Appendix B) will help making the distributions more symmetric. We also saw that even though the standard deviations are not significantly different, the group with the highest average also has the highest standard deviation. This is typical for data with heavy right-hand tails, and standard deviations for log-transformed data will often tend to be (even) more similar. Hence we define

$$y_i^* = \log_{10}(y_i)$$

and repeat all of the above assumptions and calculations with y_i replaced by y_i^*.

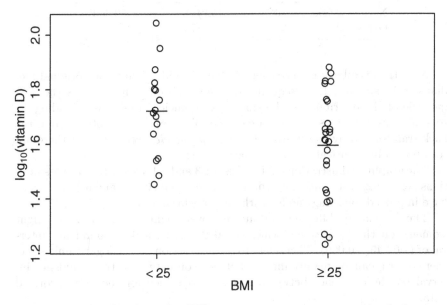

Fig. 3.1.3. The logarithmic S25OHD in two stature groups, cutpoint body mass index= 25.

The estimates for the means of the logarithmically transformed variables are shown in Table 3.1.5, together with the medians and the standard deviations.

Table 3.1.5. Summary statistics for $\log_{10}$(S25OHD) according to BMI.

Group	Number	Average	Median ($\widehat{M}$)	SD
Normal weight	16	1.720	1.719	0.164
Overweight	25	1.593	1.614	0.193

We note that the averages agree even better with the medians for the logarithmically transformed variables than for the original observations, as shown in Table 3.1.1. This means that transforming with the logarithm has produced distributions that are more symmetric than before. The standard deviations are again quite similar although now the largest group also has the largest variation. If we back-transform the averages and the medians to the original scale (e.g., $10^{1.720} = 52.481$), we get Table 3.1.6.

Table 3.1.6. Back-transformed summary statistics for S25OHD, according to BMI

Group	Number	Geometric Average	Median (M)
Normal weight	16	52.481	52.360
Overweight	25	39.174	41.115

Note that the back-transformed medians are identical to the original medians (this is simply a consequence of the definition of medians as the 50% quantile of the distribution; the small discrepancies are due to rounding errors and interpolations due to an even sample size). On the other hand, the back-transformed averages are called the *geometric averages* and these are seen not to be identical to the ordinary averages.

The graphical illustrations in Figures 3.1.3 and 3.1.4 show that the assumptions regarding distributional symmetry and equality of standard deviations have improved following the logarithmic transformation.

The estimated difference in means (overweight versus normal weight women), on the logarithmic scale, is -0.127, with a 95% confidence interval of $(-0.245, -0.009)$. This refers to a construction on the logarithmic scale, therefore we cannot readily interpret it nor compare it to the confidence interval for the difference between means, as obtained for the untransformed data.

Instead, because averages and medians are very similar on this logarithmic scale, we may also interpret this difference as a difference between logarithms of medians on the untransformed scale; that is,

$$\log_{10}(\widehat{M_1}) - \log_{10}(\widehat{M_0}) = \log_{10}\left(\frac{\widehat{M_1}}{\widehat{M_0}}\right) = -0.1268$$

and hence

$$\frac{\widehat{M_1}}{\widehat{M_0}} = 10^{-0.1268} = 0.75.$$

This means that we estimate the overweight women to have a 25% lower median S25OHD compared to the normal weight women. The confidence interval becomes $(10^{-0.245}, 10^{-0.009}) = (0.57, 0.98)$, so that we cannot rule out that overweight women may have a substantially (43%) lower S25OHD than nor-

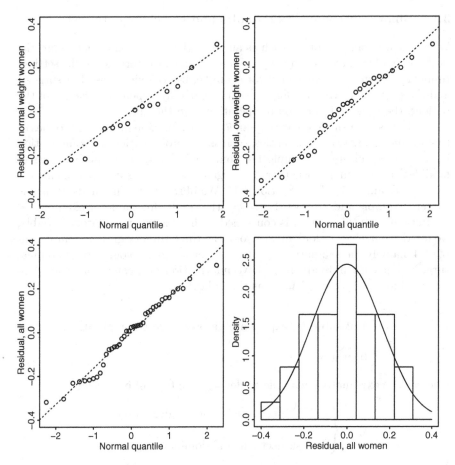

Fig. 3.1.4. Residual plots for model check after log transformation.

mal weight women, but at the same time, we also cannot rule out that there is hardly any difference at all (only 2% lower).

Digression. The paired t-test

Throughout this section we have assumed that the $n = n_0 + n_1$ observations come from different subjects and this led to the *unpaired t*-test (3.1.6). When the two groups to be compared arise by observing the same subjects twice (e.g., before and after an intervention), data are paired and the relevant method of comparison is the *paired t*-test . We return to that situation in Section 5.4. ◇

3.1.2 Binary outcome: (2×2)-tables and the chi-square test

When the outcome is binary, such as an event that may or may not occur, the probability of occurrence may depend on certain characteristics of the setting. In medical terms, the event may, for example, be complications after surgery, and the probability that a complication occurs may depend on the age of the patient, the type and duration of operation, and the like.

In the case of a single binary explanatory variable, the problem simplifies to that of comparing two probabilities, such as the probabilities of a complication in two surgery groups (Example 1.4 from Section 1.5) or the probabilities of fetal death, according to whether the pregnant woman has experienced a fever episode (Example 1.2 from Section 1.1). We illustrate the methods using the surgery example and afterwards present the results for the fever example.

Inasmuch as this section is concerned with a binary explanatory variable, we restrict ourselves to looking at two of the three surgery groups from Example 1.4, namely the 485 patients undergoing either gynecological or abdominal surgery. For each individual, we have information on postsurgery complications, a binary outcome, defined as the indicator

$$y_i = \begin{cases} 1, \text{ if subject } i \text{ experienced a postsurgery complication,} \\ 0, \text{ otherwise} \end{cases}$$

whereas the explanatory variable x_i denotes the type of operation

$$x_i = \begin{cases} 0, \text{ if subject } i \text{ had gynecological surgery,} \\ 1, \text{ if subject } i \text{ had abdominal surgery.} \end{cases}$$

We may summarize our information in a two-by-two table, for example with the surgery types as rows and the outcome (complication, yes or no) as columns, see Table 3.1.7.

Table 3.1.7. Complications in relation to operation type.

Operation Type	Complications No	Yes	Total	%
Gynecological	235	5	240	2.1
Abdominal	210	35	245	14.3
Total	445	40	485	8.2

Note from this table that in the gynecologic group, we have 5 complications out of 240 individuals, corresponding to only 2.1%, whereas in the abdominal group, we have 35 complications out of 245, that is, 14.3%. These numbers suggest that abdominal surgery is more subject to complications than gynecological surgery, but before we can safely conclude this, we have to convince ourselves that such a discrepancy would not often arise by chance alone. To do so, we need a statistical model.

Each y_i is a binary variable, therefore the distribution of the variable is fully determined by specifying its mean value, which is also the probability of a 1-outcome, that is, the probability of a complication

$$E(y_i) = \text{pr}(y_i = 1).$$

We assume that these failure probabilities are identical for all patients with the same covariate value, that is, all patients undergoing gynecological surgery will have identical probabilities of a postsurgery complication (p_0, say) and all patients undergoing abdominal surgery will similarly have the same probability (p_1, say) for postsurgery complications (although probably one that differs from the previous, p_0) .

Our model thus specifies the two mean values

$$\text{pr}(y_i = 1) = \begin{cases} p_0 \text{ if } x_i = 0 \text{ (gynecological patients)}, \\ p_1 \text{ if } x_i = 1 \text{ (abdominal patients)}. \end{cases} \tag{3.1.11}$$

The task is to estimate these two failure probabilities and compare them in order to determine whether (and to which extent) the probability of complications depends on type of surgery.

Because patients belonging to the same group are considered identical (or interchangeable) with respect to the risk of postsurgery complication, it is natural to sum up the number of failures in each group

$$S_0 = \sum_{i:x_i=0} y_i = 5$$

$$S_1 = \sum_{i:x_i=1} y_i = 35;$$

that is, S_0 is a sum of $n_0 = 240$ binary observations and S_1 a sum of $n_1 = 245$ binary observations. We may summarize Table 3.1.7 in terms of theoretical quantities in two different ways as shown in Table 3.1.8.

The notation in the left-hand table respects the fundamental asymmetry of the problem: we study the probability of a complication as a function of the type of operation and not the other way around.

However, a more widely used notation is the one to the right. This notation is very convenient for certain formulas to follow below, but it is not suitable for supporting the intuition of the problem, inasmuch as it treats outcome and explanatory variable in a symmetric fashion.

Table 3.1.8. Typical notation for a two-by-two table.

	Complications					Outcome		
Group	No	Yes	Total		Group	0	1	Total
0	$n_0 - S_0$	S_0	n_0	or	0	n_a	n_b	$n_a + n_b = n_0$
1	$n_1 - S_1$	S_1	n_1		1	n_c	n_d	$n_c + n_d = n_1$
					Total	$n_a + n_c$	$n_b + n_d$	n

Estimation

From the general likelihood theory in Section 2.3.1, we have the estimated failure probabilities

$$\widehat{p}_0 = \frac{S_0}{n_0} = \frac{5}{240} = 0.021$$

$$\widehat{p}_1 = \frac{S_1}{n_1} = \frac{35}{245} = 0.143,$$

that is, the observed proportions of postsurgery complications in each of the two groups. At first glance, these two estimates look quite different, and in fact, they do provide us with enough information to safely conclude that complications are more common for abdominal patients, as we show below. However, the very same estimates might have been found just by chance in a smaller study and only the relatively large size of the present study allows us to interpret the result as a real difference between the two groups.

The problem of quantifying the difference between complication probabilities in the two surgery groups is, however, not entirely straightforward. Even though we use the term difference, we do not necessarily imply that $p_1 - p_0$ is the relevant measure of discrepancy. Whereas such an estimated difference may be useful for health economists, alternative expressions may be more suited as patient information or for scientific purposes. More specifically, patients may think in terms of risk ratios, whereas important mathematical conveniences are connected to the use of odds ratios, as briefly mentioned in Section 1.3. We focus on this latter approach here and only briefly comment upon the other possibilities.

The logit transformation of a probability was defined in Section 1.3 as the logarithm of the odds

$$\text{logit}(p) = \log\left(\frac{p}{1-p}\right).$$

Using this scale to perform comparisons between groups offers the following advantages

- With probabilities p strictly between 0 and 1, the odds $p/(1-p)$ will be strictly positive and unbounded above, and its logarithm, the log(odds), will have no range restrictions.
- The discrepancy between two groups is not limited in value, that is, it may be arbitrarily large (positive or negative).
- The difference simply changes sign, when we switch groups in the comparison.
- The difference remains unchanged if we switch to consider the opposite event (except for a change in sign).
- The scale allows linear dependence on quantitative covariates (discussed in the next chapter).

In the surgery Example 1.4, we define the logits

$$\ell_i = \text{logit}(\text{pr}(y_i = 1)) = \begin{cases} \text{logit}(p_0) \text{ if } x_i = 0 \text{ (gynecological patients)} \\ \text{logit}(p_1) \text{ if } x_i = 1 \text{ (abdominal patients)} \end{cases}$$
(3.1.12)

and may now write the model as a regression model with logit link

$$\ell_i = \text{logit}(p_0) + (\text{logit}(p_1) - \text{logit}(p_0))x_i = a + bx_i,$$
(3.1.13)

where we have defined new parameters as

$$a = \text{logit}(p_0),\ b = \text{logit}(p_1) - \text{logit}(p_0).$$

Here the intercept a is to be interpreted as the log(odds) of a complication for the gynecological group. The regression parameter b is the change in logits when the explanatory variable increases one unit (i.e., from 0 to 1), to be interpreted as the difference in logits between the abdominal and the gynecological group.

Using this logit scale, the comparison of the probabilities of complication in the two surgery groups becomes

$$b = \text{logit}(p_1) - \text{logit}(p_0)$$
(3.1.14)

(3.1.15)

$$= \log\left(\frac{p_1}{1-p_1}\right) - \log\left(\frac{p_0}{1-p_0}\right) = \log(\text{OR}),$$
(3.1.16)

where the odds ratio OR is defined as

$$\text{OR} = \left(\frac{p_1}{1-p_1}\right) \bigg/ \left(\frac{p_0}{1-p_0}\right) = \frac{p_1(1-p_0)}{(1-p_1)p_0}.$$

The quantity may be estimated by simply inserting the estimates of p_0 and p_1 to give

$$\widehat{\text{OR}} = \frac{\hat{p}_1(1 - \hat{p}_0)}{(1 - \hat{p}_1)\hat{p}_0} \tag{3.1.17}$$

or, using the notation from Table 3.1.8,

$$\widehat{\text{OR}} = \frac{n_a n_d}{n_b n_c}.$$

For the surgery example we get

$$\widehat{\text{OR}} = \frac{0.143(1 - 0.021)}{0.021(1 - 0.143)} = 7.83$$

suggesting that the odds of getting a complication are almost eight times higher following an abdominal surgery compared to a gynecological surgery. However, this is only our best guess and it is associated with a standard deviation that reflects the sample size.

In order to construct a 95% confidence interval for this estimate, we note that on the logit scale, a symmetric confidence interval is not contraindicated. We may therefore use an approximate standard deviation for $\text{logit}(\hat{p}_j)$, given as

$$\text{SD}(\text{logit}(\hat{p}_j)) = \sqrt{\frac{1}{S_j} + \frac{1}{n_j - S_j}}, \quad j = 0, 1$$

to calculate the confidence intervals given in Table 3.1.9. Here, if the confidence interval for $\ell = \text{logit}(p)$ is from ℓ_L to ℓ_U, say, then that for

$$p = \frac{\exp(\ell)}{1 + \exp(\ell)}$$

is from

$$\frac{\exp(\ell_L)}{1 + \exp(\ell_L)} \quad \text{to} \quad \frac{\exp(\ell_U)}{1 + \exp(\ell_U)}.$$

Table 3.1.9. Probability of complications in relation to surgery type.

Surgery Type	j	$\text{logit}(\hat{p}_j)$	$\text{SD}(\text{logit}(p_j))$	CI for $\text{logit}(p_j)$	CI for p_j
Gynecological	0	-3.850	0.452	(-4.736, -2.964)	(0.0087, 0.0491)
Abdominal	1	-1.792	0.183	(-2.150, -1.434)	(0.1044, 0.1925)

Furthermore, we may calculate an approximate standard deviation for the log(odds ratio) $\hat{b}$ as

$$\mathrm{SD}(\widehat{b}) = \mathrm{SD}(\log(\widehat{\mathrm{OR}}))$$

$$= \sqrt{\frac{1}{S_0} + \frac{1}{n_0 - S_0} + \frac{1}{S_1} + \frac{1}{n_1 - S_1}} \tag{3.1.18}$$

$$= \sqrt{\frac{1}{n_a} + \frac{1}{n_b} + \frac{1}{n_c} + \frac{1}{n_d}} = 0.4874$$

and use this to calculate a symmetric confidence interval for b

$$\widehat{b} \pm 1.96 \cdot \mathrm{SD}(\widehat{b}). \tag{3.1.19}$$

This gives us the interval $(1.103, 3.014)$ and transforming back to the OR-scale, it becomes $(3.01, 20.36)$. Note that because the interval is constructed to be symmetric on the logit scale (the $\log(\mathrm{OR})$ scale), it will not be symmetric on the OR-scale. We also note that due to the relatively small number of complications, the confidence interval is rather wide and tells us that the odds of getting a postsurgery complication may be as much as 20 times bigger following an abdominal surgery as compared to a gynecological surgery. On the other hand, they may also be as low as 3.

The odds ratio derived from the logit link is invariant with respect to the choice of 0 and 1. For instance, in this example, we saw that the odds ratio for complications in the abdominal group compared to the gynecological group was 7.83. Likewise, the odds of avoiding complications in the gynecological group are 7.83 times higher than in the abdominal group.

Whether or not we can establish a difference between the groups, the quantifications above serve an important purpose. Actually, one might argue that for studies showing no convincing differences, such quantifications are even *more* important because they convey the information on the size of a possible effect that may have gone undetected because of limited information (small sample size). We return to this point in the fever example to follow.

Digression. Other contrast measures

Readers familiar with horse race betting may readily understand the concept of an odds ratio, but for many, the concept is more or less interpreted as a relative risk (or risk ratio). This is reasonable for small risks, where the approximation is

$$1 - p_0 \approx 1 \qquad \text{and} \qquad 1 - p_1 \approx 1$$

and, therefore

$$\frac{\frac{p_1}{1 - p_1}}{\frac{p_0}{1 - p_0}} \approx \frac{p_1}{p_0}.$$

For larger ps, the approximation can be very bad, as seen in the comparison in Figure 3.1.5.

Note that the relative risk corresponds to a comparison of probabilities on a log-scale (a log-link), because

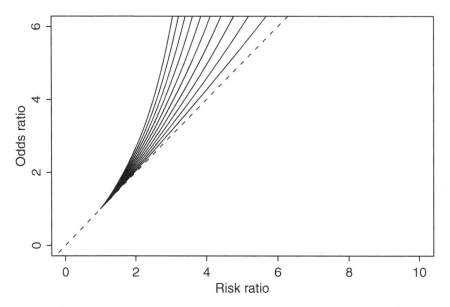

Fig. 3.1.5. The relation between odds ratio and relative risk, for values of the lowest risk equal to 0.02 to 0.2 in steps of 0.02. Lowest curve corresponds to lowest risk level.

$$\log(\text{RR}) = \log\left(\frac{p_1}{p_0}\right) = \log(p_1) - \log(p_0).$$

We may estimate the relative risk directly as the ratio of estimated probabilities; that is,

$$\widehat{\text{RR}} = \frac{\widehat{p}_1}{\widehat{p}_0} = \frac{0.1429}{0.0208} = 6.86$$

so that complications are estimated to be almost seven times as likely following an abdominal surgery as opposed to a gynecological surgery, a result, that resembles the OR above due to the relatively small failure probabilities in this study.

For the relative risk, we can construct an approximate 95% confidence interval based on an approximate standard deviation on a logarithmic scale

$$\text{SD}(\log(\widehat{\text{RR}})) \approx \sqrt{\frac{1}{S_0} - \frac{1}{n_0} + \frac{1}{S_1} - \frac{1}{n_1}}$$

$$= \sqrt{\frac{1}{n_b} - \frac{1}{n_a + n_b} + \frac{1}{n_d} - \frac{1}{n_c + n_d}}$$

and when we transform back to the relative risk itself, we get a confidence interval of (2.73, 17.21).

However appealing the above relative risk may seem, it nevertheless has certain limitations. One of these is that it is not invariant with respect to the choice of "success," that is, it depends upon what we define to be 0 and 1 in the outcome. For instance, the chance of *avoiding* a complication following a gynecological surgery as compared to an abdominal surgery is *not* 6.86, but rather

$$\frac{1 - \hat{p}_0}{1 - \hat{p}_1} = \frac{1 - 0.0208}{1 - 0.1429} = 1.14,$$

a drastically different result, interpreted to say that the probability of avoiding a complication following a gynecological surgery is only estimated to be a factor 1.14 bigger than the corresponding probability following an abdominal surgery. The reason for this discrepancy lies in the magnitude of the probabilities as such. The estimated risk of a complication in the gynecological group is only 2.1% which leaves plenty of room for a tenfold increase, whereas the probability of avoiding a complication in the abdominal group is as high as 85.7%, not leaving much room for improvement.

Whereas this choice of outcome is rarely a problem in daily life, where "good" and "bad" outcomes are almost always agreed upon, it becomes an issue in the mathematical setting because of the limited range of the relative risk. We may formulate this by noting that the log-link gives quantities that have no lower limit, but has an upper limit of 0 (we take the logarithm of a number between 0 and 1). Hence, this scale is not suited for linear models which of course do not respect such an upper bound. As we have seen above, the odds ratio, defined through a logit link, solves this problem and is hence regarded as the natural choice of link function for building linear models. This is, indeed, the main reason for choosing to work with OR rather than RR.

In many circumstances neither of the above two measures of discrepancy are used, and instead the simple difference between complication probabilities, $p_1 - p_0$, (the *risk difference*) is estimated

$$\hat{p}_1 - \hat{p}_0 = 0.143 - 0.021 = 0.122.$$

For reasonably large n, we saw in Section 2.1 that the Central Limit Theorem ensures that the Binomial distribution will tend to look like a Normal distribution. This in turn implies that the distribution of the estimate $\hat{p}$ is also approximately Normal

$$S \sim \text{Bin}(n, p) \approx N(np, np(1 - p)) \quad \text{or} \quad \hat{p} = \frac{S}{n} \approx N(p, \frac{p(1 - p)}{n}).$$

Therefore, approximate confidence limits for each of these probabilities can be calculated as

$$\hat{p} \pm 1.96 \cdot \sqrt{\frac{\hat{p}(1 - \hat{p})}{n}}, \tag{3.1.20}$$

which results in the intervals given in Table 3.1.10.

Table 3.1.10. Complications in relation to surgery type.

Surgery Type	j	n_j	S_j	$\hat{p}_j$	SD($\hat{p}_j$)	Approx. CI
Gynecological	0	240	5	0.021	0.0092	(0.0028, 0.0389)
Abdominal	1	245	35	0.143	0.0224	(0.0990, 0.1867)

In the same spirit, we may write the confidence limits for the difference in probabilities as

$$\widehat{p}_1 - \widehat{p}_0 \pm 1.96 \sqrt{\frac{\widehat{p}_1(1 - \widehat{p}_1)}{n_1} + \frac{\widehat{p}_0(1 - \widehat{p}_0)}{n_0}},$$

which in this situation amounts to the interval $(0.071, 0.174)$.

We summarize the various comparisons of the two groups in Table 3.1.11. All quantification methods agree that the discrepancy between complication risks in the two groups is substantial and sufficiently accurately estimated to allow us to infer with 95% confidence that the true (unknown) complication probabilities in the two groups differ. We infer this from the fact that the values corresponding to equality (1 for OR and RR, 0 for $p_1 - p_0$) are not included in the respective confidence intervals.

Table 3.1.11. Estimates of complications in relation to surgery type.

Type of Comparison	Estimate	Confidence Interval
Odds ratio OR	7.83	(3.01, 20.36)
Risk ratio $\frac{p_1}{p_0}$	6.86	(2.73, 17.21)
Risk difference $p_1 - p_0$	0.122	(0.071, 0.174)

The different ways of quantification of the magnitude of the discrepancy between the two groups are not in contradiction with each other but give rise to different interpretations. For instance, the difference in probabilities lies between 7.1% and 17.4%; that is, out of every two groups of 100 patients, we would expect $7 - 17$ extra complications in the abdominal group as compared to the gynecological group. Or, using the mathematically convenient logit scale, we can say, that the odds for experiencing a complication are almost 8 times bigger in the abdominal group compared to the gynecological group, although the uncertainty in this estimate indicates that the odds may well be as high as 20 or as low as 3. In Section 7.4 we study models for both relative risks and risk differences. ◇

Testing the hypothesis of equality

In Table 3.1.11, summarizing different ways of measuring the discrepancy between surgery complications, we see unanimous agreement that there is indeed greater risk of complications following abdominal surgery compared to gynecological surgery.

However, we often wish to perform a formal test for the hypothesis of identical probabilities, that is, the hypothesis

$$H_0 : p_1 = p_0 \quad (= p, \text{say}).$$

Testing this hypothesis implies that we have to compare the model considered so far with a simpler model where the two surgery groups have been lumped together as a consequence of the assumption of equal failure probabilities. In Table 3.1.7, the numbers for the combined group are shown in the last row. We note that the overall estimate of failure probability is pretty much the average of the two group-specific ones, due to the fact that the two surgery groups are of almost equal size.

From the general likelihood theory, we know that a reasonable way of testing the hypothesis of equal failure probabilities will be to compare the maximum likelihood for the model with group-specific failure probabilities to the corresponding one based on the model with only one common failure probability. This results in a ratio,

$$Q = \frac{L(\widehat{p}, \widehat{p})}{L(\widehat{p}_0, \widehat{p}_1)}$$

and as the general theory of Section 2.3.4 prescribes, we should reject the hypothesis of equal complication probabilities if Q falls below a certain value.

However, the exact distribution of Q is rather intractable and an approximation has to be relied upon. To be specific, the general theory from Section 2.3.4 tells us that for large n, "$n \to \infty$," the quantity $-2 \log Q$ will be approximately Chi-squared distributed with one degree-of-freedom. Moreover, it will asymptotically become equal to the quantity

$$z^2 = \sum \frac{(O - E)^2}{E},$$

where O, respectively, E denotes the observed, respectively, expected (under H_0) counts in each cell, and we are summing over all four cells.

Under H_0, where the two groups have the same complication probability, the expected values can be calculated by simply distributing the failures between groups according to the group sizes, see Table 3.1.12.

Table 3.1.12. Calculation of expected counts under assumption of equality, H_0.

Group	Outcome 0	Outcome 1	Total
0	$\frac{(n_a+n_b)(n_a+n_c)}{n}$	$\frac{(n_a+n_b)(n_b+n_d)}{n}$	$n_a + n_b = n_0$
1	$\frac{(n_c+n_d)(n_a+n_c)}{n}$	$\frac{(n_c+n_d)(n_b+n_d)}{n}$	$n_c + n_d = n_1$
Total	$n_a + n_c$	$n_b + n_d$	n

In the example the values are shown in Table 3.1.13.
Hence, the above statistic z^2 may be calculated as

Table 3.1.13. Expected counts in the two surgery groups, assuming equal probabilities of a complication.

Surgery Type	Expected		
	No	Yes	Total
Gynecological	220.21	19.79	240
Abdominal	224.79	20.21	245
Total	445	40	485

$$z^2 = \frac{(235 - 220.21)^2}{220.21} + \frac{(5 - 19.79)^2}{19.79} + \frac{(210 - 224.79)^2}{224.79} + \frac{(35 - 20.21)^2}{20.21}$$

$$= 0.99 + 11.06 + 0.97 + 10.83 = 23.86.$$

Because z^2 was asymptotically equal to $-2 \log Q$, which was known to have an asymptotic Chi-squared distribution with one degree-of-freedom, thus this also applies to z^2 itself. Therefore, if the criteria for the approximation to work sufficiently well are satisfied, the quantities $-2 \log Q$ or z^2 are considered significant (at a 5% level) if they exceed 3.84. The value of 23.86, which we have here, corresponds to an extremely low P-value of 1.036×10^{-6}, indicating a genuine difference between the complication probabilities for the two types of surgery.

A rule of thumb is that the approximation may be reasonably trusted whenever all expected values are above 5. In our situation, the smallest expected value is 19.79 for complications in the gynecological surgery group, so we may trust the approximation and therefore the conclusion above. For comparison purposes, the likelihood ratio test results in $-2 \log Q = 26.66$, that is, a somewhat larger value, leading of course to the same conclusion.

The statistic z^2 may be rewritten in the computationally simple form

$$z^2 = \frac{n(n_a n_d - n_b n_c)^2}{(n_a + n_b)(n_a + n_c)(n_b + n_d)(n_c + n_d)}.$$

Following up the discussion from Section 3.1.1 we notice that the significant (at the 5% level) difference between p_0 and p_1 is in accordance with the observation that the 95% confidence intervals for these two parameters do not overlap (Table 3.1.10).

Digression. Tests for small samples

In small samples, the approximation to the Chi-squared distribution may be improved by using a *continuity adjusted* version of z^2 defined as

$$z^2_{\text{adj}} = \frac{n(|n_a n_d - n_b n_c| - \frac{n}{2})^2}{(n_a + n_b)(n_a + n_c)(n_b + n_d)(n_c + n_d)},$$

which here gives 22.27, that is, a slightly smaller value than the unadjusted value. The reasoning behind this improved approximation has to do with the approximation of a continuous distribution (the Normal) to a discrete distribution (the Binomial).

Because, in large samples, z^2 and z^2_{adj} are indistinguishable and because, in small samples, the approximation using the Chi-squared distribution is better for z^2_{adj}, one could argue that the continuity-adjusted version of the test statistic should always be used.

In the case of truly small samples (one or more expected counts below 5), even this adjustment method cannot be trusted and we have to use exact methods based directly on the Binomial distribution. The exact comparison of two Binomial probabilities is known under the name "Fisher's exact test" after the famous British statistician R. A. Fisher. The method involves computation of probabilities of all possible two-by-two tables with the same margins as the observed table. The P-value corresponding to the hypothesis H_0 of identical probabilities is then the sum of the probabilities of all those tables showing more evidence against H_0 than the observed one. In this case, such tables are those that have even more than 35 of the 40 complications occurring in the abdominal group, or the ones that reverse this situation and have a more extreme distribution of complications in the opposite direction. Such an exact test may require heavy computations for large sample sizes (when, fortunately, it is not needed, because the approximative methods will work), especially when the covariate has more than two levels, as in Section 3.2.2.

In the present situation, we get these probabilities summing to 5.44×10^{-7} which is therefore the exact P-value. ◇

In the surgery example, we have seen that the conclusion concerning comparison of groups is extremely clear: there is indeed a significant difference between the complication probabilities for gynecological and abdominal patients, a difference that will most often be quoted as an odds ratio of 7.83, with confidence interval from 3.01 to 20.36. We note that even though the evidence of a difference between the groups is overwhelming, the confidence interval indicates quite a large uncertainty as to the size of this difference. We stress that stating this confidence interval is crucial for interpretation of the results.

Reporting the confidence interval of the odds ratio (or some other measure of discrepancy between two groups) becomes even more important in situations where we find no significant difference between the groups. This is due to a fundamental asymmetry in the testing of statistical hypotheses: when a hypothesis is rejected, we may conclude that groups are different, but when we fail to reject a hypothesis, we *cannot* conclude that the groups are equal, only that the present sample size was not able to detect any significant difference.

Fetal death

In Example 1.2, we looked at fetal deaths as the binary outcome in relation to the number of fever episodes during early pregnancy (cf. Table 1.1.2). If we dichotomize this covariate according to whether a fever episode has occurred at all, we get Table 3.1.14.

Table 3.1.14. Fetal death according to experience of fever in early pregnancy.

	Fever Episodes		
Fetal Death	No	Yes	Total
No	9595	2064	11659
Yes	98	21	119
Total	9693	2085	11778

As already noted in Example 1.2, the probability of fetal death is close to 1% whether or not the woman has experienced a fever episode, so obviously, there will be no significant association between fever episodes and fetal death. In fact, the test statistic z^2 here yields the value 0.0003, with an associated P-value of 0.99.

However, even a P-value so close to 1 (i.e., no indication whatsoever of a difference between groups) should not stand alone, especially not in small sample situations. A high P-value cannot be taken as an indication of absence of differences, merely as absence of *evidence* of a difference. We need to supplement with confidence intervals for the appropriate quantities, as given in Table 3.1.15.

Table 3.1.15. Association between fever episodes and fetal death.

Type of Comparison	Estimate	Confidence Interval
Odds ratio OR	0.996	(0.620, 1.600)
Risk ratio $\frac{p_1}{p_0}$	0.996	(0.623, 1.592)
Risk difference $p_1 - p_0$	-0.0000	(-0.0048, 0.0048)

We note that there is a tiny difference in observed risk in the two groups, in the direction opposite to the expected. However, as the confidence intervals show, we cannot rule out that the odds of fetal death could be 60% increased in the group experiencing fever episodes! Fetal death is a very rare fatality, therefore this coincides very closely with the interpretation in terms of relative risk: we cannot rule out that there might be a 59% increased risk of fetal death following fever episodes during early pregnancy. However, such an increased risk would amount to less than one half percent (the upper endpoint of the confidence limit for the difference in probability is 0.48%) of the total population of pregnant women.

Digression. McNemar's test

Throughout this section we have assumed that the $n = n_0 + n_1$ observations come from different subjects and this led to the Chi-square test, z^2. When the two groups to be compared arise by observing the same subjects twice (e.g., before and after an intervention), data are paired and the relevant method of comparison is *McNemar's test*. We return to that situation in Section 5.4. ◊

Digression. Case-control studies

We have everywhere in this section (as well as in most other sections of the book) assumed that sampling is *prospective* in the sense that subjects are ascertained for the study before the possible occurrence of the event of interest. For binary data, a frequently used design, in particular for *rare* outcomes, is the case-control design where subjects are sampled conditionally on having ("cases") or not having ("controls") experienced the outcome. We return to case-control studies in Section 7.4.2. ◊

3.1.3 Survival time outcome: the 2-sample logrank test

When the outcome variable y is a survival time, as in the PBC3 study, Example 1.3, the data will inevitably contain *censored* observations. Thus, as discussed earlier, the dataset from the PBC3 study contains 4 patients who were lost to follow-up before the end of study and another 255 who were alive without a liver transplantation at the end of study. For those 259 patients only a lower limit for the time to treatment failure was observed and, therefore, data cannot be described using averages (as in Section 3.1.1) or counts/percentages (as in Section 3.1.2). Table 3.1.16 shows an attempt to use averages anyway.

Table 3.1.16. Average observation times in years (and numbers of patients) by treatment group and failure status in the PBC3 trial in liver cirrhosis.

| | Treatment Failure | | |
Treatment	No	Yes	Total
Placebo	2.86	1.80	2.58
	(127)	(46)	(173)
CyA	2.77	2.02	2.58
	(132)	(44)	(176)
Total	2.81	1.91	2.58
	(259)	(90)	(349)

As expected, the average observation times for patients experiencing a treatment failure are considerably smaller than those for the patients with censored observation times. The averages for the patients with a treatment failure are likely to underestimate the true mean times to treatment failure (because we are more likely to observe the short durations). On the other hand, the size of the average observation times (for failures as well as for censorings) in each treatment group (both equal to 2.58 years) will depend strongly on the fraction of censored observations in the dataset and, furthermore, these averages will underestimate the true mean values because the censored observation times are known to be smaller than the unobserved, true failure times. Using counts or percentages is not optimal, either. Table 3.1.17 shows the number of patients with observation times less than 2 years.

Table 3.1.17. Number (%) of observation times less than two years by treatment group and failure status in the PBC3 trial in liver cirrhosis.

| | Treatment Failure | | All | |
Treatment	No	Yes	Observation Times	Patients
Placebo	40	27	67	173
	(23%)	(16%)	(39%)	(100%)
CyA	41	24	65	176
	(23%)	(14%)	(37%)	(100%)
Total	81	51	132	349
	(23%)	(15%)	(38%)	(100%)

Here, the total percentages of observation times less than two years (39 and 37 in the two treatment groups, respectively) are not reasonable estimates of the two year failure probabilities because the majority of the observations are censored. Counting only the observed failures before two years ($27/173 = 16\%$ for placebo, $24/176 = 14\%$ for CyA), on the other hand, will likely underestimate the true failure probabilities.

For survival times y we therefore need another way of describing the distribution and, typically, data in a group are summarized using an estimate of the survival function $S(t) = \text{pr}(y > t)$ for relevant values of time t. In this section we first describe the *Kaplan–Meier estimator* $\widehat{S}(t)$ for the survival function. As a measure of discrepancy between the distributions in the two groups we introduce the hazard ratio, briefly mentioned in Section 1.3, and we show how to compare the two distributions using the *logrank* test.

In Section 1.3, we briefly introduced the *hazard rate* $h(t)$ with the interpretation that, when $dt > 0$ is small,

$$h(t)dt \approx \text{pr}(t < y < t + dt \mid y > t).$$

Thus, $h(t)$ specifies the instantaneous risk of treatment failure per time unit. The hazard rate may, equivalently, be written as

$$h(t) \approx -\frac{S(t+dt) - S(t)}{dt} \frac{1}{S(t)}$$

and, using the rules of calculus, the precise definition ("letting $dt \to 0$") is

$$h(t) = -S'(t)\frac{1}{S(t)}$$

or

$$h(t) = -(\log(S))'(t).$$

From this it follows that the *cumulative hazard* is

$$H(t) = \int_0^t h(u)du = -\log(S(t)) \tag{3.1.21}$$

or, equivalently, the survival function may be written as

$$S(t) = \exp(-H(t)).$$

The Kaplan–Meier estimator

We consider the PBC3 study with the binary covariate:

$$x_i = \begin{cases} 0 \text{ if individual } i \text{ is in the placebo group} \\ 1 \text{ if individual } i \text{ is in the CyA group.} \end{cases}$$

To describe the distribution of the time y to treatment failure in these two x-subgroups we define the survival functions

$$\mathrm{pr}(y_i > t) = \begin{cases} S_0(t) \text{ if } x_i = 0 \\ S_1(t) \text{ if } x_i = 1. \end{cases} \tag{3.1.22}$$

We may then, as an alternative to (3.1.22), specify the model via the hazards, $h_0(t)$ for the placebo group, and $h_1(t)$ for the CyA group.

To introduce the notation for defining the Kaplan–Meier estimator $\widehat{S}(t)$ we consider one treatment group and define

$$0 < t_1 < t_2 < \cdots < t_N$$

to be the distinct ordered times of observation (either time to treatment failure or to right-censoring) in that group and we let

$$d(t_1), d(t_2), \ldots, d(t_N)$$

be the observed numbers of treatment failures at these time points. (If all times of observation are different then these will all be either 0 or 1 and N will be the number of subjects in the group considered.) Finally, we let

$$R(t_1), R(t_2), \ldots, R(t_N)$$

be the numbers of patients at risk at the times of observation; that is, $R(t_j)$ is the number of patients from the group with an observation time $\geq t_j$ (the "risk set").

Based on these data we estimate $S(t)$. The basic idea leading to the Kaplan–Meier estimator is to build recursively using the fact that for $t_{j_2} > t_{j_1}$ we have $\mathrm{pr}(y > t_{j_2}) = \mathrm{pr}(y > t_{j_2} \mid y > t_{j_1})\mathrm{pr}(y > t_{j_1})$. We estimate the conditional probability $\mathrm{pr}(y > t_j \mid y > t_{j-1})$ of surviving beyond t_j given survival beyond the previous observation time t_{j-1} simply as the relative frequency

$$\frac{R(t_j) - d(t_j)}{R(t_j)} = 1 - \frac{d(t_j)}{R(t_j)}.$$

This means that if the time point t is $< t_j$ and $\geq t_{j-1}$ then

$$\widehat{S}(t) = \left(1 - \frac{d(t_1)}{R(t_1)}\right) \times \cdots \times \left(1 - \frac{d(t_{j-1})}{R(t_{j-1})}\right)$$

or in shorthand notation using the "product symbol" $\prod$:

$$\widehat{S}(t) = \prod_{t_j \leq t} \left(1 - \frac{d(t_j)}{R(t_j)}\right). \tag{3.1.23}$$

This is a decreasing step function with steps at the observed times of treatment failure. Notice the way in which the censored observations are used. A person with a censored time of observation t is part of the risk set $R(t_j)$ for all times $t_j \leq t$ where, if that patient had experienced a treatment failure, this would have been observed. A censored observation does not give rise to a step in (3.1.23). A condition for using the censored observations in this way is that the only information available for a person censored at t is that the true time to treatment failure for that person exceeds t. That is, a situation where censored observations are known to belong to patients with a particularly good prognosis or to patients with a particularly bad prognosis (e.g., if seriously ill patients were forced out of the study) is not allowed. This crucial condition on the censoring mechanism is known as *independent censoring*. If censoring is caused by patients being alive at the closing date of a follow-up study then the assumption of independent censoring is usually not controversial. However, if many patients leave the study prematurely then one must be more suspicious and it is advisable always to collect information on why patients leave a study

.

The standard deviation of $\widehat{S}(t)$ may be evaluated using the simple formula $\widehat{S}(t)\sqrt{(1 - \widehat{S}(t))/R(t)}$, or using *Greenwood's formula*

$$\mathrm{SD}_G(\widehat{S}(t)) = \widehat{S}(t) \sqrt{\sum_{t_j \leq t} \frac{d(t_j)}{R(t_j)(R(t_j) - d(t_j) + 1)}}. \tag{3.1.24}$$

As an example, for the placebo group at $t = 366$ days, $\widehat{S}(t) = 0.9110$. Greenwood's formula (3.1.24) gives 0.0220 and the simpler formula gives almost the same value: $0.9110 \cdot \sqrt{(1 - 0.9110)/145} = 0.0226$. The simple formula has the advantage that the standard deviation can be estimated from the value of $\widehat{S}(t)$ once the number at risk, here $R(t) = 145$, is also known. Therefore, this information is sometimes added to the Kaplan–Meier plot (cf. Figure 3.1.6).

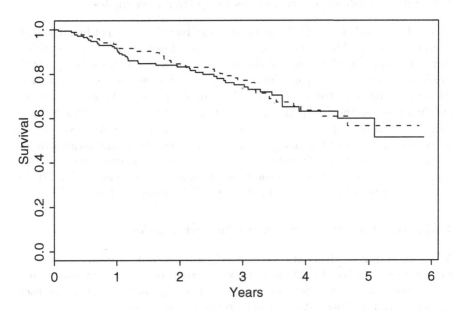

Fig. 3.1.6. Comparison of survival curves for CyA (dashed) and placebo (solid) treated patients with PBC. The numbers $R(t)$ at selected timepoints are:

t (Years)	1	2	3	4	5
Placebo	145	105	69	28	7
CyA	147	110	68	27	6

The simple, "naive" 95% confidence limits obtained from one of these standard deviation estimates are $\widehat{S}(t) \pm 1.96 \cdot \mathrm{SD}(\widehat{S}(t))$. These may have poor properties when $S(t)$ is close to 0 or 1 (cf. the discussion in Section 3.1.2). Better limits are obtained considering the *log(cumulative hazard)* or *log(−log(survival))* scale which has no upper or lower limits. For this scale, obtained by using the "cloglog" link , the standard deviation is given by

$$\mathrm{SD}(\log(-\log(\widehat{S}(t)))) = \mathrm{SD}(\widehat{S}(t))/[-\log(\widehat{S}(t))]$$

and a symmetric 95% confidence interval for the log cumulative hazard rate transforms to the following (asymmetric) interval for $S(t)$,

$$(\widehat{S}(t))^{L(t)} \leq S(t) \leq (\widehat{S}(t))^{U(t)}, \tag{3.1.25}$$

where $U(t) = 1/L(t)$ and $L(t) = \exp\big(1.96 \cdot \mathrm{SD}(\widehat{S}(t))/[-\log(\widehat{S}(t))]\big)$.

Using Greenwood's estimate of the standard deviation of $\widehat{S}(366)$ for the placebo group, the naive 95% confidence interval is (0.868, 0.954) whereas (3.1.25) yields (0.857,0.945) (because $a(366) = 1.662$), so in this case the difference is not great.

Estimating median survival times and other percentiles

As mentioned in Section 2.2.3, the median survival time may not be estimated simply as the "middle observation" because of censoring. However, recalling that the median is the value for the outcome for which there is both a 50% probability of observing a smaller and a larger value, we see that the median M has the property that $S(M) = 0.5$. We can, therefore, estimate the median survival time as the timepoint where $\widehat{S}(t)$ crosses 0.5. For the PBC3 data, neither of the Kaplan–Meier curves in the two treatment groups crosses this value, so the rates of treatment failure are too low to permit estimation of median times to treatment failure. However, the lower quartiles may be estimated as the timepoints where the Kaplan–Meier curves cross the level 0.75: 3.2 years for the CyA group and 3.0 years for the placebo group.

Estimating the ratio between two hazard functions

When analyzing survival data one is usually interested in supplementing plots of estimated survival functions in various groups of patients by computing statistics summarizing differences between the groups and by testing whether the survival time distributions in the groups are identical.

To summarize the differences between two survival curves in a simple way a proportional hazards model is frequently studied, that is the model

$$h_1(t) = c \cdot h_0(t) \quad \text{for all } t. \tag{3.1.26}$$

Proportionality between the hazard rates can alternatively be formulated as

$$S_1(t) = S_0(t)^c;$$

that is, the survival function for group 1 is obtained by raising that for group 0 to the power c (the hazard ratio). This implies, in particular, that the survival functions do not cross when there are proportional hazards. Finally, the proportional hazards assumption may be written as the *Cox regression* model for the log(hazard rate), $l_i(t) = \log(h_i(t))$, for individual i

$$l_i(t) = \log(h_0(t)) + bx_i, \tag{3.1.27}$$

where $b = \log(c)$.

If the model (3.1.26) holds, at least approximately, then it will be informative to present an estimate of c, the constant ratio between the two hazards, which is a natural measure of the "excess" mortality in one group compared to the other. Note that the proportional hazards relation may, alternatively, be expressed in terms of cumulative hazards as

$$H_1(t) = cH_0(t).$$

It can be checked graphically whether the assumption of proportional hazards is tenable by plotting an estimate of $H_1(t)$ versus an estimate of $H_0(t)$ for all values or for selected values of t. The points in such a diagram should then approximate a straight line through the point $(0,0)$ with slope c. Figure 3.1.7 shows the plot for the PBC3 data and proportional hazards does not seem to be contraindicated.

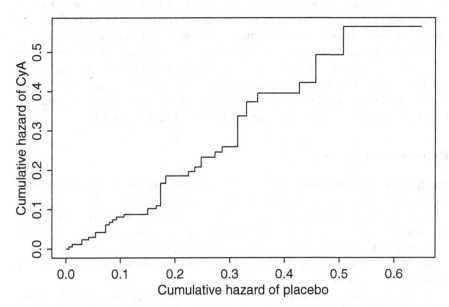

Fig. 3.1.7. Cumulative hazard for CyA patients plotted against that for placebo-treated patients with PBC.

It can be shown that the maximum likelihood estimator for c is the solution $\hat{c}$ to the equation

$$O_1 = \sum_{j=1}^{D} d(t_j) \frac{cR_1(t_j)}{R_0(t_j) + cR_1(t_j)}. \tag{3.1.28}$$

Here, $t_1 < t_2 < \ldots < t_D$ denote the different times of treatment failures in the two groups of patients and $d(t_j)$ is the total number of treatment failures observed at time t_j; that is, $d(t_j) = d_1(t_j) + d_0(t_j)$ where $d_1(t), d_0(t)$ are the numbers of treatment failures at t in the CyA and the placebo group, respectively. Furthermore, $R_1(t)$ and $R_0(t)$ are the numbers of patients known to survive without liver transplantation at least until time t in treatment groups 1 and 0, respectively, and O_1 is the observed number of treatment failures in group 1. For later use we also define $R(t) = R_1(t) + R_0(t)$ to be the total number of patients "at risk" just before time t. The contribution to the likelihood function for an uncensored time to treatment failure t is the *density function* evaluated in t (Section 2.3.4). The contribution for a censored time to treatment failure t is the *survival function* evaluated in t because all we know about the true unobserved time y_i to treatment failure in that case is that $y_i > t$, the probability of which is given by the survival function.

For the PBC3 data we find $\widehat{c} = 0.943 = \exp(-0.0585)$ close to the null value of 1 and with a 95% confidence interval $(0.624, 1.426)$ indicating that there is no significant difference in survival between the two treatment groups. However, the wide CI suggests that the CyA-treated patients may have a hazard which can be 38% smaller or 43% larger than that in the placebo group. The confidence interval is obtained by estimating a standard deviation (found as explained in Chapter 2; see (2.3.2)) for the log(hazard ratio) estimate $\widehat{b} = -0.0585$, and transforming a symmetric 95% confidence interval for b: $\widehat{b} \pm 1.96 \cdot SD(\widehat{b})$ by the exponential function (Appendix B). The Wald test is $W = (-0.0585/0.211)^2 = 0.077, P = 0.78$; the same value is obtained for the likelihood ratio test. The results are summarized in Table 3.1.19.

Pseudo-observations

For quantitative outcomes (Section 3.1.1) various scatterplots and residual plots were useful for assessment of the model fit and for binary outcome data we illustrate similar techniques in Section 4.1.2. For survival data, $\widehat{S}(t)$ predicts the failure status $I(y_i > t)$ at time t for all individuals i. Without censoring, this failure status would be observed for all i and for all values of t and graphical methods for binary outcome data could be used for each t or for selected values of t.

For censored data the failure status $I(y_i > t)$ can be replaced by its *pseudo-observation* defined as follows (for the PBC-3 study). To evaluate how much each individual i affects the estimated survival probability (i.e., the overall Kaplan–Meier estimator $\widehat{S}(t)$ based on all $n = 349$ patients), individual i is temporarily deleted from the sample and the Kaplan–Meier estimator, say $\widehat{S}_{(-i)}(t)$, based on the remaining $n - 1 = 348$ patients is computed. The pseudo-observation, $\widehat{S}_i(t)$ for patient i at time t is now defined as

$$\widehat{S}_i(t) = n\widehat{S}(t) - (n-1)\widehat{S}_{(-i)}(t). \tag{3.1.29}$$

Using (3.1.29) the pseudo-observation for every individual can be calculated. If the dataset contains no censored observations at all then $\widehat{S}_i(t)$ will equal the observed failure status $I(y_i > t)$. For a closer discussion concerning definition and uses of pseudo-observations, see for example Pohar Perme and Andersen

(2008) or Andersen and Pohar Perme (2010).

A further evaluation of the proportional hazards assumption in Model (3.1.27) may now be obtained by plotting *pseudo-residuals* from the model, that is, the pseudo-observation $\widehat{S}_i(t)$ minus the predicted survival probability (say, $p_i(t)$) which is $\widehat{S}_0(t)$ if i is a placebo-treated patient and $\widehat{S}_0(t)^{\widehat{c}}$ if i is a CyA-treated patient. We usually standardize the residual by dividing this difference by an approximate standard deviation $\sqrt{p_i(t)(1 - p_i(t))}$. In Figure 3.1.8 this is done at the quintiles of the observed times of treatment failure: 0.71, 1.18, 2.16, 3.19 years. The distribution of these pseudo-residuals is not simple. The negative residuals at a given time point t correspond to those patients failing before t, the actual value depending on the exact time of failure. The origin of a positive residual at time t is either a patient still at risk at t or a patient censored before t. However, the average of the pseudo-residuals may be useful to study and we see that these averages at the four selected timepoints are close to zero, thereby giving no indication of deviations from the proportional hazards assumption.

The 2-sample logrank test

In the present section we still consider the PBC3 study with its two treatment groups in which the survival functions are $S_1(t)$ and $S_0(t)$. We wish to compare these two functions, that is, to test the hypothesis

$$H_0 : \ S_1(t) \ = \ S_0(t) \quad \text{for all } t.$$

We discuss a simple *nonparametric* test for H_0, that is, a test which is not based on an assumption of the survival functions having a particular shape.

Digression. Nonparametric tests

The arguments for using nonparametric tests are usually that nonparametric methods rely on fewer assumptions than parametric models and hence are more robust. Being more robust, however, does not mean that the methods are universally applicable and certainly not that they are optimal. Even though the statistics are nonparametric in the sense that their approximate distribution (under the hypothesis of identical survival time distributions in the two groups of patients) can be derived no matter the shape of the survival time distributions, they are usually designed to be able to detect particular deviations from this hypothesis (cf. the discussion in Section 3.1.1). In other words, the various tests have different *power* against different alternative hypotheses, a fact which we may express by saying that *"different tests evaluate differences differently!"*

It should be noticed that classical nonparametric tests such as the Wilcoxon test cannot be used when there are censored observations although modifications to these tests have been developed for this situation (e.g., Andersen et al., 1993, Ch. 5). ◇

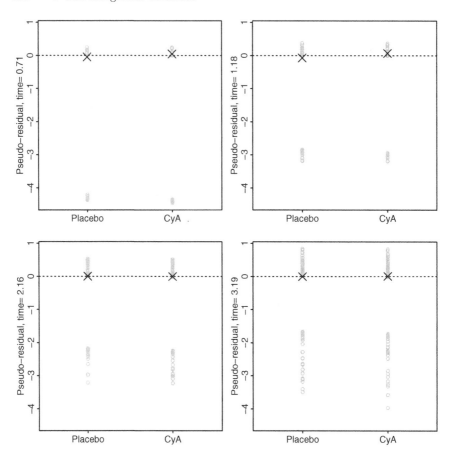

Fig. 3.1.8. Pseudo-residuals from a proportional hazards model for CyA- and placebo-treated patients with PBC. The crosses denote average values.

In the following we introduce the *logrank test* which is sensitive against deviations from the null hypothesis given by the Cox proportional hazards model (3.1.27): the logrank test examines the hypothesis $b = 0$ in this model. In fact it is the *score test* (cf. Section 2.3.3) based on this model. The main reasons why this test has become standard in survival analysis (instead of using parametric models) are that standard parametric models using, for example, the *log-Normal* or *Weibull* distributions, often do not provide a satisfactory fit to survival data and that the logrank test is almost as powerful as a parametric test against proportional hazards. In Section 7.5 we briefly discuss some parametric models for survival data.

The basic idea in the logrank test is easy to explain and at the same time the derivation of the test gives a flavor of its properties. At each time of failure, a two-by-two table can be set up summarizing the changes that happened at that time. Let us consider the PBC3 data at $t = 366$ days where $d_0(366) = 1$ patient failed in the placebo group and $R_0(366) = 145$ patients were still at risk. In the CyA group no patients failed at that time $(d_1(366) = 0)$ and $R_1(366) = 147$ patients were still at risk. At this time t we consider data as shown in Table 3.1.18.

Table 3.1.18. Contributions to the 2-sample logrank test at $t = 366$ days in the PBC-3 trial in liver cirrhosis.

	Placebo	CyA	Total
Failed	$d_0(t) = 1$	$d_1(t) = 0$	$d(t) = 1$
Survived	$R_0(t) - d_0(t) = 144$	$R_1(t) - d_1(t) = 147$	$R(t) - d(t) = 291$
At risk just before	$R_0(t) = 145$	$R_1(t) = 147$	$R(t) = 292$

The idea behind the logrank test is to calculate an "expected" number of deaths in group 0, $e_0(t)$, and in group 1, $e_1(t)$, at each time (t) of failure given the total number $d(t) = d_0(t) + d_1(t)$ of failures observed at time t and the numbers of patients at risk at time t in group 0, $R_0(t)$, and in group 1, $R_1(t)$, when (under the hypothesis H_0) the two groups have identical failure risks. Therefore, following the derivations in Section 3.1.2, we let

$$e_0(t) = d(t)\frac{R_0(t)}{R(t)} \qquad (3.1.30)$$

and

$$e_1(t) = d(t)\frac{R_1(t)}{R(t)}.$$

Notice that, inasmuch as $R(t) = R_0(t) + R_1(t)$, we always have that

$$e_0(t) + e_1(t) = d(t).$$

In the example, Equation (3.1.30) simply states that when the number $d(t) = 1$ of failures was observed at time $t = 366$ days and when $R_0(t) = 145$ out of the total number $R(t) = 292$ of the patients at risk at that time belonged to group 0 then we expect that the fraction

$$\frac{R_0(t)}{R(t)} = \frac{145}{292}$$

of the $d(t) = 1$ deaths took place in group 0, and hence that the fraction

$$\frac{R_1(t)}{R(t)} = \frac{147}{292}$$

of the failures took place in group 1.

The idea behind the logrank test is to add the observed number of deaths and the expected number of deaths for instance in group 1 from each of the D two-by-two tables, that is, to calculate the quantities

$$O_1 = \sum_{j=1}^{D} d_1(t_j)$$

and

$$E_1 = \sum_{j=1}^{D} e_1(t_j).$$

Here O_1, as above, is the total number of observed failures in group 1 whereas E_1 may be interpreted as the total "expected" number of failures in group 1 under the hypothesis. Thus the difference $O_1 - E_1$ is a measure of the (positive or negative) excess mortality in group 1 compared to what one would expect if the survival were the same in both groups. It can now be shown that by normalizing the squared difference $(O_1 - E_1)^2$ by a variance V, where

$$V = \sum_{j=1}^{D} v(t_j)$$

and

$$v(t_j) = d(t_j) \cdot \frac{R_0(t_j)R_1(t_j)(R(t_j) - d(t_j))}{(R(t_j))^2(R(t_j) - 1)} \tag{3.1.31}$$

is the variance (of $d_i(t_j)$) from the two-by-two table at time t_j, the *logrank test statistic*

$$X_{\mathrm{lr}}^2 = \frac{(O_1 - E_1)^2}{V} \tag{3.1.32}$$

is approximately Chi-squared distributed with one degree of freedom under the null hypothesis. Large values of X_{lr}^2 are significant and the approximation with the Chi-squared distribution improves when the observed numbers O_1 and O_2 are large.

Equation (3.1.32) shows that a large value of X_{lr}^2 is obtained if the difference between the observed and the expected number of deaths is large compared to the variance V. Because $O_1 - E_1 = \sum d_1(t_j) - \sum e_1(t_j) = \sum (d_1(t_j) - e_1(t_j))$ such a large difference is obtained if, in the majority of the two-by-two tables, either a larger or a smaller number of failures is observed compared to the expected number. If, on the other hand, there are more deaths than expected for small values of time and less than expected for large values of time then the difference $O_1 - E_1$ may be close to 0 showing that the logrank test is insensitive in situations where the tendency changes. This will, for instance, be the case when the survival curves cross within the time interval considered.

It should be noted that $O_0 + O_1 = E_0 + E_1$ and, therefore, the same test statistic would result from considering $O_0 - E_0$ in (3.1.32). For the PBC3 data the observed and expected numbers are given in Table 3.1.19. The value of V is 22.48 leading to $X_{lr}^2 = 0.077$.

The logrank test statistic is frequently presented in a different form:

$$X_{lr,c}^2 = \frac{(O_0 - E_0)^2}{E_0} + \frac{(O_1 - E_1)^2}{E_1} \tag{3.1.33}$$

which is easier to compute than (3.1.32) as it is based solely on the observed and expected numbers of deaths in the two groups (and not on the separately calculated variance V). It can be shown that we always have the inequality

$$\frac{(O_1 - E_1)^2}{V} \geq \frac{(O_0 - E_0)^2}{E_0} + \frac{(O_1 - E_1)^2}{E_1}.$$

Thus, the statistic $X_{lr,c}^2$ given by (3.1.33) is *conservative* and will always give larger P-values than the "correct" version (3.1.32). This will, particularly, be the case if the censoring patterns are markedly different in the two groups.

For the PBC data we found above that $O_0 = 46, O_1 = 44, E_0 = 44.7, E_1 = 45.3$, and $X_{lr}^2 = 0.077$. With three decimals $X_{lr,c}^2$ takes the same value leading to an insignificant P-value of 0.78. The similarity between the two versions of the test in this example is owing to the fact that this is a randomized study where most censoring is caused by patients being alive at the closing date of the trial. Recall that the same values were obtained for both the Wald test and the likelihood ratio test.

Digression. A simple, explicit hazard ratio estimator

When, in later chapters, we extend (3.1.27) to more general regression models we use the maximum likelihood estimator and its associated standard deviation throughout. However, for the simple 2-sample situation studied in this section a simpler and explicit estimator for the hazard ratio c is given by

$$\tilde{c} = \frac{O_1/E_1}{O_0/E_0}. \tag{3.1.34}$$

For the PBC data we find, based on the observed and expected numbers of treatment failures given above, that (3.1.34) gives the value $\tilde{c} = 0.944$ close to the maximum likelihood estimator. A confidence interval for $\tilde{c}$ may be based on the following standard deviation estimate for $\tilde{b} = \log(\tilde{c})$,

$$SD(\tilde{b}) = \sqrt{\frac{1}{O_0} + \frac{1}{O_1}}.$$

A symmetric confidence interval for b leads to a 95% confidence interval for c from $\tilde{c}/\exp(1.96 \cdot SD(\tilde{b})) = 0.624$ to $\tilde{c} \times \exp(1.96 \cdot SD(\tilde{b})) = 1.427$, again close to that based on the maximum likelihood estimate; see Table 3.1.19. ◇

Table 3.1.19. Analysis of the treatment effect in the PBC-3 study.

	CyA	Placebo	Total
Patients	176	173	349
Observed failures	44	46	90
Expected	45.3	44.7	90
Hazard ratio $\widehat{c}$	0.943	1	
	(0.624, 1.426)		
Hazard ratio $\widetilde{c}$	0.944	1	
	(0.624, 1.427)		
LR test	0.077		
Wald test	0.077		
Logrank test X_{lr}^2	0.077		
Logrank test $X_{\mathrm{lr,c}}^2$	0.077		

The proportional hazards assumption

The survival experience in the two treatment groups can always be summarized using the survival curves (cf. Figure 3.1.6). To obtain a one-number summary of the difference between the two curves, we imposed the proportional hazards assumption in the Cox regression model (3.1.27) and used the hazard ratio $c = \exp(b)$. The proportional hazards assumption is restrictive, the hazard ratio may be misleading if the model fits poorly, and methods to check the assumption are crucial. However, the desire to get a one-number summary for the difference between two groups is not unique for survival data. For quantitative outcome data, (Section 3.1.1), we used the difference between mean values as the corresponding summary, and this may be equally misleading if the positions of the two distributions to be compared are poorly described by their means.

Digression. A note on notation

To describe the Kaplan–Meier estimator, the Cox estimator for the hazard ratio, and the logrank test, we introduced the special notation used above. A notation more in line with other sections of the book would be to represent the outcome observed for individual i as

$$(y_i, d_i(y_i)). \qquad (3.1.35)$$

Here y_i is the time of observation and $d_i(y_i) = 1$ if y_i is a failure time and $d_i(y_i) = 0$ if y_i is a censoring time. In subsequent chapters, we frequently use the notation in (3.1.35). ◇

3.2 Categorical covariate with more than two levels

When the covariate is dichotomous, the situation may be described as the comparison between two groups, and as we have seen above, the conclusion can be stated as a certain measure of discrepancy between the two groups, equipped with a confidence interval.

For the quantitative outcome in the example in Section 3.1.1, we found an estimate of either difference in — or ratios of — vitamin D status for groups defined according to body mass index (overweight versus normal weight). In the example in Section 3.1.2 we found an estimate of the odds ratio for complication in the two surgery groups, and for the survival data in Section 3.1.3, the key result was an estimated hazard ratio between the Cyclosporin A-treated and the placebo-treated patients with primary biliary cirrhosis.

In all of these situations, there was a correspondence (although not always exact) between testing the hypothesis of equality between the two groups, and interpreting a confidence interval for the relevant parameter.

When shifting to a categorical covariate with more than two levels, we are dealing with the comparison of three or more groups, so that now we do not have a single difference between groups and also no longer an equivalence between test of equality of groups and construction of confidence intervals.

Whereas overall tests of equality between three or more groups is conceptually simple to derive by generalizing ideas from Section 3.1, the pairwise comparison between any two groups and the construction of confidence intervals for measures of discrepancy between pairs of groups create some fundamentally new issues for consideration, namely those of chance significance due to many tests of individual hypotheses (multiple comparisons).

In this section x denotes a categorical covariate, and the value x_i may, for instance, specify the treatment received by the ith patient. We refer to individuals with the same value of x as belonging to the same group. Our model specifies the linear predictor to have separate values for each such group.

If we have a total of $k + 1$ different groups, labeled $0, 1, \ldots, k$, it is often convenient to specify $k + 1$ dummy variables, as described in Section 1.2, Equation (1.2.6):

$$I(x_i = j) = \begin{cases} 1 \text{ if subject } i \text{ belongs to group } j \\ \\ 0 \text{ otherwise} \end{cases} \quad j = 0, 1, \cdots, k.$$

If c_j denotes some characteristic of the distribution in the jth group (e.g., mean value, log(odds) of some event, log(hazard rate)), the linear predictor for the outcome y_i may then be written as

$$LP_i = \begin{cases} c_0, \text{ if subject } i \text{ belongs to group } 0 \\ c_1, \text{ if subject } i \text{ belongs to group } 1 \\ \text{... ...} \\ c_k, \text{ if subject } i \text{ belongs to group } k \end{cases}$$

or

$$LP_i = c_0 I(x_i = 0) + c_1 I(x_i = 1) + \cdots + c_k I(x_i = k) \qquad (3.2.1)$$

and because

$$I(x_i = 0) + I(x_i = 1) + \cdots + I(x_i = k) = 1$$

we may write the above Equation (3.2.1) as

$$\begin{aligned} LP_i &= c_0 I(x_i = 0) + c_1 I(x_i = 1) + \cdots + c_k I(x_i = k) \\ &\quad + (c_0 - c_0 (I(x_i = 0) + I(x_i = 1) + \cdots + I(x_i = k)) \\ &= c_0 + (c_1 - c_0) I(x_i = 1) + \cdots + (c_k - c_0) I(x_i = k) \end{aligned}$$

or, with a different parametrization

$$LP_i = a + b_1 I(x_i = 1) + \cdot + b_k I(x_i = k), \qquad (3.2.2)$$

where we have defined new parameters as

$$a = c_0, \; b_j = c_j - c_0, \; j = 1, \ldots, k.$$

In this formulation, we have treated the groups in an asymmetrical fashion, because we have chosen one of them (group zero) to be the reference group, represented by the parameter $a = c_0$, whereas the rest of the groups are represented by their discrepancy to this reference group, on a specific scale; that is, $b_j = c_j - c_0$. In practical situations, the choice of reference group will often be noncontroversial: a control group, a group of normal subjects (compared to some genetic variant), nonsmoking individuals, the largest group, and so on. In some situations, however, the choice may be more arbitrary, and it is important to realize, that even if a change of reference group will affect the parameters (they will get a new interpretation, and the estimates will differ from the previous ones with an amount that equals the discrepancy between the two alternative reference group candidates), the model itself (and in particular the test of no effect of x) will be invariant to the choice of reference group and hence all conclusions will remain the same.

The above equation (3.2.2) is seen to be linear in the parameters b_j and hence the model belongs to the class of linear regression models. Note that the exact interpretation of this linear predictor depends on the nature of the outcome through the link function.

Digression. Relation to multiple regression

We note that even though the above model has only one explanatory variable (the group x), the linear model above takes the form of a *multiple regression model* (described in full in Chapter 5), with the derived variables $I(x_i = 1), \ldots, I(x_i = k)$ as covariates or explanatory variables. Furthermore, with the parametrization in (3.2.2) (a reference group and contrast to this reference group), the resulting parameter estimates are *correlated* (a concept dealt with in more detail in Chapter 5). Intuitively, this correlation can be explained as follows. If the reference group has, for example, a low level ($c_0 = a$ small), the remaining groups will tend to be larger than this ($b_1, \ldots, b_k$ all large). ◇

The results from estimation in a model specified as in (3.2.2) implies estimation of the parameter a (with the interpretation as the level for the reference group 0) and, most important, the parameters $b_1, \ldots, b_k$ (with the interpretation as discrepancies between each single group and the reference group).

Testing the overall hypothesis of equality between all groups simultaneously is seen to correspond to testing all b_js to be 0 simultaneously. Whereas this is by no means uninteresting, it still in many cases does not answer the fundamental research question of similarities and dissimilarities between various treatment groups. Thus there is a need for posthoc tests or multiple comparisons, where groups are compared pairwise or in various subsets.

Multiple comparisons

If we compare all groups one by one to the reference group, we make a total of k comparisons, but if we perform pairwise comparisons between all $k + 1$ groups, we make a total of $K = k(k + 1)/2$ comparisons. Each time we test a hypothesis, we have a small risk of a type I error (a false significance, i.e., declaring a difference to be present when, in fact, there is no difference). As discussed in Section 2.3.3 this corresponds to the significance level, usually 5%. This means that, if we test a series of K *true* hypotheses, we have a probability of 95% of a correct answer for each of these. Assuming all tests were independent, this means that the probability of obtaining the correct conclusion for all hypotheses is 0.95^K.

Even though 95% is a high level of security, the number 0.95^K will decrease quickly with $k + 1$ (the number of groups to be compared), or with K, the number of hypotheses to be tested, as illustrated by Figure 3.2.1. This is the problem of mass significance, implying a high risk of detecting a false significance (a type I error).

Still assuming the tests to be independent, and all hypotheses of equality to be true (i.e., no difference between any groups), we may correct for this mass significance simply by lowering the level of significance to obtain an overall level of significance of α (usually $\alpha = 0.05$), that is, choose the significance level as α_K, so that

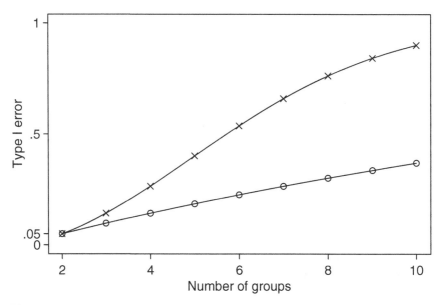

Fig. 3.2.1. Type I error rate for multiple comparisons. Upper curve refers to pairwise comparisons of all groups, lower curve to reference group comparisons.

$$1 - (1 - \alpha_K)^K = \alpha, \quad \text{that is,} \quad \alpha_K = 1 - (1 - \alpha)^{1/K}. \tag{3.2.3}$$

or the simple approximate solution

$$\alpha_K \approx \frac{\alpha}{K}. \tag{3.2.4}$$

The method of Equation (3.2.3) is known as the *Sidak correction*, whereas the simple approximation of equation (3.2.4) is known as the *Bonferroni correction* . It follows from the derivation above, that the Sidak correction gives the exact significance level α, provided that the model assumptions are met and the tests are independent. We say that we control the experimentwise error rate (EERC) under the complete null hypothesis of all means being equal. Actually, we have obtained more than this. Consider the situation where one or more of the means differ from the rest, so that the complete null hypothesis is no longer true. What can we then say about the risk of detecting false differences? It is easily seen, that the two methods of significance level correction as presented above still keep this probability at an upper bound of α (because we now need to control for a smaller number of comparisons in the above formulas) and we say that we have in fact controlled the maximum experimentwise error rate (MEER) under any partial null hypothesis as well.

The above considerations tell us how to judge whether we have significance, because they state the appropriate adjusted threshold for the P-value.

However, they do not provide a P-value for each of the hypotheses. The P-value obtained by a simple comparison of two groups will be too low and has to be adjusted upwards so as to avoid too many false significances. The obvious adjustment corresponding to the Bonferroni correction would seem to be to simply multiply the P-value by the number of comparisons made. This is in fact what is often done in practice, but it is immediately clear that this cannot be an exact procedure because we may easily get a result above 1 (which is clearly nonsense for a probability). Instead, we could use the Sidak correction and quote the adjusted P-value $1 - (1 - P)^K$ (which can never be larger than 1). However, for small P-values (which is after all our main concern), simple multiplication with the number of hypotheses under consideration works quite satisfactorily. The effect of this safeguard procedure is clearly to reduce power, which is intuitively reasonable, inasmuch as "you cannot play it both ways:" with a fixed amount of information (data), you can only reduce the risk of a type I error by increasing the risk of a type II error, or vice versa. For definitions of errors of type I and II, see Section 2.3.3.

What is being said about hypothesis tests may be said in a similar fashion about confidence intervals. Each confidence interval is constructed to have an (approximate) coverage of 95%. If this confidence interval is the only one under consideration, we can say that the coverage is indeed 95% but if we construct many such confidence intervals, the probability that they will *all* cover the respective true parameters will be less than 95%, and it will be appreciably less if many intervals are involved. In the spirit of the above considerations regarding lowering of the significance level, we should adjust the confidence intervals by using alternative quantiles. For constructing two-sided 95% limits, we use the 97.5% quantile, but if K simultaneous intervals are to be constructed, we should instead use the $(1 - \alpha_K/2)$ quantile, where α_K is an adjusted significance level according to some rule.

Considering the pairwise comparisons of a number of groups, we do have a problem, though, because the tests performed are not independent. This can be seen intuitively from the fact that if two groups look alike, they both resemble a third group equally much. This dependence between test statistics implies that an exact way of retaining an overall significance level of a pre-specified size α does not exist. The methods suggested above are still valid in the sense that they do control the EERC and even the MEER, but they are *conservative*, meaning that the resulting significance level may be well below the desired level α, which again has the consequence that true differences will be harder to detect (we have low power). It is not an easy task to correct for this dependency, but approximate solutions have been suggested in various contexts, and we look into these possibilities in the appropriate subsections to follow, with most details for quantitative data.

One useful piece of advice in the planning stage of an experiment is to avoid many categories for the covariates of primary interest, if at all possible. Comparing many groups simultaneously will lead to weak overall tests of significance (when testing whether several regression coefficients equal zero simultaneously, some nonzero parameters may be disguised among many zero parameters) and some groups may not be detected to deviate from the mainstream. Pairwise comparisons will often be uninformative in these situations, with wide confidence limits, due to the necessary correction for multiple comparisons. If many groups have to be included in the investigation, the protocol should include statements regarding importance of various comparisons, so that fishing expeditions may be replaced by confirmative analyses.

3.2.1 Quantitative outcome: One-way analysis of variance

In Section 3.1.1 we revisited Example 1.1 and compared the S25OHD levels for normal weight women with overweight women and found a marginally significant difference, indicating a slightly inferior vitamin D status for overweight women.

The outcome, S25OHD, was quantitative, and the comparison between overweight and normal weight women resulted in a quantification of the difference in mean S25OHD levels, with confidence interval, and in a t-test for testing identity of the two means.

We are concerned here with a similar situation, only with more than two groups involved, and we look at the overall test of equality between the groups as well as the comparison between specific groups, taking proper precautions to avoid mass significance, as outlined in Section 3.2 above.

This setup is often denoted as the *one-way analysis of variance* situation, a somewhat strange name, which is explained below.

To illustrate the ideas in this section, we use Example 1.5 from Section 1.5, concerned with the accumulated lymphatic absorption of fatty acids in 40 rats, subdivided into five groups that received diets with different dairy products, labeled I–V.

A graphical presentation of this absorption is seen in Figure 3.2.2. We note that the distribution of acid absorption is sufficiently symmetrical to justify the calculation of averages and standard deviations, although the amount of information for making this judgement is rather limited. Following the lines of Section 3.1.1, we let y_i denote the outcome (fatty acid absorption) for the ith rat, and let x_i denote the corresponding dairy product, defined as

$$x_i = \begin{cases} 0, \text{ if rat } i \text{ was fed with cream cheese, I} \\ 1, \text{ if rat } i \text{ was fed with sour cream, II} \\ 2, \text{ if rat } i \text{ was fed with cream, III} \\ 3, \text{ if rat } i \text{ was fed with mixed butter, IV} \\ 4, \text{ if rat } i \text{ was fed with butter, V} \end{cases}$$

We assume all the y_is to be independent with mean values given by

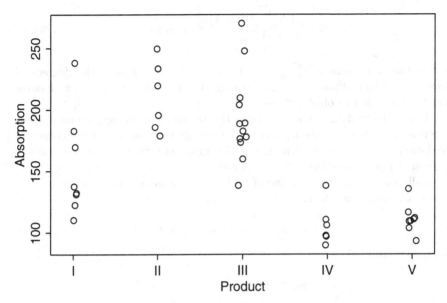

Fig. 3.2.2. Absorption of fatty acids for five dairy products, I: cream cheese, II: sour cream, III: cream, IV: mixed butter, V: butter.

$$E(y_i) = \begin{cases} m_0 \text{ if } x_i = 0 \text{ (cream cheese)} \\ m_1 \text{ if } x_i = 1 \text{ (sour cream)} \\ m_2 \text{ if } x_i = 2 \text{ (cream)} \\ m_3 \text{ if } x_i = 3 \text{ (mixed butter)} \\ m_4 \text{ if } x_i = 4 \text{ (butter)} \end{cases} \quad (3.2.5)$$

and identical standard deviations. Summary statistics are presented in Table 3.2.1.

Table 3.2.1. Summary statistics for fatty acid absorption according to diary product.

Product	j	n_j	Average $(\widehat{m}_j)$	SD $(\widehat{s}_j)$
Cream cheese	0	8	153.02	41.905
Sour cream	1	6	210.40	28.212
Cream	2	12	193.04	36.275
Mixed butter	3	6	106.38	17.200
Butter	4	8	111.13	12.034

The pooled estimate of standard deviation is given by a generalization of Equation (3.1.4)

$$\widehat{s} = \sqrt{\frac{\sum_{j=0}^{4}(n_j - 1)s_j^2}{\sum_{j=0}^{4}(n_j - 1)}} = 30.817, \qquad (3.2.6)$$

where the denominator $\sum_{j=0}^{4}(n_j - 1) = n - 5 = 35$ denotes the degrees of freedom in the estimation of the common standard deviation, and n denotes the total number of observations.

From Figure 3.2.2, as well as from the summary statistics, we note a difference in the level of absorption in the five groups, but also a difference in variation. We investigate whether these immediate findings can be said to represent true differences between groups.

Following the general outline of Section 3.2 above, the mean value may be written in regression form as

$$E(y_i) = a + b_1 I(x_i = 1) + \cdots + b_k I(x_i = k). \qquad (3.2.7)$$

with the parameters

$$a = m_0, \; b_j = m_j - m_0, \; j = 1, \ldots, k,$$

and with dummy variables $I(x_i = j)$ defined as 1, if subject i belongs to group j and 0 otherwise. In the example we have $k = 4$.

Traditionally, the research question leading to a design of this type is whether there are any real differences between groups. This can be formulated as the hypothesis that all groups have the same distribution. Typically, the focus is primarily on an overall (omnibus) test for equality of all means simultaneously, that is, a test for the hypothesis of all regression coefficients b_j being equal to zero simultaneously:

$$H_0 : m_0 = m_1 = \cdots = m_k$$

or

$$H_0 : b_1 = b_2 = \cdots = b_k = 0.$$

The overall hypothesis is that all regression coefficients are zero, thus it is intuitively reasonable that we have to look at the size of the estimates $\widehat{b}_j$ in order to quantify how close these are to zero. However, due to the correlation between these, it is not simple to write up an intuitive test statistic and we instead argue using as a basis the general situation described in Section 2.3.3. The issue here is to compare two competing models, one specifying five different mean values and the simpler one specifying only one common mean. The residual sums of squares from these two models may be written as

$$SS_W = \sum_{i=1}^{n}(y_i - \widehat{a} - \widehat{b}_1 I(x_i = 1) - \cdots - \widehat{b}_k I(x_i = k))^2 = \sum_{i=1}^{n}(y_i - \widehat{m}_{j(i)})^2,$$

respectively,

$$SS_T = \sum_{i=1}^{n}(y_i - \bar{y})^2,$$

where the subscripts W and T represent the *within group* variation (sum of squared deviations from group-specific averages), respectively, the *total* variation (sum of squared deviations from overall averages corresponding to the model with identical means).

These two sums of squares reflect the unexplained variation in each of the two models (or the model and the hypothesis). If they are almost identical, the hypothesis is reasonable, but if SS_T is much larger than SS_W, we must reject the hypothesis.

The difference between the two may be calculated as

$$SS_T - SS_W = \sum_{i=1}^{n}(\hat{m}_{j(i)} - \bar{y})^2 = SS_B,$$

where the subscript B represents the *between group* variation (sum of squared deviations between group-specific averages and overall average).

Based on a Normal distribution assumption, the likelihood ratio test statistic is given by

$$Q = \left(\frac{SS_W}{SS_T}\right)^{n/2}$$

and general theory tells us to consider the test statistic $-2\log Q$. Furthermore, it tells us that for large samples, this will have an approximate Chi-squared distribution with degrees of freedom equal to the difference in number of mean value parameters in the two models; that is, $df = (n-1) - (n-k-1) = k$.

For Normally distributed data (i.e., when the observations are Normally distributed within each group), we need not use the asymptotic version of the likelihood ratio test, but may instead look at another transformation of Q:

$$F = \left(\frac{n-k-1}{k}\right)\frac{1 - Q^{2/n}}{Q^{2/n}} = \frac{MS_B}{MS_W}, \tag{3.2.8}$$

where MS_B and MS_W are the mean squares, defined by dividing the sums of squares by their respective degrees-of-freedom, that is, the mean squares between groups,

$$MS_B = \frac{SS_B}{k}$$

and the mean squares within groups,

$$MS_W = \frac{SS_W}{n-k-1}.$$

We note that the test statistic (3.2.8) for testing equality of means is a ratio between two variances, the variance between groups and the variance within groups, and under the assumption of equal means given by H_0, these two variances ought to be identical. We would therefore expect the ratio to be close to one, the closeness depending upon the amount of information (i.e., the degrees of freedom). It can be shown that under H_0 the distribution of F is $F(k, n - k - 1)$. We reject the hypothesis of equal means if F is large, that is, if the variation between groups is too large compared to the variation within groups.

At this point, the origin of the name *analysis of variance* should be clearer, because we compare two estimates of variance, which ideally should be identical under H_0. The reason for the term *one-way* is that we only have one classification criterion in this case, namely dairy product. If we had also included the sex of the rat in our analysis, we would have been in a *two-way analysis of variance* situation with a possibility to determine the effect of gender as well as dairy product. We treat this situation in Section 5.1.1 as a special case of a multiple regression model, namely one with two categorical explanatory variables.

In our example, we get the quantities as presented in Table 3.2.2, and the two alternative test statistics become

Table 3.2.2. Decomposition of the variation in the fatty acids Example 1.5

Variation	SS	df	MS
Total		39	
Within group	33239.12	35	949.69
Between groups	64960.46	4	16240.12

$$-2 \log Q = 43.33 \sim \chi^2(4),\ P < 0.0001$$
$$F = 17.10 \sim F(4, 35),\ P < 0.0001$$

agreeing on an overwhelmingly significant rejection of the hypothesis of equality of all five means.

Traditionally, the F-test as derived above, is shown as part of an *analysis of variance table*, showing the decomposition of the variation with associated degrees of freedom, much as the information in Table 3.2.2. In general, we do not want to present such tables inasmuch as we do not believe that they add any important information. It is included here only to illustrate the way in which the test statistic is derived.

Digression. The case $k = 1$

Note that in the case of only two groups, $k = 1$, the F-statistic reduces to the square of the test statistic (3.2.12) in accordance with the fact that the square of a t-distributed quantity with df degrees-of-freedom has an $F(1, df)$-distribution. Using a Normal approximation to the t-distribution reflects that for large df, the $F(1, df)$-distribution will look approximately like a Chi-squared distribution with a single degree-of-freedom. $\diamond$

Now that we have established beyond much doubt that the five dairy products differ with respect to accumulated lymphatic absorption, a very natural question arises as to which groups differ from which.

We may estimate the parameters of model (3.2.7) using the least squares method (derived from the likelihood principle for Normally distributed data) to obtain $\widehat{a} = \bar{y}_0$ and $\widehat{b}_j = \bar{y}_j - \bar{y}_0$ with mean value

$$\mathrm{E}(\widehat{b}_j) = \mathrm{E}(\bar{y}_j - \bar{y}_0) = m_j - m_0 = b_j$$

and a standard deviation estimated by

$$\mathrm{SD}(\widehat{b}_j) = \mathrm{SD}(\bar{y}_j - \bar{y}_0) = \widehat{s}\sqrt{\frac{1}{n_0} + \frac{1}{n_j}}. \qquad (3.2.9)$$

As a direct generalization of the results from Section 3.1.1, the Central Limit Theorem ensures that for large samples, $\widehat{b}_j = \bar{y}_j - \bar{y}_0$ will have an approximate Normal distribution, and an approximate 95% confidence interval for b_j may therefore be calculated as

$$\widehat{b}_j \pm 1.96 \cdot \mathrm{SD}(\widehat{b}_j) = \bar{y}_j - \bar{y}_0 \pm 1.96 \cdot \mathrm{SD}(\bar{y}_j - \bar{y}_0), \qquad (3.2.10)$$

where the term $\mathrm{SD}(\widehat{b}_j) = \mathrm{SD}(\bar{y}_j - \bar{y}_0)$ is given by (3.2.9). The estimates are shown in Table 3.2.3.

For small samples, this construction of confidence limits based on an asymptotic Normal distribution will result in a smaller coverage than the nominal 95% and we should instead use the appropriate t-quantile.

The upper 2.5% quantile in the t-distribution with 35 degrees of freedom is 2.030, thus the confidence limits should therefore be calculated as

$$\bar{y}_j - \bar{y}_0 \pm 2.030\widehat{s} \cdot \sqrt{\frac{1}{n_0} + \frac{1}{n_j}}. \qquad (3.2.11)$$

This construction ensures confidence limits with an individual coverage of 95%, but the chance that all confidence intervals simultaneously include the true value will be less (cf. the discussion in Section 3.2). Following the Bonferroni or Sidak approach to correction for multiple comparisons, we should adjust the significance level from $\alpha = 0.05$ to $\alpha/4 = 0.0125$ (Bonferroni) or to

Table 3.2.3. Parameter estimates in the fatty acids Example 1.5.

Product	Parameter	Estimate	SD	95% Confidence Interval
Cream cheese	$a = m_0$	153.02	10.90	(130.91, 175.14)
Sour cream vs. cream cheese	$b_1 = m_1 - m_0$	57.37	16.64	(23.58, 91.16)
Cream vs. cream cheese	$b_2 = m_2 - m_0$	40.01	14.07	(11.46, 68.57)
Mixed butter vs. cream cheese	$b_3 = m_3 - m_0$	-41.90	15.41	(-73.18, -10.61)
Butter vs. cream cheese	$b_4 = m_4 - m_0$	-46.64	16.64	(-80.43, -12.86)

the more exact $1 - (1 - \alpha)^{1/4} = 0.0127$ (Sidak) . The corresponding quantile should therefore be 2.63 instead of 2.030.

This situation of comparing k means to a single control group may be performed also using the procedure suggested by Dunnett which takes correlation between the individual difference estimates $\widehat{b}_j$ into account. Dunnett's test keeps the MEER to a level not exceeding the nominal level of $\alpha = 0.05$.

In order to show the effect of these corrections, we have calculated the various intervals resulting from two (cream and butter) of the four comparisons to the control group receiving cream cheese (group 0). The estimates are

$$\widehat{b}_2 = \bar{y}_2 - \bar{y}_0 = 40.01, \ \widehat{b}_4 = \bar{y}_4 - \bar{y}_0 = -46.64$$

and the four different types of confidence limits are shown in Table 3.2.4.

Table 3.2.4. Comparisons to a reference group in the fatty acids Example 1.5

Method	Cream vs. Cream Cheese	Butter vs. Cream Cheese
Individual comparisons		
Normal approx.	(12.44, 67.58)	(−72.10, −11.70)
t approx.	(11.46, 68.57)	(−73.18, −10.61)
Comparisons to reference		
Bonferroni/Sidak	(2.97, 77.05)	(−82.47, −1.32)
Dunnett	(3.99, 76.03)	(−81.36, −2.44)

The confidence limits constructed above may be used for assessing differences between the various groups to the reference group. A group can be declared significantly different from the reference group if zero is not included in the corresponding confidence interval. In analogy with the above construction of a confidence interval (and following from our general theory of maximum likelihood in the case of a Normal distribution assumption) we may also look at the intuitively interpretable Wald-type test statistic

$$t = \frac{\widehat{b_j}}{\text{SD}(\widehat{b_j})} = \frac{\bar{y}_j - \bar{y}_0}{\text{SD}(\bar{y}_j - \bar{y}_0)}. \tag{3.2.12}$$

For large samples, this quantity will have an approximate $N(0,1)$ distribution, whereas for smaller samples, we should instead use the t-distribution. This gives us tests for comparing individual groups to the reference group.

Comparing all groups pairwise

In the above model, we estimated a total of $k + 1$ parameters, the mean for the reference group, a and k regression parameters b_j. These regression parameters represent the comparison of k groups with a single control group, and we have discussed ways of correcting for these k comparisons in order to obtain confidence limits which have a certain simultaneous coverage.

In the present example, the reference group was chosen more or less arbitrarily and we might be interested in even more pairwise comparisons than the ones considered so far. In the absence of preplanned comparisons, we may simply want to compare all groups to each other in a pairwise manner, resulting in a total of $K = k(k+1)/2 = 10$ comparisons. If we make a Bonferroni (or a Sidak correction) for all of these comparisons, the relevant quantile to use would correspond to $\alpha_K = 0.005$ (or $\alpha_K = 1 - (1 - 0.05)^{1/10} = 0.0051$), which in a t-distribution with 35 degrees of freedom is 3.00. The corresponding adjustment of a P-value would be to multiply it by a factor 10, which of course weakens our possibility of finding the true differences (lower power).

Table 3.2.5. Comparison of all groups in the fatty acids Example 1.5.

method	Cream vs. Cream Cheese	Butter vs. Cream Cheese
A single comparison		
t approx.	(11.46, 68.57)	(−73.18, −10.61)
All pairwise comparisons		
Bonferroni/Sidak	(−2.13, 82.15)	(−88.06, 4.27)
Tukey-Kramer	(−0.43, 80.45)	(−86.20, 2.40)

We note a drastic inflation of the confidence interval when correcting for all pairwise comparisons. The Bonferroni/Sidak intervals are 47.6% wider than the traditional intervals based on individual t-distributions. We can do somewhat better (in terms of narrow confidence intervals and higher power) by applying instead the *Tukey–Kramer correction*. This is based on the standardized maximum difference between the group means and generally yields a significance level (MEER; see Section 3.2) closer to the nominal (and never larger than this) as compared to the Bonferroni/Sidak procedure (meaning that it is generally less conservative). Here, we note that the intervals shrink by approximately 4% and hence provide slightly tighter bounds while still controlling the MEER. For a more detailed discussion on methods for multiple comparisons following a one-way analysis of variance, see, for example, Miller (1981)

The assumption of Normality

Just as in the two-sample situation of Section 3.1.1, the above results regarding confidence limits and test statistics are approximate unless we have Normally distributed data within each group. However, for reasonably large samples, deviations from Normality are not so crucial, at least if they are not too systematic. Obvious deviations from symmetry (heavily skewed distributions) make comparisons of means and standard deviations doubtful because these quantities do not characterize skewed distributions. Thus, we have to demand the distributions to be reasonably symmetric in order for mean and standard deviation to make sense, and it is therefore necessary to get an idea of the distributional shape.

Following the procedure from Section 3.1.1, we make a visual inspection of the residuals

$$r_i = y_i - \widehat{y}_i = y_i - \widehat{m}_{j(i)}.$$

In Figure 3.2.3, we have collected a sample of such possible plots. These graphical displays, in particular the quantile–quantile plot, show a tendency towards a heavy right tail.

If the assumption of Normality is far from fulfilled, we may instead perform a nonparametric test of identity of the distribution of fatty acid absorption for the five dairy products. For comparing five groups as here, the most traditional test is the Kruskal–Wallis test, but using this, we merely get the conclusion that the five dairy products cannot be assumed to act identically, $P < 0.0001$, based on a Chi-squared distributed test statistic of 27.85 with four degrees of freedom.

We might now proceed to make nonparametric pairwise comparisons between groups, again properly adjusted to avoid mass significance, but inasmuch as such tests provide no quantifications and confidence limits, we would rather try to improve model assumptions through transformation, as shown briefly below.

The assumption of equal standard deviations

The derivation of confidence limits and test statistics outlined above relies on the traditional assumption of identical standard deviations in all groups. If

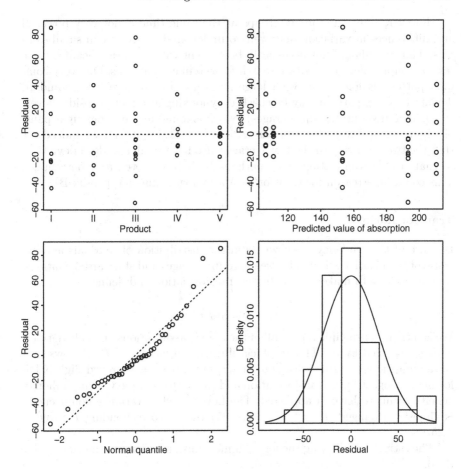

Fig. 3.2.3. Residual plots for model check in the fatty acids Example 1.5.

this assumption is not reasonably fulfilled, we may modify the 95% confidence interval for $b_j = m_j - m_0$ using a formula equivalent to (3.1.8). A Welch test statistic relaxing the assumption of equal standard deviations also exists using reciprocal variances as weights in the analysis (cf. Section 3.1.1). This test statistic here takes the value $F = 26.03 \sim F(4, 15.22)$ which is highly significant ($P < 0.0001$) to confirm our previous conclusion.

We may note from Figure 3.2.2 that the assumption of equal variances seems to be not entirely reasonable, because two groups appear to have a larger variation than the remaining. We can make a formal test for variance homogeneity in several ways, the most commonly used being the Levene's test and Bartlett's test.   For robustness reasons we prefer to use the Levene's test (least sensitive to deviations from Normality), which is based on an anova-type model for the squared residuals. We get a test statistic of $1.32 \sim F(4, 35)$ giving a P-value of 0.28 and hence no indication of variance inhomogeneity.

However, comparing many groups at the same time is not very powerful and differences in variation may well go undetected, especially in small samples. Thus, we should not necessarily be content with an insignificant Levene test but supplement this with a search for sytematic patterns. One very common pattern is for groups with large averages also to have large standard deviations. This pattern may be checked by looking at a plot of residuals versus predicted values (group averages), which is found in the upper-right panel of Figure 3.2.3. From this plot (as well as from Table 3.2.1), we indeed see that the two groups with the low averages also have small standard deviation, so that standard deviations may perhaps be better quoted as a percentage. This could be a reason for transformation by logarithms (Appendix B).

Transformation

Because of the tendency to skewness in the distribution of residuals and because of the positive relation between group averages and standard deviations, we may choose to make a logarithmic transformation and define

$$y_i^* = \log_{10}(y_i).$$

We can then in principle repeat all of the above, assumptions and calculations, with y_i replaced by y_i^*. The graphical illustration in Figure 3.2.4 shows that the assumptions regarding distributional symmetry have improved slightly following the logarithmic transformation and the pattern in the variance inhomogeneity seems to have disappeared. The Levene test of variance homogeneity is almost unchanged, $F = 1.40 \sim F(4,35)$ with a corresponding P-value of 0.25.

The estimates following the logarithmic transformation are shown in Table 3.2.6.

Table 3.2.6. Parameter estimates in the fatty acids Example 1.5 after logarithmic transformation.

Product	Parameter	Estimate	SD	95% Confidence Interval
Cream cheese	$a = m_0$	2.172	0.0270	(2.117, 2.227)
Sour cream vs. cream cheese	$b_1 = m_1 - m_0$	0.148	0.0413	(0.064, 0.232)
Cream vs. cream cheese	$b_2 = m_2 - m_0$	0.107	0.0349	(0.036, 0.178)
Mixed butter vs. cream cheese	$b_3 = m_3 - m_0$	−0.128	0.0382	(−0.206, −0.051)
Butter vs. cream cheese	$b_4 = m_4 - m_0$	−0.150	0.0413	(−0.233, −0.066)

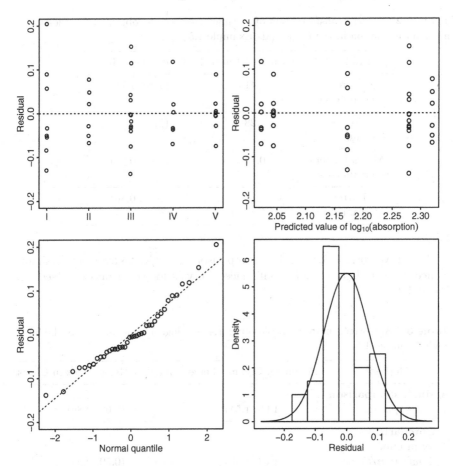

Fig. 3.2.4. Residual plots for model check following logarithmic transformation of outcome in the fatty acids Example 1.5.

As explained in Section 3.1.1, the interpretation of group differences changes when we make a logarithmic transformation. Instead of quoting ordinary differences on the original units as in Table 3.2.6, we should quote relative differences, in percentages. We calculate these percentages by transforming back with the appropriate antilogarithm (here using the estimate as a power to base 10, because we used a base 10 logarithm). Here, we get the estimated relative differences as seen in Table 3.2.7. As an example, for the cream group, we get a fatty acid uptake which is a factor 1.28 larger than that of cream cheese, whereas for mixed butter, the uptake is only 0.74 times that of cream cheese, that is, 26% smaller. The confidence limits for this latter estimate are seen to be $(0.62, 0.89)$ indicating that the uptake for mixed butter may be as much as 38% smaller than that for cream cheese, but also, that it may only be 11% smaller.

Table 3.2.7. Back-transformation of parameter estimates, obtained from logarithmic transformation in the fatty acids Example 1.5.

Product	Estimated Ratio	95% Confidence Interval
Sour cream vs. cream cheese	1.41	(1.16, 1.71)
Cream vs. cream cheese	1.28	(1.09, 1.51)
Mixed butter vs. cream cheese	0.74	(0.62, 0.89)
Butter vs. cream cheese	0.71	(0.58, 0.86)

When we correct for multiple comparisons in order to avoid mass significance, we get slightly wider confidence intervals for these ratios, as seen in Table 3.2.8.

Table 3.2.8. Correction for multiple comparison in logarithmic analysis of the fatty acids Example 1.5.

Method	Cream vs. Cream Cheese	Mixed Butter vs. Cream Cheese
A single comparison		
t approx.	(1.09, 1.51)	(0.62, 0.89)
Comparisons to cream cheese only		
Bonferroni/Sidak	(1.04, 1.58)	(0.59, 0.94)
Dunnett	(1.04, 1.57)	(0.59, 0.93)
All comparisons		
Bonferroni/Sidak	(1.01, 1.63)	(0.57, 0.97)
Tukey–Kramer	(1.02, 1.61)	(0.58, 0.96)

The vitamin D example revisited

We now return to the vitamin D example, this time with three groups, because we subdivide the overweight group into two (a redefined overweight group and an obese group) by introducing a second cutpoint of 30. The regression model relating vitamin D level y_i for the ith woman to her body mass index x_i then becomes

$$E(y_i) = a + b_1 I(25 \leq x_i < 30) + b_2 I(x_i \geq 30). \qquad (3.2.13)$$

Figure 3.2.5 shows the scatterplot of vitamin D levels in these three groups. From this, we note the same tendency for heavy-tailed distributions as was the case in the fatty acids Example 1.5 and in our previous analysis of the vitamin D example in Section 3.1.1, and we therefore proceed by analyzing logarithmic observations.

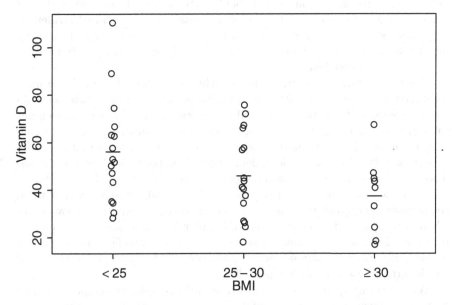

Fig. 3.2.5. The S25OHD in three stature groups, cutpoints BMI= 25 and 30.

The statistical model for logarithmic vitamin D levels is now exactly the same as for the example above on fatty acids, except that we only have three and not five groups.

The overall hypothesis of identical means is

$$H_0 : m_0 = m_1 = m_2$$

and we get the test statistic

$$-2\log Q = 6.26 \sim \chi^2(2), \quad P = 0.044$$
$$F = 3.13 \sim F(2, 38), \quad P = 0.055.$$

Although these two tests do not formally agree on a rejection of the hypothesis of equal means, this must be seen as a formality, because the P-values come close to the significance level for both tests.

In Section 3.1.1 we found a P-value of 3.6% when comparing two body mass groups (overweight and obese women in one single group, compared to normal weight women, on a logarithmic scale). W here maintain the trend in the association between body mass index and S25OHD, therefore it may at first glance seem contradictory to get a less significant result now (formally even insignificant as judged by the F-test)

This seeming paradox comes from a misinterpretation of an insignificant result. As was pointed out in Section 2.3.3, an insignificant result does *not* indicate that the groups are equal, but only that we *do not have sufficient evidence* of a difference, and this is by no means the same thing! Evidently, very small studies will most often fail to provide significant results for any hypothesis, and this can hardly be taken as evidence of equality, but rather as an absence of conclusion.

The logical next question might be: why do we have less evidence now, compared to the situation with only two groups? The answer to this has to do with the power of tests, that is the ability to detect real differences. Remember the fact that when we perform a test we are in fact comparing two competing models for our data: the most general one (our initial model) and the more specific one (the simplified model, defined by our hypothesis). Because the two models are nested, the most general one will always give the best fit, but it also uses the largest number of parameters. In general, we may say that when the number of parameters in the two models is very different, we get low power whereas comparing two models that only differ by one single parameter, will result in a high power. Of course, sample size also has an effect on power, but this is quite another discussion which has been touched upon in Section 2.3.3 and is further discussed in Section 6.3.

When testing equal means for the vitamin D example, we compare a model with three mean values to a model with only a single mean value (i.e., a difference of two parameters), whereas in the t-test situation (with only two groups based on body mass index), we compare two models differing by only a single parameter. Therefore, comparing three groups simultaneously is not as powerful as comparing only two groups and we expect to have a harder time establishing a difference, even if there actually is one.

This gives us some valuable information concerning design of experiments: if we are interested in comparing two specific groups, we should not carelessly design an experiment comparing more than these two groups.

A tempting solution to this problem of low power seems to be to compare the three groups in a pairwise manner, that is, perform three comparisons among the three groups. As we have discussed above, such multiple comparisons should, however, be adjusted for the risk of mass significance, whereby power is again lost. Hence, there is no way to retrieve power from a poorly designed study unless specific subhypotheses have been specified in advance

In the present situation with three ordered groups, we may have specified in advance that we wanted to compare only successive differences, that is, the difference between normal weight and overweight women and the difference between overweight and obese women. If this is the case, we will only have to perform two pairwise comparisons and therefore only adjust the P-values by a factor two.

After back-transformation to ratios, we get the results presented in Table 3.2.9.

Table 3.2.9. Multiple comparisons in logarithmic analysis of the vitamin D Example 1.1.

Method	Overweight vs. Normal weight	Obese vs. Overweight
Individual comparisons	0.806 (0.598, 1.086)	0.809 (0.569, 1.150)
Adjusted for two comparisons	0.806 (0.571, 1.137)	0.809 (0.540, 1.214)

The results suggest an approximate 20% reduction in vitamin D level from one weight category to the next, although with quite a bit of uncertainty.

Another approach for comparing the three ordered BMI groups is to assign a *score* to each category (see, e.g., Figure 1.2.1) and to apply instead a *trend test*. We illustrate such an approach in Sections 4.1.2 and 4.1.3 in connection with other examples .

3.2.2 Binary outcome: The $2 \times (k + 1)$-table

In Section 3.1.2, we looked at Example 1.4 from Section 1.5, concerning complications following different types of surgery. We compared two of the three groups and found a significantly elevated risk of complications following abdominal surgery as compared to gynecological surgery. In this section, we include also the third kind of surgery patients, the orthopedic patients, and the total data are shown in Table 3.2.10, together with estimated probabilities of complications.

Table 3.2.10. Complications in relation to operation type.

Operation Type	Complications No	Yes	Total	Risk
Gynecological	235	5	240	0.021 (0.009)
Abdominal	210	35	245	0.143 (0.022)
Orthopedic	200	6	206	0.029 (0.012)
Total	645	46	691	0.067 (0.009)

We again define the outcome variable as the indicator of postsurgery complication for the ith patient:

$$y_i = \begin{cases} 1 \text{ if subject } i \text{ experiences a postsurgery complication} \\ 0 \text{ otherwise,} \end{cases}$$

whereas the explanatory variable x_i denotes the type of operation, now with three levels, of which we again choose the gynecological group as our reference:

$$x_i = \begin{cases} 0 \text{ if subject } i \text{ had gynecological surgery,} \\ 1 \text{ if subject } i \text{ had abdominal surgery,} \\ 2 \text{ if subject } i \text{ had orthopedic surgery.} \end{cases}$$

Recall that, inasmuch as y_i is a binary variable, the distribution is fully determined by its mean value, the probability of a complication

$$\text{E}(y_i) = \text{pr}(y_i = 1).$$

The model specifies each surgery group to have a specific mean value

$$\text{pr}(y_i = 1) = \begin{cases} p_0 \text{ if } x_i = 0 \text{ (gynecological patients)} \\ p_1 \text{ if } x_i = 1 \text{ (abdominal patients)} \\ p_2 \text{ if } x_i = 2 \text{ (orthopedic patients)} \end{cases} \tag{3.2.14}$$

and following the approach from Section 3.1.2 we define the logits of these probabilities

$$\text{logit}(p_j) = \log\left(\frac{p_j}{1 - p_j}\right).$$

With dummy covariates defined as indicators of belonging to group 1 and 2, as outlined in Section 3.2 and used in Section 3.2.1, we can write up the model as a regression model with logit link as

$$\ell_i = \text{logit}(\text{pr}(y_i = 1)) = a + b_1 I(x_i = 1) + b_2 I(x_i = 2), \tag{3.2.15}$$

where we have defined new parameters as

$$a = \text{logit}(p_0), \ b_1 = \text{logit}(p_1) - \text{logit}(p_0), \ b_2 = \text{logit}(p_2) - \text{logit}(p_0).$$

Here, the intercept a is the logit for the gynecological group. The regression parameters b_j denote the changes in logits from the reference group of gynecological patients to either the abdominal or the orthopedic group, that is, log(odds ratios); see Equation 3.1.16.

From Table 3.2.10, we see that the complication risks in the gynecological and orthopedic groups are pretty much the same (2–3%), whereas the risk is remarkably higher among abdominal patients (14.3%).

Following the lines of Section 3.2.1, the usual approach in a situation such as this is to perform an overall test of equality for all three groups. The hypothesis is that the risk of complication does not depend on type of surgery; that is,

$$H_0 : p_0 = p_1 = p_2 \quad (= p, \quad \text{say}).$$

As was described in Sections 2.3.4 and 3.1.2, the likelihood ratio statistic for testing this hypothesis

$$Q = \frac{L(\widehat{p}, \widehat{p}, \widehat{p})}{L(\widehat{p_0}, \widehat{p_1}, \widehat{p_2})}$$

may be used in the form $-2 \log Q$, but now that we are comparing three groups, this will for large samples have an approximate Chi-squared distribution with two degrees of freedom.

It is common to use instead the approximation

$$z_2 = \sum \frac{(O - E)^2}{E} \approx -2 \log Q,$$

where O and E denote the observed, respectively, expected, number of counts in each cell (calculated under H_0), and we are summing over all six cells. The observed and expected numbers of complications are shown in Table 3.2.11.

Table 3.2.11. Observed (O) and expected (E) numbers of complications in relation to operation type.

| Operation Type | Complications | | | | Total |
| | No | | Yes | | |
	O	E	O	E	
Gynecological	235	224.0	5	16.0	240
Abdominal	210	228.7	35	16.3	245
Orthopedic	200	192.3	6	13.7	206
Total	645	645.0	46	46.0	691

In our situation, we get $z_2 = 35.67$ whereas $-2 \log Q = 34.32$. Thus both quantities clearly indicate that the hypothesis of equal complication probabilities does not fit the observed data particularly well. In fact, the corresponding P-value is less than 0.0001, so that the observed distribution of complications is very unlikely to occur in situations with three identical complication probabilities.

We recall that the Chi-squared approximation is reasonable when all expected values (expected number of complications in each cell under the null hypothesis) are at least five, as is indeed the case here. Otherwise, we may use Fisher's exact test as mentioned in Section 3.1.2. This will here result in the P-value 4.03×10^{-8}, confirming our overall conclusion of a significant difference among the three groups.

In view of this overwhelmingly significant result, we may proceed to evaluate pairwise differences between surgery groups. As pointed out in Section 3.2, comparing groups in a pairwise manner may too often (i.e., more often than predetermined by the significance level) lead to false detection of discrepancies as well as too narrow confidence intervals for the relevant contrasts. To avoid this mass significance problem, we should make proper corrections of the significance level in the construction of confidence limits as well as in the evaluation of test statistics.

Some attempts to handle multiple comparisons for binary outcomes have been taken (e.g., Horn and Vollandt, 2000). Here, we stick to the general Bonferroni/Sidak corrections which can always be used but are based on an independence assumption for the comparisons and hence give conservative conclusions.

In this situation, we have to correct for three pairwise comparisons, so we adjust from a significance level of $\alpha = 0.05$ to $\alpha_3 = 0.017$ by using 2.39 as the corresponding quantile for construction of confidence intervals of the form

$$\widehat{b}_j \pm 2.39 \cdot \mathrm{SD}(\widehat{b}_j), \tag{3.2.16}$$

where $\log(\widehat{OR}) = \widehat{b}_j$ and $\mathrm{SD}(\widehat{b}_j)$ are given by formulas analogous to Equations (3.1.17) and (3.1.18). Transforming back to confidence intervals for the odds ratio, we get the results in Table 3.2.12.

Table 3.2.12. Odds ratio estimates in the surgery Example 1.4.

Method	Abdominal vs. Gynecological	Orthopedic vs. Gynecological	Abdominal vs. Orthopedic
Individual comparisons			
Normal approx.	7.83 (3.01, 20.36)	1.41 (0.42, 4.69)	5.56 (2.29, 13.49)
Comparisons to reference			
Bonferroni/Sidak	7.83 (2.44, 25.16)	1.41 (0.32, 6.12)	5.56 (1.88, 16.42)

We note the inflation of the confidence intervals due to correction for three simultaneous comparisons, although in this situation, the conclusions remain the same.

Digression. A word of warning

It might be tempting to pool the two low-complication surgery groups and subsequently establish a significance between this pooled group and the high-complication abdominal surgery group. This is, however, not advisable, because such a hypothesis is data-driven and only one of many possible hypotheses that could be considered for these data. The additional problem here is that we cannot identify the pool of such possible hypotheses and consequently we cannot adjust for the mass significance problems that arise. ◇

3.2.3 Survival time outcome: The $(k+1)$-sample logrank test

The results from Section 3.1.3 are easily extended to the case where a survival time outcome is related to a single categorical explanatory variable with $k+1$ levels. More specifically we discuss the use of the Kaplan–Meier estimator, $\widehat{S}_j(t)$, for the survival function $S_j(t) = \mathrm{pr}(y > t)$ in group j and revisit estimation of the hazard ratios in relation to a chosen reference group as a measure of discrepancy between the groups. Finally we introduce the $(k+1)$-sample logrank test for comparison of the $S_j(t)$ for $j = 0, \ldots, k$. We also briefly discuss the problem of multiple comparisons for this situation.

As an example we again use the PBC3 study with the explanatory variable $x_i =$ bilirubin for patient i. We divide x_i into quintiles (cf. Section 1.3); that is, we have $k = 4$ and define the group, j, to which patient i belongs by:

$$j = \begin{cases} 0 \text{ if } x_i \leq 10.3 \\ 1 \text{ if } x_i \in (10.3, 16] \\ 2 \text{ if } x_i \in (16, 26.7] \\ 3 \text{ if } x_i \in (26.7, 51.4] \\ 4 \text{ if } x_i > 51.4. \end{cases}$$

The Kaplan–Meier survival curves for the five groups are shown in Figure 3.2.6 which suggests that survival deteriorates with increasing values of serum bilirubin.

Proportional hazards

To quantify differences among the groups we study a Cox proportional hazards model and introduce the hazard functions for the $k+1$ groups by defining the hazard for patient i as $h_j(t)$ if patient i belongs to group $j = 0, 1, \ldots, k$. The proportional hazards model may now, following (3.1.26) be formulated as

$$h_j(t) = c_j \cdot h_0(t), \ j = 1, \ldots, k, \text{ for all } t. \tag{3.2.17}$$

To rewrite equation (3.2.17) as one regression model (such as (3.1.27)) we follow the previous two sections using k *indicator* or *dummy* variables so that the proportional hazards model for the $k + 1 = 5$ groups becomes

$$l_i(t) = \log(h_0(t)) + b_1 I(x_i \leq 10.3) + b_2 I(10.3 < x_i \leq 16) + \cdots + b_4 I(x_i \geq 51.4), \tag{3.2.18}$$

where $l_i(t) = \log(h_i(t))$ is the log(hazard rate) for individual i and $b_j = \log(c_j), j = 1, \ldots, k$.

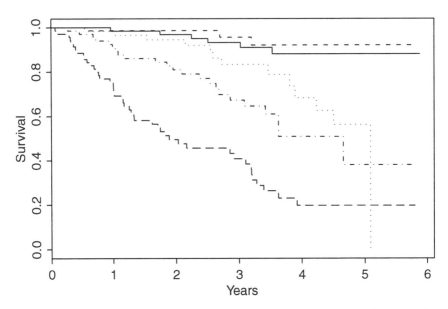

Fig. 3.2.6. Survival curves for patients with PBC in quintile groups of serum bilirubin: first quintile (solid), second (upper dashed), third (dotted), fourth (dotted-dashed), fifth (lower long-dashed).

The maximum likelihood estimators $\widehat{c}_1, \ldots, \widehat{c}_k$ for the hazard ratios $c_1, \ldots, c_k$ are solutions to equations like (3.1.28) and we use such estimators for general Cox regression models discussed in subsequent chapters. The estimates are shown in Table 3.2.14.

Digression. A simple hazard ratio estimator

For the present situation with a single categorical explanatory variable, a simpler estimator is given as

$$\widetilde{c}_j = \frac{O_j/E_j}{O_0/E_0} \tag{3.2.19}$$

(cf. (3.1.34)). Furthermore, the standard deviation of $\widetilde{b}_j = \log(\widetilde{c}_j)$ can be evaluated as

$$\text{SD}(\widetilde{b}_j) = \sqrt{\frac{1}{O_0} + \frac{1}{O_j}}.$$

For the PBC3, data the hazard ratios estimated from the Os and Es are given in Table 3.2.14. ◇

To evaluate the assumption of proportional hazards we follow the approach of Section 3.1.3: that is, we plot the estimated cumulative hazards for the groups 1 to 4 against that of the baseline group (group 0) (cf. Figure 3.2.7). These plots appear to be reasonably linear, thus no systematic deviations from proportional hazards are indicated.

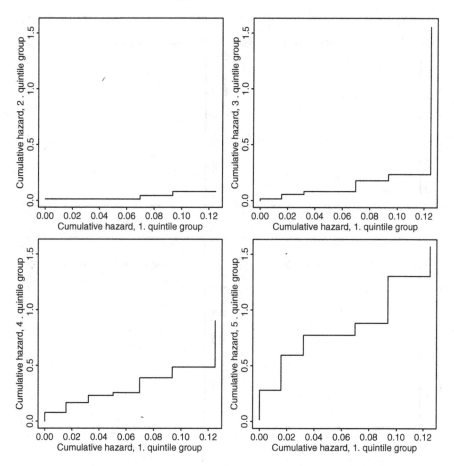

Fig. 3.2.7. Cumulative hazard for PBC3 patients in second, third, fourth, and fifth bilirubin quintile plotted against that for the first quintile.

Furthermore, still following Section 3.1.3, we plot pseudo-residuals from the proportional hazards model (see Figure 3.2.8). Recall that the negative values for the plot at a time point t correspond to patients with a failure time less than t. Because average residual values are close to 0, the figure suggests that proportional hazards are not contraindicated.

The logrank test

To compare the $k + 1 = 5$ survival functions for the five bilirubin groups in the PBC study, that is, to test the hypothesis

$$H_0 : \; S_0(t) \; = \; \ldots \; = \; S_k(t) \text{ for all } t,$$

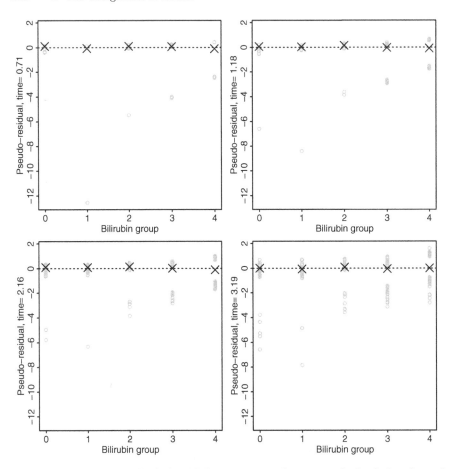

Fig. 3.2.8. Pseudo-residuals for PBC3 patients in first, second, third, fourth, and fifth bilirubin quintile plotted for four values of time. Crosses indicate average values.

we follow the derivation in Section 3.1.3 to introduce the $(k+1)$-sample logrank test. In the proportional hazards model this test examines the hypothesis $b_1 = \cdots = b_k$ of identical hazards in all groups versus the alternative that at least one b_j is different from 0.

We introduce notation similar to that used for the 2-sample case and let $t_1 < t_2 < \ldots < t_D$ denote the different times of treatment failures for all patients. We let $d(t)$ be the total number of treatment failures observed at time t; that is, $d(t) = d_0(t) + d_1(t) + \cdots + d_k(t)$ where $d_j(t), j = 0, \ldots, k$ is the number of treatment failures at t in group j. Finally, $R_j(t)$ is the number of patients known to survive at least until time t in patient group j and $R(t) = R_0(t) + \cdots + R_k(t)$ is the total number of patients in the risk set just before time t.

At each time of failure, a 2-by-$(k+1)$ table can be set up summarizing what happened at that time; see Table 3.2.13.

Table 3.2.13. Contributions to the $(k+1)$-sample logrank test at time t.

Group	0	1	...	k	Total
Failed	$d_0(t)$	$d_1(t)$	...	$d_k(t)$	$d(t)$
Survived	$R_0(t) - d_0(t)$	$R_1(t) - d_1(t)$	...	$R_k(t) - d_k(t)$	$R(t) - d(t)$
At risk just before	$R_0(t)$	$R_1(t)$	...	$R_k(t)$	$R(t)$

The $(k+1)$-sample logrank test is based on calculating an "expected" number of deaths, $e_j(t)$, in each group j at each time t of failure given the total number $d(t)$ of failures observed at time t and given the numbers of patients $R_j(t)$ at risk at time t in group j when (under the hypothesis H_0) the $k + 1$ groups have identical failure risks. This expected number, following (3.1.30), is given as

$$e_j(t) = d(t)\frac{R_j(t)}{R(t)}. \tag{3.2.20}$$

As for the 2-sample case we add the observed numbers of deaths and the expected numbers of deaths in each group j from each of the (D) $2 \times (k+1)$ tables; that is, the quantities

$$O_j = \sum_{u=1}^{D} d_j(t_u)$$

and

$$E_j = \sum_{u=1}^{D} e_j(t_u)$$

are calculated. Here O_j is the total number of observed failures in group j and E_j has an interpretation as the total "expected" number of failures in group j under the null hypothesis and the difference $O_j - E_j$ is a measure of the excess mortality in that group compared to what one would expect if the survival were the same in all groups.

A $(k+1)$-sample logrank test may now, following (3.1.33), be defined by

$$X^2_{\text{lr,c}} = \sum_{j=0}^{k} \frac{(O_j - E_j)^2}{E_j} \tag{3.2.21}$$

and under H_0, $X^2_{\text{lr,c}}$ is approximately Chi-squared distributed with k degrees of freedom.

An alternative form of the test in the spirit of (3.1.32) is more frequently used. That version, in fact the score test (Section 2.3.4) based on the proportional hazards model (3.2.18) requires inversion of a $(k \times k)$-matrix. As for the 2-sample situation, however, the simple version (3.2.21) is conservative if the censoring patterns in the groups to be compared are markedly different.

Table 3.2.14. Number of patients, observed and "expected" numbers of treatment failures and hazard ratio estimates in serum bilirubin quintile groups in the PBC3 trial in liver cirrhosis.

	\multicolumn{5}{c}{Serum bilirubin (μmol/L)}		
Interval	$\leq$10.3	10.3–16	16–26.7	26.7–51.4	>51.4	Total
Mean	(7.66)	(13.26)	(20.23)	(37.32)	(148.83)	
Patients	70	73	66	70	70	349
Treatment failures	6	3	13	23	45	90
"Expected"	23.26	20.34	16.78	16.89	12.73	90
Hazard ratio $\widehat{c}_j$	1	0.57	3.07	5.46	14.44	
95% CI		(0.14,2.28)	(1.17,8.08)	(2.22,13.45)	(6.13,34.01)	
Hazard ratio $\widetilde{c}_j$	1	0.57	3.00	5.28	13.70	

For the PBC3 data, the observed and expected numbers are given in Table 3.2.14 and the simple version of the logrank test is 112.5. For comparison, the more complicated statistic in this case takes the value 113.8 and the likelihood ratio test statistic is 94.9. All are highly significant ($P < 0.001$) when evaluated in the $\chi^2(4)$-distribution. Note the similarity between the two versions of the logrank test owing to the fact that the censoring patterns in the five groups are very similar.

Multiple comparisons

For survival data with a categorical covariate, adjustment for multiple comparisons is usually performed (if at all), using the Bonferroni/Sidak correction. In the current PBC3 example with bilirubin quintile groups, all pairwise comparisons are not warranted. If pairwise comparisons are, at all, to be carried out then comparing only neighboring categories is probably the most obvious approach. However, for a (semi-)quantitative variable, such as bilirubin quintile groups, a test for the effect of the covariate on the outcome may instead be performed using the one-degree-of-freedom *trend test* discussed in the next chapter (Section 4.1.3).

3.3 Exercises

Exercise 3.1. Use the tryptase dataset 3 from Example 1.12 for investigating the difference in baseline tryptase for men and women.

1. Show that men have an average tryptase 1.00 above that of women. Find the standard deviation of this estimate and construct a 95% confidence interval.

2. Draw a histogram for the tryptase values, separately for the two sexes. Comment upon the adequacy of an assumption of Normality for tryptase values.

3. Make a logarithmic transformation of tryptase and compare the means of these transformed values for men and women. Show that the difference can be formulated as "Median tryptase values for men are 19.1% higher than for women" and find a 95% confidence interval for this percentage.

4. Can we conclude that men have a higher level than women? What is the P-value for this comparison?

Exercise 3.2. Use the tryptase dataset 3 from Example 1.12 for investigating whether baseline tryptase is related to the degree of illness (as specified by the ASA classification).

1. Make a two by four table of counts for gender and ASA group.
   In the following we collapse categories 3 and 4 of ASA.

2. Do we see any overall difference in untransformed baseline values among the three ASA groups? What is the P-value for a test of identical means?

3. Make residual plots (residuals plotted against predicted values and histogram of residuals) and comment upon the appearance of these. Is it reasonable to assume a common SD for the three groups? Do we have a reasonably symmetrical distribution for the residuals?

4. Make a logarithmic transformation (e.g., $\log_{10}$) and perform the analyses and model checks again. Comment on the comparison between the two approaches. What is the conclusion?

5. Find a 95% confidence interval for the difference between ASA class 2 and 3–4, with Bonferroni adjustment. Is it reasonable to lump categories 2–4 into one? If so, perform a revised analysis comparing the resulting two ASA groups.

Exercise 3.3. Baseline tryptase is considered "elevated" if it is above 11.4. Use the tryptase dataset 3 from Example 1.12 for investigating the probability of this event.

1. Estimate the probability (with confidence interval) of an elevated tryptase value, for each sex separately. Show that the Chi-squared test statistic for comparison of these two is 0.51 and find the associated P-value. Can we detect a difference between men and women?

2. Calculate the confidence interval for the difference between these sex-specific probabilities, with a 95% confidence interval. Formulate the conclusions in words.

3. Show that the relative risk of an elevated tryptase value for men compared to women is 1.28, with a confidence interval of (0.65, 2.53). Find the

corresponding odds ratio for this comparison and compare to the value of the relative risk.
4. Make a three by two table with classifications according to ASA group (categories 3 and 4 taken together) and elevated tryptase (no/yes).
5. Estimate the probability (with confidence interval) of an elevated tryptase value, for each ASA group and look at the pattern of these estimates. Do we see any differences or tendencies?

Exercise 3.4. Use the tryptase dataset 3 from Example 1.12 for the assessment of an age effect in baseline tryptase values.

1. Compare the distribution of baseline tryptase values for patients below and above 60 years of age. In particular, test whether the mean values are identical for the two groups.
2. Compare the results with those obtained by performing the analysis on logarithmic values.

Exercise 3.5. The tryptase dataset 2 from Example 1.12 contains information on tryptase values reported for cases with suspicion of allergy (reaction tryptase).

1. Do we see evidence of different reaction tryptase levels for the three different ASA classification groups (collapsing groups 3 and 4)?
2. Can we rule out a difference of 30% between ASA 1 and 2?
   Calculate the difference between the reaction tryptase values and the subsequent baseline values (untransformed as well as on a logarithmic scale) and answer the following question.
3. Show that men have a larger difference than women and that this may be formulated as a mean difference (between differences) of 6.8. Calculate the corresponding confidence interval.
4. Make a logarithmic transformation of tryptase values, the baseline as well as the reaction, and calculate the individual differences between these. Use these to estimate the ratio of reaction tryptase and baseline tryptase for each sex separately. How can we express the discrepancy between these two ratios?
5. Make a scatterplot of differences versus type of surgery. How can we proceed to compare these surgery groups?

Exercise 3.6. The tryptase dataset 2 from Example 1.12 contains information on the result of an allergy test (the variable "positive" which may be 0 or 1).

1. Make a two by two table relating the result of the allergy test to age groups below and above 60. Estimate the difference between the probabilities of a positive test, as well as the relative risk and the odds ratio. Remember to quote confidence intervals also.

2. Investigate similarly whether the probability of a positive test is related to the ASA classification group. How can we report such a possible dependence?

3. Do we have evidence that the probability of a positive allergy test is related to whether the reaction tryptase value was elevated (>11.4)?

Exercise 3.7. The tryptase dataset 2 from Example 1.12 contains information on the type of allergic reaction, classified into four groups. Collapse the two groups with highest levels (life-threatening reactions and cardiac arrest).

1. Make a three by two table relating the reaction class to the subsequent result of an allergy test (the variable "positive") and estimate the difference of the probabilities of a positive test, using reaction class 1 as reference group.

2. Show that the Chi-square statistic for comparing these three probabilities is 8.07, and find the corresponding P-value. Can we conclude that there is a difference among the three groups?

3. Show that the estimate of the odds ratio for a positive test in reaction class 3–4 compared to reaction class 1–2 is 1.93. Find the confidence interval for this quantity.

4. Investigate whether the type of reaction is related to age group or ASA classification group.

Exercise 3.8. Use data from the fever in pregnancy Example 1.2 to describe and compare the distribution of birthweight between women with or without fever in early pregnancy.

1. Estimate the mean difference in birthweight for the two groups, with 95% confidence interval.

2. Comment on the possibility of making a logarithmic transformation of birthweight.

Exercise 3.9. Use data from the fever in pregnancy Example 1.2 to compare the risk of fetal death between women with and without previous abortions. Show that the Chi-square statistic for comparing these two probabilities is 0.006. Find the corresponding P-value and make a conclusion.

Find the estimate of the odds ratio for fetal death for a woman with previous abortions compared to a woman without previous abortions. Calculate the 95% confidence interval for this quantity and reformulate your conclusion, if necessary.

Exercise 3.10. In Exercise 3.7 we looked at dataset 2 from Example 1.12, and more specifically at the type of allergic reaction, classified into three groups, obtained by collapsing the two groups with highest levels (life-threatening reactions and cardiac arrest).

1. Make a three by two table relating the reaction class to gender. Calculate relevant percentages.

2. Do we see a genuine gender difference in the severity of the allergic reactions?

Exercise 3.11. Use data from the CSL1 Example 1.7 to compare the survival for patients treated with prednisone and placebo.

1. Limit the follow-up period to two years after treatment and define the binary outcome "died before two years" (yes/no). Make the two by two table relating this outcome to treatment. How do the censored patients appear in this table?
2. In order to distinguish between survivors and censored patients, make instead an outcome variable with three categories: dies, censored, and survives, again for the first two years of observation. Make the corresponding two by three table and comment.
3. Would it be sensible to make any formal comparisons between treatment based on either of these two tables?
4. Compare the two treatment groups using the whole observation period. Do we see a significant difference between the two Kaplan–Meier curves?

Exercise 3.12. Use data from the PBC-3 Example 1.3 to compare the survival functions for male and female patients.

1. Estimate the hazard ratio with 95% confidence limit and state your conclusion.
2. Perform a model check of the assumption of proportional hazards.

Exercise 3.13. Use data from the fever in pregnancy Example 1.2 to describe and compare the distribution of birthweight among women with parity 0 or above 0.

1. Show that birthweight is significantly higher for women with previous children as compared to women with no previous children.
2. Find the estimated difference in birthweight for these two groups, with 95% confidence interval.

Exercise 3.14. Use the CSL data from Example 1.7 to compare the distribution of ascites in each of the two treatment groups.

1. Make a three by two table and calculate relevant percentages.
2. Comment on the relevance of calculating a Chi-squared test for identical distributions of ascites in the two groups.

Exercise 3.15. Use data from the CSL1 Example 1.7 to compare the survival functions for varying degree of ascites.

Exercise 3.16. Use data from the PBC-3 Example 1.3 to compare the survival functions for groups with albumin values defined as five quintile groups.

Exercise 3.17. Use the surgery data from Example 1.4 to compare the duration of anesthesia in the three surgery groups.

1. Show that the difference in duration for the abdominal and gynecological patients is estimated to be approximately 39 minutes, with an SD of 5.5. State the confidence interval and test the hypothesis of equal mean duration in these two groups, adjusting for multiple comparisons.
2. Perform the same comparison, only on a logarithmic scale for the duration, and formulate the conclusion.

Exercise 3.18. Use the surgery dataset to compare the level of TOF-ratio for the three groups defined by the neuromuscular blocking agent.

1. Do we see any significant differences?
2. Find a confidence interval for the difference between Atracurium and Vecuronium and decide whether it is reasonable to collapse these two groups. If so, then compare the resulting two groups.
3. How could we improve the comparison of these three groups? See Exercise 5.7 in Chapter 5.
4. Explain why it does not make sense to perform a logarithmic transformation of this outcome.

One quantitative covariate

In this chapter we study models with a single quantitative covariate, that is, a covariate measured on a numerical scale. Some quantitative variables are *continuous*, meaning that they can take on any value (in principle infinitely many but in practice at least "many" values) in some interval, finite or infinite. Typical examples could be age and body mass index. The number of fever episodes for a pregnant woman is not a continuous variable, but still obviously quantitative. Ordered categorical variables, such as (underweight, normal weight or overweight) can also be thought of as quantitative variables, if each category can be assigned a meaningful score.

The typical models considered in this chapter assume the effect of the covariate to be continuous in the sense that relevant properties of the outcome (the mean, the expected probability of a success, or the survival function, according to the nature of the outcome) are expected to change gradually with the covariate, so that any two units differing in their covariate value will also differ in the expected value of the outcome. These models constitute one of the two building blocks of all regression models with a linear predictor.

In the previous chapter, we discussed the other building block of linear regression models, namely models including a single categorical covariate. These models typically involved comparisons of groups, for example, characterized by partitioning body mass index into separate intervals, as in Example 1.1. When the number of groups is large, the groups will typically be small and the model treating each such group as a separate entity becomes unstable due to the large number of parameters. If, for instance, we have a random sample of an adult population and wish to establish a relation between blood pressure and age, we could divide the sample into age groups and compare these with the analysis of variance techniques as described in the previous chapter. We are then faced with the dilemma of making the groups sufficiently narrow, so that they become almost homogeneous (and hence numerous and sparse, with many parameters in the model) or limit the number of groups, thereby implicitly making an assumption about a constant blood pressure over, for example, decades of a life span.

When the groups arise from a partition of an underlying continuous scale, a natural solution to this dilemma is to imagine the construction of numerous, very narrow, homogeneous groups. Each of these will be very sparse, and if covariate values are unique in the sample, in the limit they will consist of only a single observation. The simplifying approach is now to make a further assumption about the characteristics of all these groups, namely to specify the linear predictor to be a specific continuous function of the covariate values, characterized by only a few parameters. In its simplest form, the predictor could be specified as a linear function of the covariate, that is, a constant linear increase or decrease, involving only one parameter apart from the general level of the outcome. This is the starting point of the present chapter.

We have divided the chapter into two main sections, the distinction being the complexity of the relation between the linear predictor and the covariate. Section 4.1 is concerned with the simplest models where the quantitative co-variate (or some simple transformation of this, such as the logarithm) enters directly in the linear predictor, giving rise to the classical forms of simple linear regression, logistic regression, and Cox regression. In Section 4.2 we study models where the relation between the linear predictor and the quanti-tative covariate is nonlinear in a way that calls for construction of several new covariates derived from the original one, typically involving partition into in-tervals (groups), polynomial effects, and the combination of these in the form of splines. Remember from Section 1.4.2 that the term "linear predictor" refers to a construct that is linear in the unknown parameters. Therefore, in spite of the nonlinear nature of the relation between outcome and covariate in Sec-tion 4.2, we are in fact still dealing with linear predictors. This is important because all models with a linear predictor can be fitted quite simply using the same type of general software.

Section 4.1 is divided into subsections according to the nature of the out-come. However, as was also the case in the previous chapter, it turns out that the basic ideas are the same whatever the nature of the outcome; only the techniques differ according to the mathematics of the models. In Section 4.2 subdivision according to outcome type is not performed.

The models in Section 4.1 are conceptually much simpler than the ones in Section 4.2, but the assumption of a direct linear relation between covariate and predictor is not one to be taken lightly. If it is not fulfilled to a reasonable extent, the model will be inappropriate and perhaps totally useless.

Therefore, a check of the linearity assumption should be an integral part of any analysis involving quantitative covariates, along with checks of other parts of the model (which we have already encountered; cf. Chapter 3). We may follow two general strategies. One is graphical, displaying the lack of fit for each individual observation and searching for patterns in these deviations (residuals). The other is numerical, focusing on an extension of the model relaxing the linearity assumption and judging whether this leads to a signifi-cantly improved fit. The precise nature of the methods depends on the nature of the outcome and is therefore discussed in the appropriate subsections.

Closely related to the model check is the discussion of model stability or robustness based on regression diagnostics. This topic is new to this chapter because of the quantitative nature of the covariate which may give rise to very influential observations (typically the ones with extreme values of the covariate). Note the distinction between an *outlier* (an observation that is numerically farther away from its expected value than considered reasonable) and an *influential observation* (an observation that has an unduly large impact on the conclusion of the analysis). Influential observations may be detected by a leave-one-out technique, that is, by studying the change in estimated parameter values resulting from omitting each single observation at a time. Although no precise threshold for importance is given, the relative importances may offer substantial insight and create new ideas.

4.1 Linear effect

This section discusses models where the linear predictor is a direct linear function of the covariate itself (or some simple transformation of this), that is, where

$$\mathrm{LP}_i = a + bx_i. \tag{4.1.1}$$

Here the parameter a denotes the intercept (the value of the linear predictor when the covariate x is zero), and the parameter b denotes the slope of the linear relationship (the expected difference in the linear predictors for two individuals differing one unit in x).

Note that this model may be inadequate for x_i itself, but useful for a *transformed* covariate: $x_i^* = f(x_i)$ where $f(\cdot)$ is a completely specified transformation, for example, the logarithm $f(x) = \log(x)$ or the inverse $f(x) = 1/x$.

This section is divided into subsections according to the nature of the outcome y_i, which may be quantitative (ordinary linear regression, the least squares method), binary (logistic regression), or a survival time (Cox regression), respectively.

Describing the linear predictor as a simple linear function of the covariate is an obvious first step in many applications, because all smooth continuous functions may be approximated by a linear function, at least locally (i.e., for a limited range of covariate values). This is, however, no guarantee that such a model will fit the data, and check of this assumption is mandatory in order to prevent erroneous and misleading conclusions.

The check of linearity is part of the general model checking, which as already mentioned, follows two general strategies, a graphical and a numerical, the precise nature of which depends on the type of outcome. We mostly focus on graphical methods, displaying the lack of fit for each individual observation and searching for patterns in these deviations (residuals or "pseudo"-residuals; see Section 3.1.3). In the search for patterns in scatterplots or residual plots, a strong tool is the concept of *smoothing*. Various forms of smoothing have been developed, but a common feature is that observations corresponding to covariate values in the vicinity of each other are pooled to form a local average and that these averages are combined to give a hint of the common trend in the association, if any (e.g., Hastie and Tibshirani, 1990, Ch. 2–3).

If x_i has few possible values, for example, if the covariate is ordered categorical, then the test for linearity is particularly simple. This is because model (4.1.1) is then *nested* in the model treating x_i as a categorical variable (as in Chapter 3). However, inference in this case may depend critically on the scores attached to each category. Special attention is devoted to that situation in Sections 4.1.2 and 4.1.3.

4.1.1 Quantitative outcome: Simple linear regression

In Section 3.1.1, we compared the vitamin D level for Irish women, in groups defined by body mass index (BMI). Specifically, we defined two groups using the threshold 25 kg/m^2 and in Section 3.2.1, we extended this to three groups using an additional threshold of 30 kg/m^2.

When comparing vitamin D status in such groups, the within-group variation is regarded as biological variation in vitamin D for women having the same body stature. However, even within each group, the body mass indices may be quite different. In the normal weight group, a woman may have a body mass index of 19 kg/m^2 but equally well of 24 kg/m^2, whereas in the group of obese women, the lower threshold for body mass index is 30 kg/m^2 with no upper threshold to limit the degree of overweight. If the expected vitamin D is related to body mass index in a continuous way, any two individuals differing in body mass index will also differ in their expected vitamin D level, even if they belong to the same body mass index group. This heterogeneity within groups makes it more difficult to detect the possible systematic differences between stature groups. Expressed in another way: some of the possible systematic effect of body mass index on vitamin D is erroneously regarded as noise or unsystematic variation between individuals within each group. Thus, grouping of a quantitative covariate may not always be wise and may, indeed, lead to a substantial loss of information.

In order to study a continuous relationship between vitamin D and body mass index, a natural first step is to look at a scatterplot of the individual observations. This was already introduced in Chapter 1 for the group of Irish women, but is reproduced in Figure 4.1.1 below. We note from this figure that there is a tendency for women with a high body mass index to have a somewhat inferior vitamin D status compared to women with a low body mass index. This is in accordance with the result from Section 3.1.1 where we found that overweight women had an inferior vitamin D status compared to normal weight individuals, quantified as -13.33 nmol/l with the confidence interval $(-25.87, -0.79)$ nmol/l.

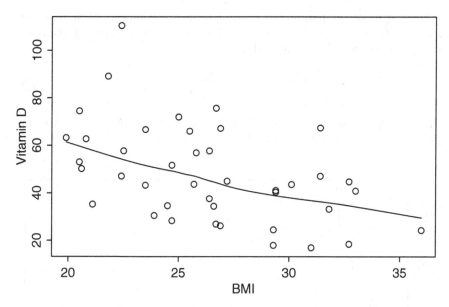

Fig. 4.1.1. Scatterplot of vitamin D concentration versus body mass index for Irish women.

Relating the vitamin D concentration to the quantitative information in body mass index may be thought of as a comparison of very many body mass groups, one for each particular value of body mass index. Each of these groups has a particular mean value of vitamin D concentration but because the number of groups is so large, we need a description of the relation between these mean values in order to get a parsimonious model. Superimposed on Figure 4.1.1 is a scatterplot smoother. This figure suggests that it is reasonable to specify the mean values to lie on a straight line, *the line of means* for varying body mass index.

If we let y_i denote the vitamin D concentration for the ith individual and let x_i denote the corresponding body mass index, we write this model as

$$\mathrm{E}(y_i) = m_i = a + bx_i \qquad (4.1.2)$$

and denote it as a *simple linear regression model*, "simple" because we only have one predictor, x. In model (4.1.2) the parameter a denotes the intercept (the expected value of y when x is zero), and the parameter b denotes the slope of the linear relationship (the expected difference in y for two individuals differing one unit in x). Note that even for cross-sectional studies such as this, where we have no longitudinal information on any single individual we still often refer to the slope as the expected change in y corresponding to a one-unit increase in x. This is so, even if we do not necessarily assume a causal effect of x.

Estimation of the parameters a and b from Equation (4.1.2) may be performed by the method of least squares, which consists in minimizing the *residual sum of squares* (RSS) , defined as

$$\text{RSS} = \sum_{i=1}^{n}(y_i - \widehat{y}_i)^2 = \sum_{i=1}^{n}(y_i - \widehat{a} - \widehat{b}x_i)^2, \tag{4.1.3}$$

residuals here being the vertical distance from the observation y_i to the line $\widehat{y}_i = \widehat{a} + \widehat{b}x_i$, as shown in Figure 4.1.2.

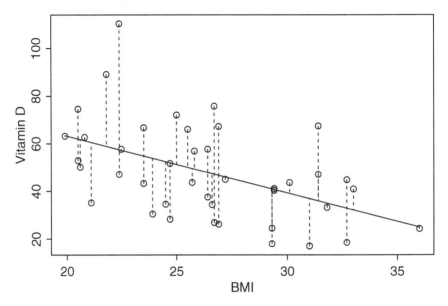

Fig. 4.1.2. Definition of residuals for regression of vitamin D on BMI.

The least squares method is derived from the maximum likelihood principle when the observations are Normally distributed with equal standard deviations (variance homogeneity) , but it can be shown to be sensible even when these assumptions are not fulfilled. We return to a discussion of this below, together with the assumption of linearity.

In this simple linear regression situation with only one covariate, it is possible to derive explicit formulas for the parameter estimates. In order to facilitate a subsequent discussion on design, precision, and the concept of correlation, we choose to do so.

The parameter of most interest is usually the slope b, which has the least squares estimate

$$\widehat{b} = \frac{\widehat{s}_{xy}}{\widehat{s}_x^2}, \tag{4.1.4}$$

where

$$\widehat{s}_{xy} = \frac{1}{n-1} \sum_{i=1}^{n} (x_i - \bar{x})(y_i - \bar{y})$$

is the *empirical covariance* between x and y (body mass index and vitamin D),

$$\widehat{s}_x^2 = \frac{1}{n-1} \sum_{i=1}^{n} (x_i - \bar{x})^2$$

is the empirical variance of the xs, and $\bar{x}$, respectively, $\bar{y}$ denote the average values of the observed xs and ys. Note that even though the variance of the covariate enters into the formulas, there will be no assumptions about the distributional form of these measurements. This is an important fact to keep in mind during the subsequent discussion of design, correlation, and sensitivity analysis.

The estimate $\widehat{b}$ is an unbiased estimate of the slope. Furthermore, when we can assume variance homogeneity (all observations have the same standard deviation - or variance), it can be shown to be the most efficient unbiased estimate, that is, the one with the lowest standard deviation. The standard deviation of this estimate is given by

$$\mathrm{SD}(\widehat{b}) = \frac{\widehat{s}_{y|x}}{\sqrt{n-1}\widehat{s}_x}, \tag{4.1.5}$$

where

$$\widehat{s}_{y|x}^2 = \frac{\mathrm{RSS}}{n-2}$$

is the estimated residual variance: a scaled version of the residual sum of squares (4.1.3) around the regression line.

The Central Limit Theorem ensures that, for large samples, $\widehat{b}$ will have an approximate Normal distribution, and an approximate 95% confidence interval for b may therefore be calculated as

$$\widehat{b} \pm 1.96 \cdot \mathrm{SD}(\widehat{b}) \tag{4.1.6}$$

although for moderate-sized samples, we usually replace 1.96 by the appropriate t-distribution quantile (usually somewhat above 2). In this example, we have 41 observations ($n = 41$), 2 parameters and therefore 39 degrees of freedom ($n - 2 = 39$) and the appropriate t quantile is 2.023.

We may also write a formula for the estimate of the intercept as well as its standard deviation, but inasmuch as these formulas do not contribute with any important insight, they are omitted.

For the vitamin D data we get the estimates: $\widehat{a} = 111.05(18.40)$, $\widehat{b} = -2.392(0.690)$, and $\widehat{s}_{y|x} = 17.91$. Here, a and s are measured in the units of the outcome variable (nmol/l), and b is measured in units of "outcome per explanatory variable" $((\mathrm{nmol/l})/(\mathrm{kg/m}^2))$.

The parameter a denotes the intercept. Although this does not always have a sensible interpretation (that depends on whether $x = 0$ is a sensible covariate value), it is nevertheless necessary to report this in order to use the model for predictions. In this example, it refers to the vitamin D concentration for a hypothetical individual with a zero body mass index, that is, weighing nothing. Using a simple reparametrization of body mass index, for example using the new covariate $x^* = x - 25$ and thus writing the (very same) model as

$$E(y_i) = a^* + bx_i^* \tag{4.1.7}$$

will not change the slope, but will change the intercept to

$$a^* = a + 25b,$$

now interpreted as the expected level of vitamin D for an individual with a body mass index of 25. Here, we get $\hat{a}^* = 51.244(2.948)$, leading to a 95% confidence interval of $(45.280, 57.207)$.

The parameter b is the focus of interest, denoting the slope of the linear relationship between body mass index and vitamin D concentration. Based on the above estimate, $\hat{b} = -2.392(0.690)$, we may calculate the 95% confidence interval to $(-3.788, -0.996)$. The interpretation is that the expected difference in vitamin D concentration for two individuals differing one unit in body mass index (corresponding to a weight difference of approximately three kilos for individuals of height 1.75 m) is (in round figures) 2.4 nmol/l. However, this is only our best guess and it might as well (with 95% credibility) be as much as 3.8 nmol/l or as little as 1.0 nmol/l.

The confidence interval for the slope contains only negative values (it does not include zero), thereforewe are reasonably convinced that there is indeed a (negative) relationship between body mass index and vitamin D.

A formal test for no relation between body mass index and the level of vitamin D may be performed using the Wald Test $W = (-1.952/0.657)^2 = 8.82$ which according to the general theory of Section 2.3.4 follows an approximate Chi-squared distribution with a single degree-of-freedom and leads to a P-value of 0.003, that is, a clear indication of a relation between body mass index and vitamin D, under the assumption of linearity. In this simple situation we may also choose to use the t-test: $t = (-1.952/0.657) = -2.97$, which in the case of a Normally distributed outcome follows a t-distribution with 39 degrees of freedom and yields a P-value 0.005. The same P-value is obtained from the $F(1, 39)$-distributed statistic $t^2 = 8.82$.

Confidence and prediction limits

Based on the parameter estimates above, we may construct predicted values for the outcome (vitamin D concentration) for a whole series of values of body mass indices, with confidence limits. The predicted value of vitamin D for the ith individual is given by the straight line

$$\widehat{y}_i = \widehat{a} + \widehat{b}x_i \tag{4.1.8}$$

and the standard deviation of this prediction may be calculated and used to construct confidence limits.

All these predicted values will of course lie on a straight line (as specified by our model) and the lower and upper confidence limits become symmetric curves around this line, as shown in the left panel of Figure 4.1.3. The limits are most narrow around the average body mass index and become wider as we move towards either small or large values of body mass index. The width of the limits is inversely proportional to the square root of the number of observations, so when the sample size becomes large, the limits narrow and may eventually become indistinguishable from the line itself.

Confidence limits may be used as a visualization of the evidence of a relationship between two variables, or they may be used for an immediate comparison between two such relationships in subgroups (we show an example of this in Section 5.2.2). It is important, however, that they may not be used for diagnosing single individuals, inasmuch as they do not reflect the biological variation around the regression line.

For diagnostic purposes, we should instead use the prediction limits, as seen in the right-hand panel of Figure 4.1.3. These limits are constructed to include 95% of future observations (using an assumption of Normality for the biological variation) and may therefore be used as a diagnostic tool to identify individuals with an uncommon level of vitamin D as compared to their body mass index. The width of these reflects the biological variation around the regression line as well as the uncertainty of the line itself. This means that including a lot of individuals in the investigation will cause these limits to narrow, but only to a certain extent, because a large sample size has no impact on the biological variation of vitamin D for individuals with a common body mass index (variation around the regression line). We notice that these limits are almost straight lines. This is because the biological variation is of larger magnitude than the uncertainty of the estimated line (due to a relatively large sample size).

The prediction limits may be thought of as a continuous collection of reference regions, one for each value of body mass index, that is, reference regions "moving along" the regression line.

Check of model assumptions

The results and interpretation of a simple linear regression relies (to different extents) on various assumptions. Some of these have been discussed previously, in Chapter 3 (variance homogeneity, Normality) whereas linearity is new. Another new consideration deals with examination of the influence of individual observations.

The most fundamental assumption is of course that of linearity between the outcome (vitamin D concentration) and the covariate (body mass index).

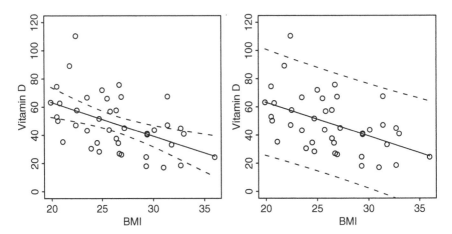

Fig. 4.1.3. Confidence and prediction limits (reference region), vitamin D concentration versus body mass index.

If this is not a reasonable approximation, the results become uninterpretable and therefore useless. We may judge this linearity assumption by looking at the scatterplot Figure 4.1.1. If this scatterplot had shown clear evidence against linearity we should not have proceeded with the analysis but rather tried to modify our model to describe the actual relationship. We present an example of this later in this section.

In some situations, a small systematic curvature may go undetected, especially if the range of the covariate is large and observations are abundant. The visual inspection of the original scatterplot should therefore be supplemented by a residual plot, showing residuals (vertical distances form observations to line; cf. Figure 4.1.2) against the covariate. In later chapters where we have two or more covariates in the model, such a plot becomes mandatory because the dependencies in the data can now no longer be displayed as a simple scatterplot.

The residual plot in question is shown in the upper-left panel of Figure 4.1.4. Deviations from linearity between vitamin D and body mass index will display themselves as curved shapes in such a residual plot. We do not see any such clear tendencies from the smoothing, therefore we conclude once again that linearity is reasonable in this situation.

If we detect a clear deviation from linearity, it would make little sense to continue making conclusions from the present model. Instead, a remedy may be to perform a transformation of the outcome, the covariate, or both. Alternatively, a nonlinear relation could be formulated (cf. Section 4.2 and Appendix B).

A requirement for the least squares method to produce the optimal estimates (in the sense of a small SD) is variance homogeneity, that is the assumption that all residuals have the same standard deviation. A trained

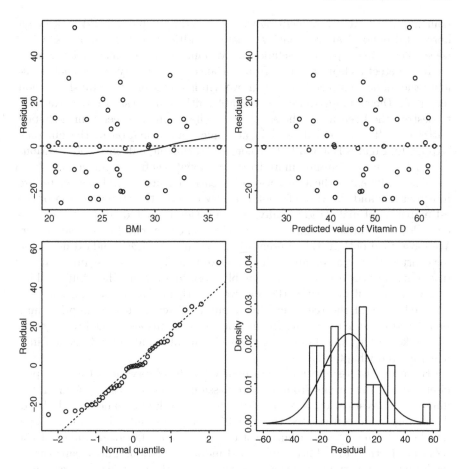

Fig. 4.1.4. Model check for vitamin D concentration versus body mass index.

eye may judge this assumption directly from the scatterplot in Figure 4.1.1 or
Figure 4.1.2 by noting whether the observations form a band of approximately
constant width around the regression line. More often, a residual plot is used,
and even though we may use the same plot as described above, it is more
common (for reasons that become clear in the next chapter concerned with
multiple covariates) to display the residuals against the predicted values of the
outcome $\widehat{y}_i$, as shown in the upper right panel of Figure 4.1.4. Because we only
have a single covariate, there is a one-to-one correspondence between values of
the covariate and predicted values of the outcome (given by the line), and the
residual plots discussed thus far contain exactly the same information. Apart
from a linear transformation of the horizontal axis (here involving a change of
direction), the two plots will always be identical. However, a deviation from
the assumption of variance homogeneity will not show itself as curves but
rather as trumpet- or funnel-shaped patterns. If the assumption of variance

homogeneity is well in agreement with the data, the plot should look like a horizontal band of approximately constant width. This is more or less what we see here, therefore we conclude that variance homogeneity is reasonable.

If we detect a clear deviation from variance homogeneity, it does not invalidate the model completely although we will lose efficiency. A transformation may make the assumption more reasonable, although one should take care not to destroy the linearity at the same time. The commonly seen funnel-shaped pattern is often remedied by a logarithmic transformation of the outcome (Appendix Figures B.3 and B.4), whereas scrutinizing influential observations may help in understanding more irregular deviations from homogeneity.

The fulfillment of the assumption of linearity ensures that the estimates are interpretable and the variance homogeneity ensures that the precision of the estimates is optimal. Traditionally, this precision is quoted either as the standard deviation of the estimate or as a confidence interval for the parameter. We have done both in this presentation. When using the standard deviation for construction of a confidence interval, we must be able to assume that the distribution of the estimate is reasonably close to a Normal distribution. This follows directly if we assume the observations themselves to be Normally distributed (around the regression line), but in practice this assumption may be relaxed because increasing the number of observations in the investigation will make up for (small) deviations from Normality, due to the Central Limit Theorem (cf. Chapter 2).

However, the assumption of Normality for the observations (or more precisely, for the deviations around the regression line) becomes important if the aim of the investigation is to construct prediction limits as described above. These limits are constructed to cover 95% of future individual observations and hence utilize the distribution of outcome values for given values of the covariate in the form of a population standard deviation. This means that a deviation from Normality in the variation around the regression line will have a direct effect on the prediction limits and make them inaccurate and possibly useless. If a proper transformation cannot solve this problem, one should abandon the use of these prediction limits altogether.

Diagnostics

Above, we investigated the appropriateness of various model assumptions. We checked whether the assumptions underlying the linear regression model were reasonable for describing the data at hand. Now we look at the situation from a different perspective and ask whether all observations support the model to the same extent. We discuss terms such as outliers and influential observations. In this setting of a simple linear regression, these ideas are easily illustrated but they become even more important in the subsequent chapters where graphical illustrations can no longer display all data simultaneously.

An *outlier* is an observation that is numerically farther away from its expected value than considered reasonable. Whether such an observation is also *influential* depends on the sample size as well as the focus of interest. For instance, in the vitamin D example, a subject may have a moderate body mass index (e.g., 25 kg/m^2), but a very high vitamin D concentration (e.g., 130 as for the hypothetical point labeled with a star in the upper-right panel of Figure 4.1.5). Whereas this observation will tend to pull the regression line upwards, the effect is very small due to the size of the sample. Likewise, the influence on the slope is also very limited, because a body mass index of 25 kg/m^2 is close to the average value in the sample. On the other hand, if a subject with a high body mass index (e.g., 50 kg/m^2) has a moderate vitamin D concentration (i.e., not as low as expected, e.g., 80 nmol/l), she will pull the line to make it less steep, that is, exert an influence on the slope, as shown in the lower-left panel of Figure 4.1.5). This generalizes to say that an observation with an extreme value of a covariate will be a *potentially* influential observation concerning the effect of this variable. If the outcome corresponds well to this extreme value (i.e., if the subject with the extremely high body mass index has a correspondingly low vitamin D concentration, e.g., 10 as in the lower-right panel of Figure 4.1.5), it will, however, not have any particular effect on the slope itself, only on its standard deviation, which will become smaller because this subject increases the variation in the covariate. The results for these hypothetical extra observations are presented in Table 4.1.1. In this table, we have also included the results obtained from retaining a single underweight Irish woman (with body mass index 15.9) in the analysis.

Table 4.1.1. Influence of single hypothetical observations for S25OHD according to BMI (cf. Figure 4.1.5).

Panel	BMI (kg/m^2)	VitD	Intercept, $\hat{a}$	"Level," $\hat{a}^*$ at BMI $= 25$	Slope, $\hat{b}$
Upper left	—	—	111.05 (18.40)	51.24 (2.95)	−2.392 (0.690)
Upper right	25	130	116.98 (22.07)	53.32 (3.50)	−2.546 (0.829)
Lower left	50	80	68.02 (16.08)	50.14 (3.35)	−0.715 (0.586)
Lower right	50	10	102.03 (14.00)	51.01 (2.92)	−2.041 (0.510)
With under-weight woman	15.9	39.2	98.76 (17.39)	49.95 (2.92)	−1.952 (0.657)

Note that seemingly large changes in the intercept estimates occur, especially for the observation (50 kg/m^2, 80 nmol/l) in the lower-left panel of Figure 4.1.5. This is due to the fact that the intercept gives an extrapolated value of vitamin D for a hypothetical value of body mass index (zero), a value far from all observed values in the sample and therefore irrelevant. We therefore included also the more realistic parameter a^*, defined in Equation (4.1.7) as the expected level of vitamin D corresponding to a body mass index of 25 kg/m^2. This parameter is seen to be more stable.

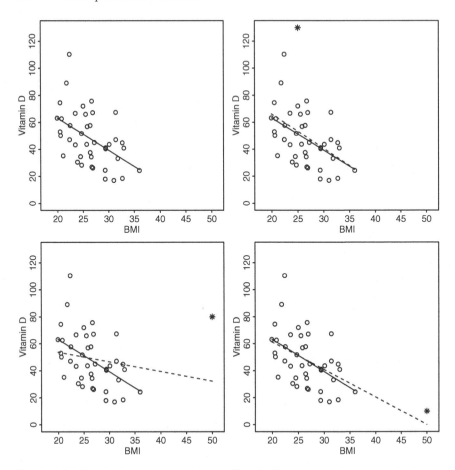

Fig. 4.1.5. Hypothetical observations in vitamin D concentration versus body mass index. Upper-left panel: the original data: all other panels: one hypothetical observation ($*$) added and new regression line shown as a dashed line.

One may investigate the influence of each individual observation simply by performing the analysis in a dataset where we omit the observation in question and observe the change from the original estimates. Omitting the ith individual from the analysis will result in new estimates, say $\widehat{a}_{(-i)}$, respectively, $\widehat{b}_{(-i)}$ and relevant measures of change, $\mathrm{dev}(a)_i$ and $\mathrm{dev}(b)_i$ are the differences, $\widehat{a} - \widehat{a}_{(-i)}$ and $\widehat{b} - \widehat{b}_{(-i)}$ normalized by the standard deviation of the estimate. The squared *influence* (or *deletion*) *diagnostics*, $(\mathrm{dev}(a)_i)^2$ and $(\mathrm{dev}(b)_i)^2$ may be combined into a single diagnostic, *Cook's distance* $\mathrm{Cook}(a,b)_i$.

In Figure 4.1.6 these diagnostic measures are shown graphically. The figure gives the impression that there may be a couple of slightly influential subjects (the largest Cook distances) characterized as having either large values of vitamin D and/or a body mass index in the lower or upper end of the population values.

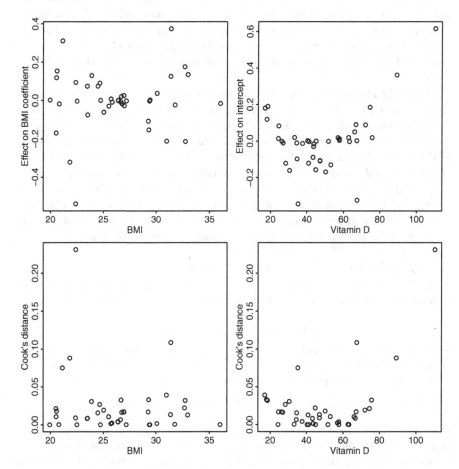

Fig. 4.1.6. Diagnostics $(\text{dev}(a)_i,\ \text{dev}(b)_i,\ \text{and Cook}(a,b)_i)$ plotted against body mass index and/or vitamin D concentration.

Identifying the reason why a subject is influential is important in order to take proper action. In particular, note that being *influential* is not a sufficient cause for omittance from the data analyses!

Observations with extreme values of the *covariate* should often be considered excluded from the analysis, no matter if they are influential or not, simply because they may give rise to an increased precision in the slope estimate which is not warranted because we have little support for the relation in these extreme regions, based on a single observation only. Note that the exclusion of such covariate values corresponds to an exclusion criterion which could have been stated before data collection and that conclusions should be limited accordingly.

On the other hand, observations with extreme values of the *outcome* variable, that is, outcome values that do not correspond well to the covariate values, cannot be removed from the analysis by just referring to exclusion criteria, because this would lead to a circular argument such as "we want to predict y but only for those y-values that correspond well to the average linear trend."

The only reasonable action in this situation is to investigate the possible causes for such an observation to deviate from the rest. A simple error of course should be corrected: a flaw or deviation from the routines or circumstances concerning this observation should be investigated further and could possibly lead to an exclusion of the observation altogether. In such a case, however, all observations should be investigated in this respect and all those that were subject to deviations from routine should be eliminated whether or not they were found to be influential or outlying. Also, the conclusions should be limited accordingly. If deviations from routine are expected to be unavoidable in practice, it does not serve as a proper reason to exclude observations.

Digression. Diagnostics and pseudo-observations

In Section 3.1.3 we introduced *pseudo-observations*. We did this based on the Kaplan–Meier estimator for the survival function, $S(t) = \text{pr}(y > t) = \text{E}(I(y > t))$, as

$$\widehat{S}_i(t) = n\widehat{S}(t) - (n-1)\widehat{S}_{(-i)}(t),$$

where $\widehat{S}_{(-i)}(t)$ was the Kaplan–Meier estimator based on the sample obtained by leaving subject i out. Pseudo-observations can be defined from any estimator, say $\widehat{c}$, of an expected value parameter, c, as

$$n\widehat{c} - (n-1)\widehat{c}_{(-i)} = \widehat{c} + (n-1)(\widehat{c} - \widehat{c}_{(-i)}).$$

It is seen that the pseudo-observation is the estimator $\widehat{c}$, based on the full sample of n observations plus the "leave-i-out-diagnostic", $\widehat{c} - \widehat{c}_{(-i)}$ (multiplied by $n - 1$). Pseudo-observations and leave-one-out diagnostics, however, tend to be used for somewhat different purposes in statistical inference. ◇

Design and correlation

The primary focus of a linear regression will typically be either estimation of the slope or prediction of outcome for a given covariate value. In either case, it is important to obtain as precise an estimate of the slope as possible. Looking at the formula (4.1.5) for the standard deviation of the estimated slope, we see that this is small when the residual variation is small and the variation in the covariate is large.

The residual variation is an intrinsic property of the subject matter that cannot be controlled by design because it reflects the biological variation in the outcome variable for subjects with a common value of the covariate. On the other hand, the variation in the covariate may sometimes be a matter of choice by the investigator.

In the vitamin D example, the covariate is body mass index. If subjects are enrolled in the study through a mechanism that allows the investigator to meet the subjects before possible enrollment, it is possible to ensure a large variation in body mass index within the study group. Likewise, if age or height were the covariate in question, subjects might be chosen with the aim of ensuring a large variation in this respect. For other types of covariates, such as the level of cholesterol, it requires a blood sample to determine the covariate which makes it less convenient for composing the study group in a particular way.

If the subjects are chosen in a nonrandom fashion in order to increase the precision of the slope estimate, it is important to note that the sample will not be representative for the outcome! For instance, if we include many overweight individuals in the vitamin D investigation, we will expect to see a vitamin D distribution shifted somewhat to the left (towards small values) as compared to the population in general. The primary object of the present study was to assess the vitamin D status in different countries, therefore this could have been fatal if no adjustment was made for BMI.

Digression. The correlation coefficient

Linear regression is concerned with evaluating and quantifying a linear relationship between two quantitative variables. However, the correlation coefficient is often used in this situation as well, and although there is a strong resemblance between the two approaches, there are certainly also important differences, unfortunately often overlooked in practical situations.

The correlation coefficient between two quantitative variables, such as vitamin D concentration (y) and body mass index (x), is a dimensionless quantity that can be estimated, symmetrically in x and y, as

$$\widehat{r} = \frac{\widehat{s}_{xy}}{\widehat{s}_x \widehat{s}_y}. \tag{4.1.9}$$

It may be seen that this coefficient can take on values between -1 and 1, and that these extremes are attained when the relationship between the two variables is exactly linear (either with a negative or a positive slope). A coefficient of 0 indicates no linear relationship between the variables.

Comparing the definition (4.1.9) to the formula (4.1.4) for the estimated slope, we see that there is a simple relationship between the two, given by

$$\widehat{r} = \widehat{b}\frac{\widehat{s}_x}{\widehat{s}_y}, \tag{4.1.10}$$

so that the correlation coefficient is simply a scaled version of the slope (or vice versa). In particular, the two quantities are zero in the same situations, and the test of zero slope is identical to the test of zero correlation.

Actually, the correlation coefficient can be interpreted as the slope of the regression line between a normalized y and a normalized x, both being normalized to have standard deviation 1 (by dividing all observations of y by $\widehat{s}_y$ and all observations of x by $\widehat{s}_x$). This implies that r may be interpreted as the expected change in y (in units of $\widehat{s}_y$) when x is changed by one (in units of $\widehat{s}_x$).

The fact that the correlation coefficient r is dimensionless and always takes on values in the range $[-1,1]$ has led to various *rules of thumb* for interpretation (in the sense of defining what is meant by a *low*, a *moderate*, and a *high* correlation, respectively). Whereas this may seem useful for practical purposes, we claim that this is often illusory and may lead to erroneous conclusions.

The problem is that the correlation coefficient is highly dependent on the chosen sampling strategy, that is, the distribution of the covariate. If subjects are chosen deliberately with the aim of providing a precise estimate of the slope of the regression line, $\widehat{s}_x$ will be large, and this has the effect of increasing the correlation. In fact, rearranging the equation (4.1.10) leads to the equation

$$1 - \widehat{r}^2 = \frac{\widehat{s}^2_{y|x}}{\widehat{s}^2_{y|x} + \frac{n-1}{n-2}\widehat{b}^2\widehat{s}^2_x}.$$

Keeping the sample size (n) as well as the intrinsic properties of the problem $(\widehat{b}, \widehat{s}^2_{y|x})$ fixed, we see from this equation, that increasing the variation $\widehat{s}^2_x$ in the covariate x makes the right hand side tend to zero which in turn makes the correlation approach either 1 or -1. This means that designing the investigation in a clever way to obtain a precise estimate of slope will inevitably lead to a high correlation (except if there is no relation whatsoever between the two quantities). Consequently the magnitude of the correlation coefficient is not useful for designed investigations.

If the variables x and y follow a bivariate Normal distribution and sampling is performed in a random fashion, the correlation has a very concise meaning. If the distribution cannot be assumed to be Normal, but we still sample randomly from a well-defined population, we may use a nonparametric version of the correlation. For quantitative data, the most commonly used nonparametric correlation is the *Spearman* correlation coefficient, which utilizes rank values for computation. In contrast, the correlation (4.1.9) is also called the *Pearson* correlation. The Spearman correlation is affected by the chosen sampling strategy in the same way as described above for the Pearson correlation and should, therefore, also be avoided in case of selective (nonrandom) sampling .

In the vitamin D example, we obtained the Pearson correlation $\widehat{r} = -0.425$. For the reasons described above, we abstain from an interpretation of this quantity, but we may test whether it deviates significantly from zero. As mentioned, this is precisely equivalent to testing for zero slope in the linear regression model, so that once again we get $P = 0.005$. The Spearman rank correlation coefficient is $\widehat{r}_S = -0.435$, equally significant $(P = 0.004)$.

Note that apart from telling us that there is a significant association between body mass index and vitamin D status, the value of a correlation does not provide much insight into the subject matter. An exception to this is the situation where we have actually been sampling randomly from a well-defined population. In this case, the squared Pearson correlation coefficient may be stated as a measure of *explained variation*, often referred to as R^2 or *the coefficient of determination*. If the sampling is anything less than completely random, this quantity will suffer from the same objections as stated for the correlation coefficient itself, and should not be used, except for internal comparisons of models for the same data.   ◇

Cell concentration of tetrahymena

Recall from Example 1.6 that in an experiment with the unicellar organism
tetrahymena grown in two different media, we were interested in determining
how cell concentration x (number of cells in 1 ml of the growth media) may
affect the cell size y (average cell diameter, measured in μm). We here look into
the relationship between y and x for the media without glucose, the graphical
presentation of which is shown in Figure 4.1.7.

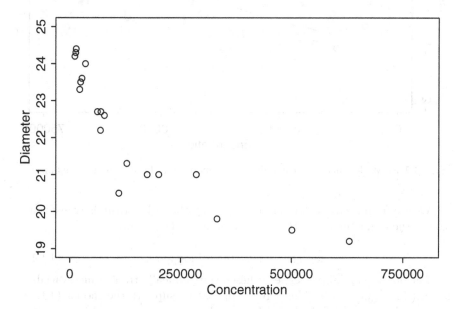

Fig. 4.1.7. Cell diameter as a function of cell concentration.

We note that the effect of an increased concentration is to decrease cell size
and that this effect diminishes for large concentrations. Such a relationship is
fairly typical for positive quantities and it may often be reasonably described
by a power relationship, such as

$$y = ax^b \tag{4.1.11}$$

of which a hyperbola is a special case, setting $b = -1$. In (4.1.11), a is a
parameter denoting the cell size for a concentration of $x = 1$, an extrapolation
to the extreme lower end of the concentration range as seen from Figure 4.1.7.

If we had performed a linear regression analysis without realizing that
the relation does not at all look linear, we would have had a plot for model

checking look like Figure 4.1.8. Note the curved shape indicating that linearity between cell diameter and concentration is not appropriate.

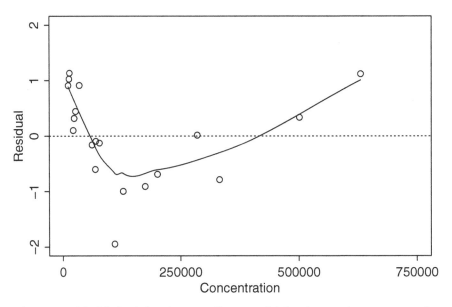

Fig. 4.1.8. Model check for the naive linear model for the tetrahymena example.

We see from the postulated model (4.1.11), that a logarithmic transformation of the diameter yields the new theoretical relationship

$$\log_{10}(y) = \log_{10}(a) + b \log_{10}(x). \tag{4.1.12}$$

The observed relation between these logarithmically transformed variables is seen in Figure 4.1.9. This figure appears to support the model (4.1.11) because the average of the logarithm of cell diameter seems to be reasonably well described as a linear function of the logarithmic cell concentration.

The model checking plots for this transformed model are shown in Figure 4.1.10, which shows a much better fit to the data inasmuch as most of the systematic trends of Figure 4.1.8 have now gone.

If we let $y_i^* = \log_{10}(y_i)$ denote the logarithm of the cell size for the ith suspension and let $x_i^* = \log_{10}(x_i)$ denote the corresponding logarithm of the cell concentration, we may now write the model in the form (4.1.2) (i.e., as $E(y_i^*) = a^* + bx_i^*$) and perform the estimation as a linear regression, estimating $a^* = \log_{10}(a)$ as the intercept and b as the slope.

We get the slope estimate to be $\hat{b} = -0.0597$ with an estimated standard deviation of 0.0041 and a corresponding confidence interval from –0.0684 to –0.0510. The intercept estimate is $\hat{a}^* = 1.635$, with an estimated standard deviation of 0.0202, and a corresponding confidence interval of $(1.5921, 1.6774)$.

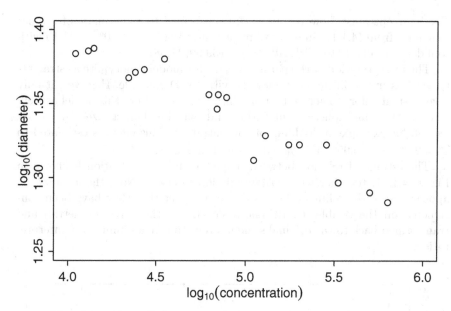

Fig. 4.1.9. Log cell diameter as a function of log cell concentration.

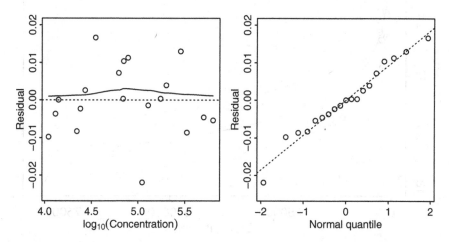

Fig. 4.1.10. Model checking for the linear model on logarithmic scale for the tetrahymena example.

The intercept must, however, be back-transformed to an estimate of the parameter a from (4.1.11) in order to make sense. We get $\hat{a} = 10^{\hat{a}^*} = 43.15$ with confidence interval $(10^{1.5921}, 10^{1.6774}) = (39.09, 47.58)$.

The interpretation of the parameters in this model is not quite as straightforward as in the linear model for the vitamin D example. However, it only takes a small effort to get quite useful interpretations from this model as well. The model is multiplicative in nature and may be characterized by the effect of, for example, a doubling of concentration. This effect is estimated to $2^{\hat{b}} = 2^{-0.0597} = 0.959$, a 4.1% reduction of diameter.

The estimated relation between diameter and concentration is shown in Figure 4.1.11, together with 95% prediction intervals. Note the asymmetric appearance of these limits. This is due to the fact that they have been constructed on the double logarithmic scale (where they are symmetric) and transformed back to the original scale in order to give an immediate interpretation.

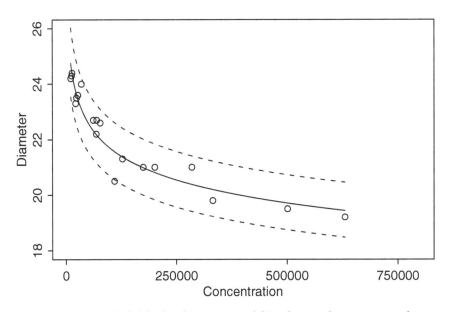

Fig. 4.1.11. Model fit for the power model in the tetrahymena example.

4.1.2 Binary outcome: Simple logistic regression

In this section we consider binary outcomes $y_1, \ldots, y_n$ whose distribution we want to relate to a single quantitative explanatory variable x with observed values $x_1, \ldots, x_n$. As an example we consider the fever in pregnancy Example

1.2 where the outcome is fetal death and where an interesting covariate is the reported weekly alcohol intake for the women in the study (cf. Table 1.3.1).

In the previous Section 4.1.1 an initial graphical representation of outcome and covariate was given as a scatterplot, Figure 4.1.1. The corresponding plot in the present example is not very useful due to the fact that the outcome is binary. However, by adding a scatterplot smoother to the graph (as we have done in Figure 4.1.12), it is seen that there is a clear tendency to higher risk of fetal death with increasing alcohol consumption. (Note that the individual y_i-values (0 or 1) are not given in the figure.)

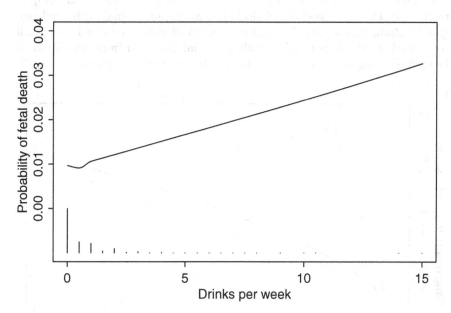

Fig. 4.1.12. Scatterplot smoother for the binary outcome y (fetal death) when plotted against the covariate x (alcohol consumption) in Example 1.2. The distribution of x is indicated along the horizontal axis.

To introduce the *simple logistic regression model* we define the failure probability

$$p_i = \mathrm{pr}(y_i = 1)$$

for individual i and the corresponding log(odds)

$$\ell_i = \log\left(\frac{p_i}{1 - p_i}\right).$$

Recall from Sections 1.3 and 3.1.2 that the log(odds) ℓ_i is unbounded. This makes a linear relationship more suitable for this transformed scale and the model is then

$$\ell_i = a + bx_i. \tag{4.1.13}$$

Here a is the log(odds) when $x_i = 0$ and b is the log(odds ratio) associated with x_i-values differing 1 unit; that is, $\exp(b)$ is the odds ratio between any two individuals whose x-values differ by 1. The basic modeling assumption in (4.1.13) is that this odds ratio does not depend on x: the log(odds) depends linearly on x. A preliminary evaluation of this assumption was already obtained in Figure 1.3.4. We may obtain further information regarding the shape of this relation by transforming the smoother from Figure 4.1.12, and in Figure 4.1.13 this smoother is displayed using the log(odds) transformation. The figure shows that, except for $x = 0$, the logit-linear relationship is reasonable. Because the effect of alcohol consumption is small, this tendency may be unimportant even though the majority of women reported no alcohol consumption. The importance of this potential deviation from linearity may be studied using the methods discussed in the next section (Section 4.2).

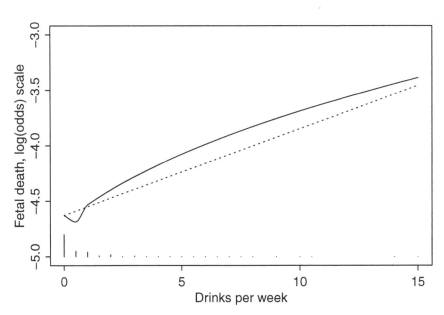

Fig. 4.1.13. Scatterplot smoother (solid curve) and fitted straight line (dashed) in log(odds) scale when the binary outcome y, fetal death, is plotted against the covariate x, alcohol consumption, in Example 1.2. The distribution of x is indicated along the horizontal axis.

The maximum likelihood estimates $\widehat{a}, \widehat{b}$ in the model (4.1.13) cannot be presented as explicit expressions. They are given as the solutions to the two equations

$$\sum_i x_i(y_i - p_i(a, b)) = 0, \quad \sum_i (y_i - p_i(a, b)) = 0, \tag{4.1.14}$$

where $p_i = p_i(a, b)$, following (4.1.13), is given by

$$p_i = \frac{\exp(a + bx_i)}{1 + \exp(a + bx_i)}. \tag{4.1.15}$$

The relationship between p_i and x_i in (4.1.15) is known as the *logistic* curve, hence the name logistic regression (see Figure 1.3.3) For the fever data the estimates $\widehat{a}$ and $\widehat{b}$ are shown in Table 4.1.2. The estimates correspond to a risk when $x = 0$ of $\exp(\widehat{a})/(1+\exp(\widehat{a})) = 0.0097$ and an odds ratio of $\exp(\widehat{b}) = 1.08$ per weekly drink.

Table 4.1.2. Logistic regression models for the log(odds), ℓ_i, of fetal death according to the individually recorded alcohol consumption x_i or a scored version of that, $s(x_i)$.

Model	$\widehat{a}$	$\widehat{b}$	W	P
$\ell_i = a + bx_i$	-4.627 (0.105)	0.078 (0.087)	0.81	0.37
$\ell_i = a + bs(x_i)$	-4.609 (0.107)	0.046 (0.099)	0.21	0.65

Note the appearance of the residuals $y_i - p_i(a, b)$ from the model in the equations (4.1.14). These residuals (inserting the estimates $(\widehat{a}, \widehat{b})$) may be used to evaluate the fit of model (4.1.13), as follows. Simply plotting the residuals against the covariate alcohol consumption will not be very informative inasmuch as the residuals will fall in two groups depending on the outcome. Adding a smoother to the plot may be helpful to see whether residuals, on average, are around 0. In Figure 4.1.14 the residuals $y_i - p_i(\widehat{a}, \widehat{b})$, as explained in Section 2.3.2 (Equation (2.3.5)), have been standardized by dividing by the standard deviation $\sqrt{p_i(\widehat{a}, \widehat{b})(1 - p_i(\widehat{a}, \widehat{b}))}$.

In Section 6.2.2 we introduce more methods for checking the fit of logistic regression models based on comparing observed and expected counts (see, e.g., Table 6.2.14).

Although no explicit expression is available for the estimated odds ratio in (4.1.13), a simple explicit score test for the hypothesis $b = 0$ of no effect of x on y is available. This so-called *trend test* statistic is given by

$$T = \frac{(\sum_i x_i(y_i - \bar{y}))^2}{\bar{y}(1 - \bar{y})\sum_i(x_i - \bar{x})^2}, \tag{4.1.16}$$

where $\bar{y} = 1/n \sum_i y_i$ and $\bar{x} = 1/n \sum_i x_i$. Under the hypothesis $b = 0$ the distribution of T is approximately $\chi^2(1)$. For the fever data, T takes the value 0.81 corresponding to $P = 0.37$, almost identical to the Wald test statistic $(\widehat{b}/SD(\widehat{b}))^2 = 0.81$. Note the similarity between (4.1.16) and the squared Pearson correlation coefficient (Section 4.1.1).

As we did in the previous section (Section 4.1.1), we now study influential observations for $\widehat{b}$. Figure 4.1.15 shows the deletion diagnostics dev$(b)_i$ plotted

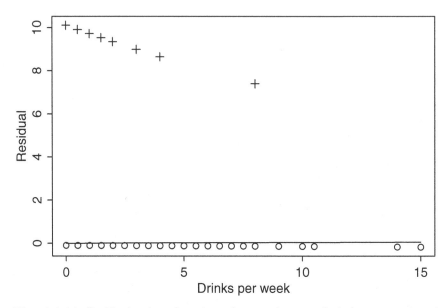

Fig. 4.1.14. Residuals plotted against the covariate x, alcohol consumption, in Example 1.2: + indicates fetal death, o indicates no fetal death. A smoother has been added to the plot.

against alcohol consumption x_i. Different symbols are used for observations with $y_i = 1$ and $y_i = 0$. The diagnostics are seen to be quite small and everywhere smaller than 0.02; that is, no observations will change the estimate by more than 2% of the standard deviation when deleted. In fact, the presence of highly influential points is not expected in very large datasets. The figure also shows the similar diagnostics for the intercept, a.

Digression. Computation of $\text{dev}(b)_i$

For linear regression of a quantitative outcome (Section 4.1.1), the deletion diagnostic $\text{dev}(b)_i$ may be computed explicitly without having to refit the model n times. For logistic regression (and for Cox regression; see Section 4.1.3), however, this is not the case and an approximation is frequently used in software implementations. We have also done so everywhere in the book. ◇

An ordered categorical explanatory variable

We now pay special attention to the situation where the quantitative covariate only takes $k + 1$ (k "small") different values. This may be the case when x is categorical with ordered categories and a *score* $s(x)$ is attached to category $j, j = 0, 1, \ldots, k$. For example, these categories may be obtained by grouping a continuous covariate into $k + 1$ intervals and attaching a score to each

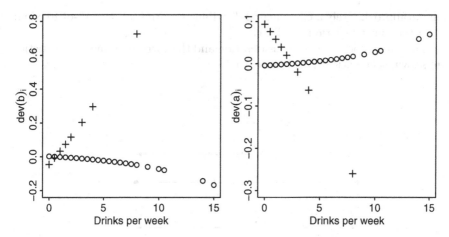

Fig. 4.1.15. Deletion diagnostics $\mathrm{dev}(b)_i$ for the effect of alcohol consumption plotted against the covariate in Example 1.2: $+$ indicates fetal death, o indicates no fetal death.

interval; for example, $s(x_i) = j$, $s(x_i) =$ midpoint in interval j, or $s(x_i) = \bar{x}_j$, the average x-value in interval j, when i belongs to interval j.

We can now obtain a simpler graph by plotting the average outcome, that is, the empirical failure probability in each group, against the score for the group. Again, it may be advantageous to transform the vertical axis using the logit function as we did in Figure 4.1.13 and also in Figure 1.3.4. That figure also suggests a modest increase in risk with increasing alcohol consumption.

In this situation we can still consider a linear logistic model

$$\ell_i = a + bs(x_i)$$

as in (4.1.13) and the interpretation of a and b is similar to that in (4.1.13). What makes this situation somewhat simpler than when x is truly quantitative is the fact that the linear logistic model $\ell_i = a + bs(x_i)$ is now *nested* in the model considered in Section 3.2.2 with separate failure probabilities $p_0, p_1, \ldots, p_k$ in the $k + 1$ categories. This, first of all, means that a simple graphical representation such as in Figure 1.3.4 is available but, furthermore, a simple test for the linear model is possible by comparing with the model with the $k + 1$ categories.

This test statistic for linearity may be obtained using the general principles of likelihood ratio tests introduced in Section 2.3.4. However, a simple approximation to this goodness-of-fit test for the linear logistic model may be obtained as the difference between the general k degree-of-freedom chi-squared statistic for the $k + 1$ categories (cf. Section 3.2.2), and the trend test statistic (4.1.16) (using the covariate $s(x_i)$). This difference

$$L = X^2 - T$$

follows approximately a Chi-squared distribution with $k-1$ degrees-of-freedom when the linear logistic model holds.

The three models under consideration and the corresponding test statistics are shown schematically in Figure 4.1.16.

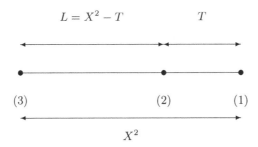

Fig. 4.1.16. Illustration of the three models where, (1) all p_js are equal, (2) logit(p_j) depend linearly on the covariate, (3) no restriction on the p_j.

As an example we once more consider the fever in pregnancy study (Example 1.2) with the covariate x_i =reported weekly alcohol consumption for woman i. In Section 1.3 we studied five groups (i.e., $k = 4$): 0, (0,1], (1,2], (2,3],and 3+ (cf. Table 1.3.1). The scores, $s(x_i)$ attached to these groups were the averages 0, 0.73, 1.85, 2.83, 4.89.

The estimates in the model with a linear effect of $s(x_i)$ are shown in Table 4.1.2. It is seen that the Wald test for no effect of the covariate is $W = (0.046/0.099)^2 = 0.21$ which evaluated in the $\chi^2(1)$-distribution gives the insignificant P-value of 0.65. The corresponding likelihood ratio test statistic is 0.20. Considering instead the model where the five alcohol groups are treated as a categorical explanatory variable, the likelihood ratio test statistic (with four degrees-of-freedom) is 0.60 and the likelihood ratio test statistic for linearity is, therefore, $0.60 - 0.20 = 0.40$. The corresponding P-value when evaluated in the $\chi^2(3)$-distribution is 0.94.

The conclusion is that the model with a linear effect of $s(x_i)$ cannot be rejected when compared to the model with alcohol as a categorical covariate, and in the model assuming a linear effect of alcohol its effect is insignificant.

For comparison, we finally present the tests where all computations can be presented explicitly. The chi-square test on 4 d.f. based on the data in Table 1.3.1 takes the value $X^2 = 0.63$, the trend test statistic (4.1.16) is $T = 0.21$, and the test for linearity then becomes $L = X^2 - T = 0.42$ close to the values based on the likelihood ratio tests.

Digression. Nomenclature

The test statistic for linearity is also known as a *test for departures from trend* although the hypothesis is the model *with* a linear trend. Similarly, the hypothesis for the trend test statistic is actually the model with *no trend*. ◇

4.1.3 Survival time outcome: Simple Cox regression

We now turn to (possibly censored) survival time outcomes $y_1, \ldots, y_n$ and the problem of relating their distribution to a single quantitative explanatory variable x with observed values $x_1, \ldots, x_n$. The motivating example is the PBC-3 study, Example 1.3, and the covariate bilirubin (cf. Table 1.3.2).

To introduce the simple *Cox proportional hazards model* for the covariate x we let $h_i(t)$ be the hazard function for individual i and recall from Sections 1.2 and 3.1.3 that because the log(hazard), $l_i(t) = \log(h_i(t))$, is unbounded this makes a linear relationship more suitable for the transformed scale and the model is then

$$l_i(t) = \log(h_0(t)) + bx_i. \tag{4.1.17}$$

Here, $\log(h_0(t))$ is the log(hazard) at time t when $x_i = 0$ and b is the log(hazard ratio) associated with x_i-values differing 1 unit; that is, $\exp(b)$ is the hazard ratio between any two individuals whose x-values differ by 1. The basic modeling assumptions in (4.1.17) are the proportional hazards assumption and the fact that the log(hazard) depends *linearly* on x (i.e. x has the same *multiplicative* effect on the hazard throughout its entire range).

The maximum likelihood estimates in the model (4.1.17) cannot be presented as explicit expressions. However, b is estimated by the solution to the equation

$$\sum_i d(y_i)(x_i - \bar{x}(y_i, b)) = 0, \tag{4.1.18}$$

where $d(y_i) = 1$ if y_i is a failure time, $d(y_i) = 0$ if y_i is a censoring time, and $\bar{x}(y_i, b)$ is a weighted average of x-values among individuals j still at risk at time y_i (i.e.; individuals for whom $y_j \geq y_i$). Here, the weights are $\exp(bx_j)$ and this weighted average is, therefore, given by

$$\bar{x}(y_i, b) = \frac{\sum_{j:y_j \geq y_i} x_j \exp(bx_j)}{\sum_{j:y_j \geq y_i} \exp(bx_j)}.$$

For the PBC-3 data the estimate $\widehat{b}$ is shown in Table 4.1.3. This estimate corresponds to a hazard ratio of $\exp(10\widehat{b}) = 1.10$ per 10 μmol/L of bilirubin, that is, a 10% increase in hazard whenever individuals differing 10 μmol/L are compared.

Like the case of binary outcomes in the previous section, a simple explicit test for the hypothesis, $b = 0$, of no effect of x on y is available. This *logrank trend test statistic*, the score test based on model (4.1.17), is given by

Table 4.1.3. PBC-3 study: Cox regression models for the log(hazard) $l_i(t)$ according to the individually recorded bilirubin level x_i or a scored version of that, $s(x_i)$.

Model	$\widehat{b}$	W	P
$l_i(t) = \log(h_0(t)) + bx_i$	0.00934 (0.000891)	109.7	<0.001
$l_i(t) = \log(h_0(t)) + bs(x_i)$	0.0150 (0.0016)	82.7	<0.001
$l_i(t) = \log(h_0(t)) + b\log(x_i)$	1.009 (0.099)	103.9	<0.001
$l_i(t) = \log(h_0(t)) + bs(\log(x_i))$	0.993 (0.109)	82.6	<0.001

$$T = \frac{(\sum_i d(y_i)(x_i - \bar{x}(y_i, 0)))^2}{\sum_i d(y_i)V_x(y_i)}, \tag{4.1.19}$$

where $\bar{x}(y_i, 0)$ and $V_x(y_i)$ are the mean and variance, respectively, of x-values among individuals still at risk at time y_i. Under the hypothesis $b = 0$ the distribution of T is approximately $\chi^2(1)$. For the PBC3 data T takes the highly significant value 160.6 yielding the same conclusion as the Wald test statistic $(\widehat{b}/\mathrm{SD}(\widehat{b}))^2 = 109.7$ (Table 4.1.3).

The differences $x_i - \bar{x}(y_i, \widehat{b})$ appearing, for example, in (4.1.18) are known as the *Schoenfeld* or *score residuals* for the Cox regression model and may be used for assessment of the proportional hazards assumption (e.g., Therneau and Grambsch, 2000, Ch. 6) . However, because of the more general nature of pseudo-residuals and because of the close resemblance of residual- and scatterplots based on pseudo-observations to graphical goodness-of-fit checking methods for quantitative and, in particular, binary outcome variables we have chosen not to illustrate the use of Schoenfeld residuals and instead concentrate on pseudo-observations.

Figure 4.1.17 shows a scatterplot of pseudo-observations against bilirubin for four time points chosen as the quintiles of the observed event times. A smoother has been added to the plot. Under the model (4.1.17), the smoothers for the four situations should be straight lines (linearity) that are parallel (proportional hazards) on the log(hazard) scale or equivalently (see Section 3.1.3) on the log(–log(survival function)) ("cloglog") scale. The fact that this does not seem to be the case (see Figure 4.1.18 where the plot of the transformed smooth curve is shown) suggests a poor fit of (4.1.17). Also, the pseudo-residuals, Figure 4.1.19, where residuals do not seem to be 0 on average, suggest a poor fit. The model, therefore, needs to be improved and we do this below using a transformation of the covariate.

An ordered categorical explanatory variable

As in the section on binary outcomes we now pay special attention to the simpler situation where the quantitative covariate only takes $k+1$ (k "small") different values, for example, when x is categorical with ordered categories and a score, $s(x_i)$ is attached to individuals i from category $j, j = 0, 1, \ldots, k$.

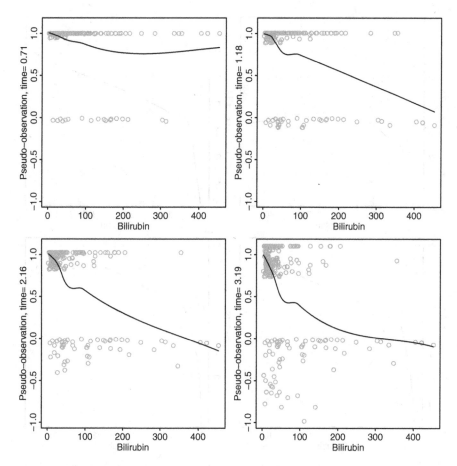

Fig. 4.1.17. Pseudo-observations and scatterplot smoother for the PBC3 study plotted against bilirubin for quintiles of observed event times.

For survival data we can consider the proportional hazards model

$$l_i(t) = \log(h_0(t)) + bs(x_i), \qquad (4.1.20)$$

where the interpretation of b is similar to that in (4.1.17), namely that $\exp(b)$ is the hazard ratio between any two individuals whose $s(x)$-values differ by 1. We continue the PBC3-example and use the scores for bilirubin from Table 3.2.14, and fitting the model (4.1.20) we get $\widehat{b} = 0.0150$ (0.0016) (Table 4.1.3). This model is nested in the model considered in Section 3.2.3 with separate survival functions in the $k + 1$ categories satisfying the proportional hazards assumption. This means that a simple test for the linear model is available by comparing with the model with the $k + 1$ categories.

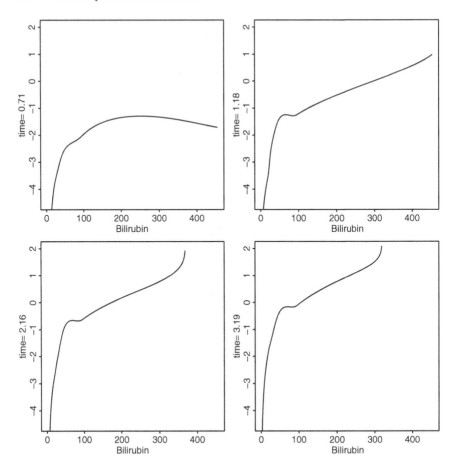

Fig. 4.1.18. Scatterplot smoother for the pseudo-observations in the PBC study plotted in cloglog scale against bilirubin for quintiles of observed event times.

This test is known as the logrank *test for linearity* and it is obtained as the difference L between the $k+1$ sample logrank test and the logrank trend test. The latter is given by (4.1.19) (using the covariate $s(x_i)$) and the numerator can be shown to take the simple form

$$\left(\sum_{j=0}^{k} s_j(O_j - E_j)\right)^2,$$

where s_j is the score attached to group j and O_j and E_j are defined in Section 3.2.3. The difference L follows approximately a Chi-squared distribution with $k-1$ degrees-of-freedom when the model with a linear effect of $s(x)$ holds, see the illustration in Figure 4.1.16. Alternative trend tests and tests for linearity, in fact used more often than the logrank tests, are the likelihood ratio tests.

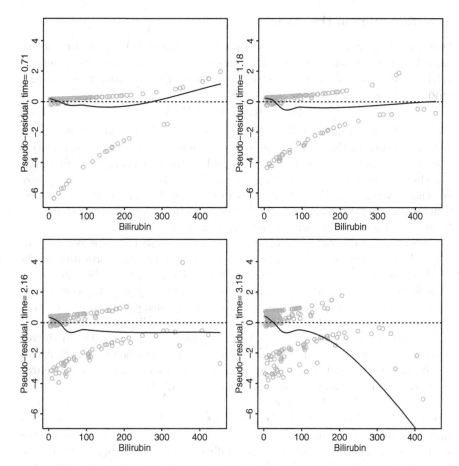

Fig. 4.1.19. Pseudo-residuals from model (4.1.17) and scatterplot smoother for the PBC study plotted against bilirubin for quintiles of observed event times.

For the PBC3 data and the five bilirubin groups considered in Section 3.2.3 we get, using the scores 7.66, 13.26, 20.23, 37.32, and 148.83 from Table 3.2.14, that the logrank trend test statistic takes the highly significant value 109.2 whereas the corresponding Wald test (Table 4.1.3) is $W = (0.0150/0.0016)^2 = 82.7$ and the likelihood ratio test is 75.9. The likelihood ratio test for linearity is then 19.0 which evaluated in the $\chi^2(3)$-distribution gives $P = 0.003$. Judged from these tests, the model with a linear effect of $s(x_i)$ is clearly rejected when compared to the model with bilirubin as a categorical covariate. In the model assuming a linear effect of bilirubin its effect is strongly significant but this linear model needs further investigation.

Transformation of the covariate

One way of improving on the fit of an assumed linear model, as already discussed in the section dealing with quantitative outcome variables, Section 4.1.1, is to transform the explanatory variable x. This amounts to studying a model such as

$$l_i(t) = \log(h_0(t)) + bf(x_i), \qquad (4.1.21)$$

for some known transformation, $f(\cdot)$, for example, $f(x) = \log(x)$ or $f(x) = 1/x$. We return to this problem in a more general setting in the next section (Section 4.2) but, based on Figure 1.3.7 and on the scatter- and residual plots based on pseudo-observations, Figures 4.1.17 and 4.1.19, we can already now see that a transformation of bilirubin in the PBC3 example with a *concave* function (i.e., a "downward bending" function whose slope decreases), like the logarithm (Figure B.1), may improve the linear fit.

We use here the *natural logarithm*, $\log(x)$, because that was done in the original publication by Lombard et al. (1993). However, interpretation of the resulting regression coefficient would be simpler if, instead, bilirubin were transformed by, for example, $\log_2(x)$. As a preliminary investigation we redefine the scores for the quintile bilirubin groups using instead the average log(bilirubin) values: 2.00, 2.58, 3.00, 3.60, and 4.84. Figure 4.1.20 shows the log(hazard ratios) log(1), log(0.57), log(3.00), log(5.28), and log(13.70) plotted against these new scores. It is seen that (apart from the nonmonotonicity for small bilirubin values) the association now seems more closely approximated by a straight line when we compare with Figure 1.3.7.

Letting $f(x_i) = \log(x_i)$ and fitting the model (4.1.21) we get $\widehat{b} = 1.009(0.099)$ (Table 4.1.3) and thereby $\exp(\widehat{b}) = 2.74$. This value has the interpretation that every time we compare two patients whose $\log(x)$-values differ by 1, or equivalently the ratio of their bilirubin values is $\exp(1) = 2.718$, the associated hazard ratio is 2.74. This somewhat awkward interpretation has to do with the use of the natural logarithm $\log(\cdot)$. Had we instead transformed bilirubin using base-2 logarithms we would have estimated the hazard ratio associated with a doubling of bilirubin. The corresponding b-estimate, however, is easily obtained from our results because it is simply given by $\widehat{b} \cdot \log(2) = 0.70$ and thereby $\exp(\widehat{b} \cdot \log(2)) = 2.01$. This result is very easy to communicate: every time bilirubin is doubled the hazard rate is doubled. The 95% confidence limits for this hazard ratio are from $\exp(1.009 \cdot \log(2) - 1.96 \cdot 0.099 \cdot \log(2)) = 1.76$ to $\exp(1.009 \cdot \log(2) + 1.96 \cdot 0.099 \cdot \log(2)) = 2.30$.

Figure 4.1.21 shows a scatterplot of pseudo-observations against logarithmic values of bilirubin for the same four time points as above. A smoother has been added to the plot. Under the model (4.1.21) (with $f(\cdot) = \log(\cdot)$), the smoothers for the four situations should be parallel straight lines on the cloglog scale; see Figure 4.1.22. Compared to Figure 4.1.17 this now looks more reasonable and also the pseudo-residuals, Figure 4.1.23, where residuals now do seem to be 0 on average, suggest a much better fit of the model after log-transformation of bilirubin.

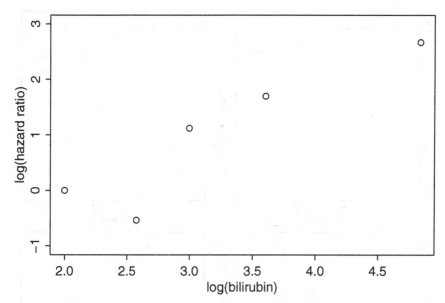

Fig. 4.1.20. Estimated log(hazard ratios) for the PBC study for quintiles of serum bilirubin plotted against average log(bilirubin) in quintile groups.

In Section 6.2.3 we discuss more ways of checking the proportional hazards assumption based on either adding time-dependent covariate effects to the model (Table 6.2.19) or using the *stratified* Cox model (6.2.2) introduced in Section 5.1.1; see (5.1.4).

Alternatively, we may treat log(bilirubin) as an ordered categorical co-variate by defining $s(x_i)$ to be the average log-bilirubin value in group $j = 0, 1, \ldots, k$, when i belongs to category j. This model, as we noted above, is nested in the proportional hazards model treating bilirubin as a categorical covariate. For the covariate scored using average log–bilirubin values we find the regression coefficient estimate $\widehat{b} = 0.993, (0.109)$ giving a Wald test statistic of $W = 82.6$ (Table 4.1.3). The corresponding score test, the logrank trend test, takes the value 102.6 and the likelihood ratio test statistic is 88.7. For the log-scores the likelihood ratio test for linearity is 6.2 and, evaluated in the $\chi^2(3)$-distribution, the P-value is 0.10, so, in this case, the linear model for log(bilirubin) is not rejected. The example illustrates the important fact that trend tests depend on the chosen scores.

Influential observations

As in Section 4.1.1 we supplement the fit of the model by studying influential points using the deviation diagnostics $\text{dev}(b)_i$ for b which show (in units of the standard deviation) how much the estimate of b changes by eliminating

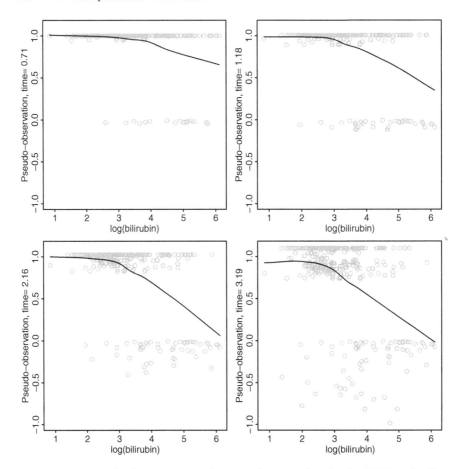

Fig. 4.1.21. Pseudo-observations and scatterplot smoother for the PBC study plotted against log(bilirubin) for quintiles of observed event times.

observation i from the sample. In Figure 4.1.24 (left panel), dev$(b)_i$ values are plotted against log(bilirubin) and, in the right panel, they are plotted against time. In the figures, three fairly large negative values (≈ -0.3) appear. It is seen that these all correspond to censored patients with rather large bilirubin values, observations that, if deleted, would increase the large positive value of $\hat{b}$ because they have survived for "too long" considering their large values of bilirubin. However, none of these observations appears to be a suspiciously large outlier.

Let us, finally, return to the untransformed bilirubin covariate. This has, as can be seen from Figures 4.1.17 and 4.1.19, a highly skewed distribution with few very large values. Such outlying covariate values have, as discussed in Section 4.1.1, the potential of being strongly influential on the estimate of

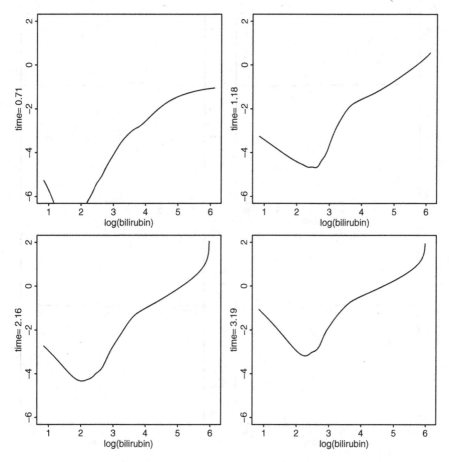

Fig. 4.1.22. Scatterplot smoother for the pseudo-observations in the PBC study plotted in cloglog scale against log(bilirubin) for quintiles of observed event times.

the effect of the covariate. Figure 4.1.25 shows the diagnostic plots without tranforming bilirubin. It is seen that some observations have a relatively large influence on the estimate (e.g., ≈ -0.5 for the patient with the largest observed bilirubin value with a treatment failure at about 1 year, and -0.6 for a patient with bilirubin about 350, censored after 2.3 years), both with somewhat larger diagnostics than seen for the log-transformed covariate.

Although there are no distributional assumptions for covariates, it is often advisable to make a transformation to make the covariate distribution more symmetric, partly to avoid very influential values. It should be kept in mind, however, that what matters most is whether the assumption of linearity for the covariate is reasonable. Fortunately, quite often, for example, a log-transformation of a highly skewed covariate at the same time reduces the

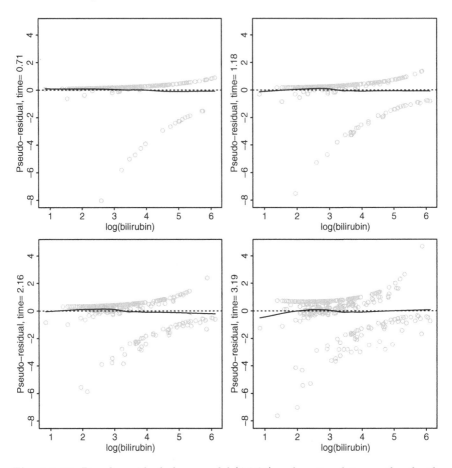

Fig. 4.1.23. Pseudo-residuals from model (4.1.21) and scatterplot smoother for the PBC study plotted against log(bilirubin) for quintiles of observed event times.

amount of influential points and improves on the linearity. Bilirubin in the PBC-3 study provides such an example.

4.2 Nonlinear effect

In the previous section we dealt with regression models with a single quantitative explanatory variable x assuming its effect on the linear predictor to be linear, possibly through transformation by a known function $f(x)$. Both models for quantitative, binary, and survival time outcome variables y were studied and in all cases the effect of x was expressed by one parameter, b. This has the simple interpretation as the difference in values of the linear predictor for individuals differing in 1 unit for x (or $f(x)$). For the three types

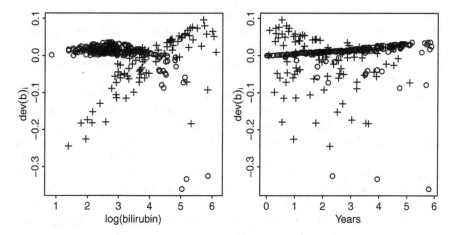

Fig. 4.1.24. Deviation diagnostics for model (4.1.21) for the PBC3 study plotted against log(bilirubin) (left panel) and against time (right panel); +: observed event times, o: censored observations.

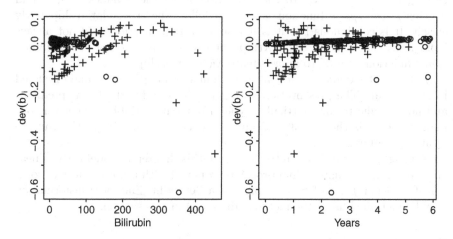

Fig. 4.1.25. Deviation diagnostics for model (4.1.17) for the PBC3 study plotted against bilirubin (left panel) and against time (right panel); +: observed event times, o: censored observations.

of outcome considered this parameter could further be interpreted as either a mean value difference, a log(odds ratio), or a log(hazard ratio).

Thus, linear effects of x are simple and easy to interpret, however, the assumption of linearity is restrictive and may give misleading results if the model specifying a linear effect fits poorly (see, e.g., Example 1.6 in Section 4.1.1). It is, therefore, of great importance both to check this assumption properly and to have alternative models that may be used when linearity fails. This is the topic of the present section where we discuss nonlinear effects of a quantitative explanatory variable. We still restrict attention to the case where only a single such covariate is considered and return to multiple regression models in the next chapter (although some of the advantages of applying the methods of the current section become more apparent for multiple regression; see Section 6.1.3).

We study two main classes of nonlinear effects, one based on a choice of intervals for x and one that is not. To get a feeling for the models used when intervals for x are studied, Figure 4.2.1 shows the linear predictor for some simulated data. Here the true model specifies the mean of y_i as $\log(x_i) - \log(6)$ (the distribution of x is uniform on the interval $(1,11)$) and this relationship is shown in the first panel together with the best fitting straight line for the 250 observations generated. In the second panel the relationship is approximated by a step function with steps between the intervals $(1,3)$, $(3,5)$, $(5,7)$, $(7,9)$, and $(9,11)$. It is seen that the step function indicates a concave relationship much like the true logarithmic function. The step function is not continuous and, therefore, often not biologically plausible. In the third panel the relationship is approximated by a piecewise linear function where the slope changes when moving from one interval to the next, that is, at the x-values 3, 5, 7, and 9. This *linear spline* function is seen to follow the true relationship fairly closely. It is continuous but it is not smooth and, therefore still not always biologically plausible. In the fourth panel a smooth function of x, a *quadratic spline* function, is used to approximate the relationship

In the next section (Section 4.2.1) such models are presented and discussed in more detail. The presentation is in general terms for the linear predictor and not specific to any particular type of outcome variable y, however, our main example is the PBC3 trial and the effect of bilirubin on the time to treatment failure.

Alhough, as noted in the introduction to this chapter, a model with a linear effect of x_i, itself, may be inappropriate, a model with a linear effect of some transformation $f(x_i)$ of x_i may provide a better fit. Such a transformation may be identified using the methods discussed in this section.

Scatterplot smoothers

The models discussed all have the property that the linear predictor can be expressed using simple explanatory variables and, as mentioned in the introduction to the current chapter, such models can all be fitted quite simply using standard software. Smooth regression functions may also be obtained using lowess or other nonparametric scatterplot smoothers (e.g., Hastie and Tibshirani, 1990, Ch. 2). We have illustrated the use of such smoothers in a number of examples (e.g., Figures 4.1.1, 4.1.12, and 4.1.17) and seen that these are useful tools when assessing assumptions of regression models. However, because the curve obtained using a scatterplot smoother does not have a simple mathematical representation, it is less useful for inference on the curve than for a description.

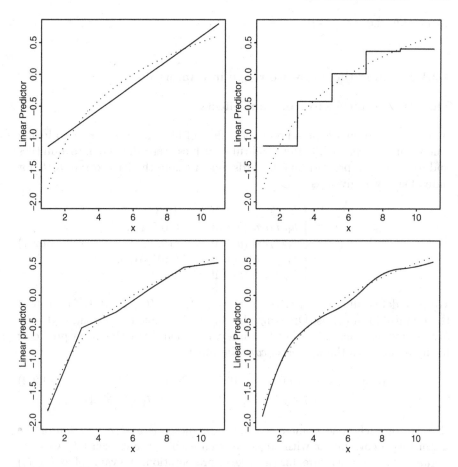

Fig. 4.2.1. Illustration of models for the linear predictor that are alternatives to the simple linear model from Section 4.1. The dotted curve represents the true relationship.

Digression. Truly nonlinear models

Let us finally mention that the nonlinear models discussed in this section all include a linear predictor; that is, the models are "linear in the parameters." However, other nonlinear models without a linear predictor exist. One example of such a model for a quantitative outcome y_i is the Gompertz model with the mean given by

$$E(y_i) = a + b \exp(cx_i).$$

For $c > 0$ such a model may be used in studies of growth curves whereas, also for $c < 0$, the model has applications in enzyme kinetics; see, for example, Seber and Wild (1989, Ch. 7–8). Inference in intrinsically nonlinear regression models is considerably more complicated than regression models with linear predictors and is not discussed further. ◇

4.2.1 Dividing the covariate range into intervals

Models with piecewise constant effects

A simple way of modeling a non-linear effect of bilirubin was, in fact, already studied in Section 3.2.3. Here, bilirubin values were divided into quintiles and we studied a proportional hazards model where the hazard rate $h_i(t)$ for individual i was given as

$$h_i(t) = \begin{cases} h_0(t) & \text{if } x_i \leq 10.3, \\ h_0(t) \exp(b_1) & \text{if } x_i \in (10.3, 16], \\ h_0(t) \exp(b_2) & \text{if } x_i \in (16, 26.7], \\ h_0(t) \exp(b_3) & \text{if } x_i \in (26.7, 51.4], \\ h_0(t) \exp(b_4) & \text{if } x_i > 51.4. \end{cases} \quad (4.2.1)$$

We now define dummy variables $I(x_i \leq 10.3), \ldots, I(x_i > 51.4)$ for each of these bilirubin intervals. Omitting the dummy variable corresponding to the desired *reference level*, here the first interval, we can write the linear predictor for individual i as the *piecewise constant* function :

$$\text{LP}_i(t) = \log(h_0(t)) + b_1 I(10.3 < x_i \leq 16) \quad (4.2.2)$$
$$+ b_2 I(16 < x_i \leq 26.7) + \cdots + b_4 I(x_i > 51.4);$$

that is, for each time point t the linear predictor is a *step function* of the quantitative covariate x with steps between each of the chosen intervals (cf. Figure 4.2.2). In the figure, for the sake of presentation, the value of $\log(h_0(t))$ has been set to 0 such that the value of the linear predictor for each step, $j = 1, 2, 3, 4$, is simply $\hat{b}_j$. The estimates for b_1, b_2, b_3, b_4 are: -0.537 (0.708), 1.120 (0.494), 1.698 (0.460), and 2.670 (0.437), respectively. The scores previously used (cf. Sections 3.2.3 and 4.1.3) have been indicated on the figure and the values of the linear predictor in these points have been connected with straight lines. This gives a rough idea about the fit of the model where x_i enters linearly. As discussed in Section 4.1.3, the model where the levels of the factor corresponding to the five intervals for bilirubin have been coded using the scores

$$s(x_i) = \begin{cases} 7.66 & \text{if } x_i \leq 10.3 \\ 13.26 & \text{if } x_i \in (10.3, 16] \\ 20.23 & \text{if } x_i \in (16, 26.7] \\ 37.32 & \text{if } x_i \in (26.7, 51.4] \\ 148.83 & \text{if } x_i > 51.4 \end{cases}$$

(and where the linear predictor is $\log h_0(t) + bs(x_i)$) is nested in the model including bilirubin as a categorical explanatory variable . Thereby, a formal goodness-of-fit test for the model including $s(x_i)$ can be carried out. In this case the likelihood ratio test statistic comparing the two models is 19.0, which evaluated in a $\chi^2(3)$ distribution gives a P-value of 0.0003, thereby clearly rejecting the linear model. The figure suggests that very low bilirubin values are associated with somewhat higher hazard rates than for the interval from 10.3 to 16. The linear predictor increases from this interval and up according to a nonlinear (concave) function.

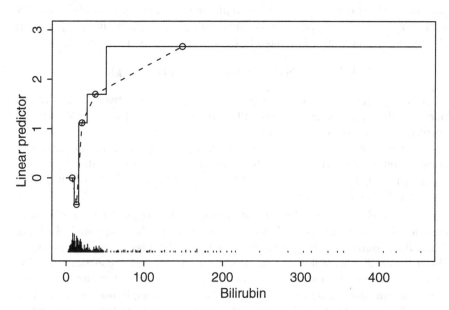

Fig. 4.2.2. Estimated linear predictor (solid curve) for the PBC study assuming an effect of serum bilirubin that is piecewise constant in quintile groups. The dashed curve joins values of the linear predictor for the scores attached to each interval of bilirubin. The distribution of bilirubin is shown on the horizontal axis.

General formulation

In general, we have the following situation: x is a quantitative covariate and k cutpoints $r_1 < r_2 < \ldots < r_k$ are studied. For individual i we define $k + 1$ dummy variables by

$$I(r_j < x_i \le r_{j+1}), j = 0, 1, \ldots, k$$

(where, formally, $r_0 = -\infty, r_{k+1} = \infty$). A model where the effect of x is piecewise constant has the linear predictor

$$\text{LP}_i = a + b_1 I(r_1 < x_i \le r_2) + \cdots + b_k I(x_i > r_k) \qquad (4.2.3)$$

if the first interval is chosen as the reference. Here, a is the value of LP for the reference interval $x \le r_1$ and for $j = 1, \ldots, k$, b_j is the difference between the linear predictor for the interval $r_j < x \le r_{j+1}$ (which is $a + b_j$) and that for the reference interval (a). The hypothesis $b_1 = \cdots = b_k = 0$ corresponds to a constant linear predictor (i.e., no effect of x on y), and may be tested by the standard k-degree-of-freedom likelihood ratio test.

Note that the same model may be parametrized differently. In (4.2.3) the b_j parameters are differences compared to a fixed reference group. An alternative parametrization may be obtained by replacing the dummy variables above by $I(x_i > r_j), j = 0, 1, \ldots, k$, that is, indicators of exceeding the left points of the respective intervals. The model (4.2.3) may then be rewritten as

$$\mathrm{LP}_i = a + b_1^* I(x_i > r_1) + \cdots + b_k^* I(x_i > r_k),$$

where the parameters b_j^* now correspond to differences between values of the linear predictor for successive intervals. The hypothesis $b_1^* = \cdots = b_k^* = 0$ still corresponds to no effect of x on y.

For the PBC3 example the alternative parametrization of the piecewise constant effect of bilirubin gives the following parameter estimates: $\widehat{b}_1^* = \widehat{b}_1 = -0.537(0.708)$, $\widehat{b}_2^* = \widehat{b}_2 - \widehat{b}_1 = 1.657(0.641)$, $\widehat{b}_3^* = \widehat{b}_3 - \widehat{b}_2 = 0.578(0.348)$, $\widehat{b}_4^* = \widehat{b}_4 - \widehat{b}_3 = 0.972(0.257)$.

The model (4.2.3) can be presented graphically by plotting the piecewise constant function against x. This corresponds to the second panel of Figure 4.2.1. If the outcome y is quantitative then this plot may be superimposed on the y versus x scatterplot and, in any case, the piecewise constant function may be compared to a scatterplot smoother. In the present example, dealing with survival data, such a plot may be based on pseudo-observations. Figure 4.2.3 shows the piecewise constant linear predictor added to the scatterplot smoother of the pseudo-observations plotted against bilirubin (cf. Figure 4.1.17). For small values of bilirubin the piecewise constant curve approximates the curve reasonably for all of the four time points. However, for large bilirubin values the fit is not good. Figure 4.2.4 presents the corresponding figure for log(bilirubin) and shows a better fit.

When scores, $s(x)$ like midpoints, are attached to each interval one may further plot the broken line connecting the values of the linear predictor for these points and thereby obtain a graphical evaluation of the fit of the model where x enters linearly. However, an obvious drawback of the model (4.2.3) is that the linear model $\mathrm{LP}_i = a + bx_i$ is not nested in it and, thereby, the model does not provide a formal test of a linear effect of x. Furthermore, the linear predictor in (4.2.3) is not a continuous function of x, a fact which will often make that model biologically implausible. Finally, x has no effect within intervals, only between intervals.

We now turn to models based on *regression splines* where these drawbacks are no longer an issue.

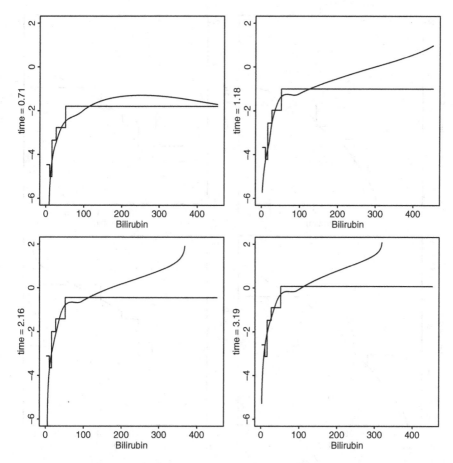

Fig. 4.2.3. The estimated linear predictor for the PBC3 study (assuming an effect of serum bilirubin which is piecewise constant in quintile groups) plotted against bilirubin together with smoothed pseudo-observations. The four panels correspond to quintiles of observed event times.

Regression splines

A model where the relation between y and x is continuous and contains the linear relationship as a special case may be based on a flexible class of functions called *local polynomials* or *regression splines*. Among these, linear regression splines are the simplest. In a model with a linear regression spline the relationship between the linear predictor and x is a broken line with breaks at each interval endpoint as depicted in the lower-left panel of Figure 4.2.1.

The model is defined by including the explanatory variables

$$x_{ij}^{+} = (x_i - r_j)I(x_i > r_j),\qquad(4.2.4)$$

$j = 0, 1, \ldots, k$, so that the linear predictor becomes

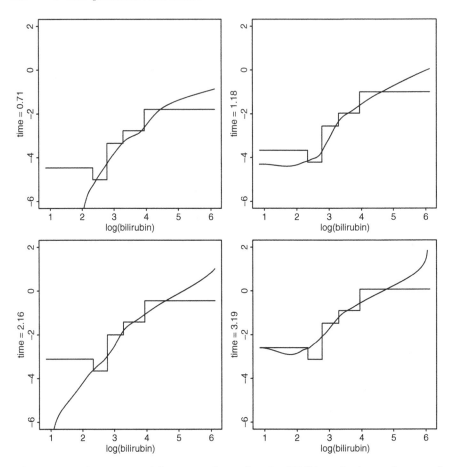

Fig. 4.2.4. The estimated linear predictor for the PBC3 study (assuming an effect of log(serum bilirubin) which is piecewise constant in quintile groups) plotted against log(bilirubin) together with smoothed pseudo-observations. The four panels correspond to quintiles of observed event times.

$$\mathrm{LP}_i = a + bx_i + b_1 x_{i1}^+ + \cdots + b_k x_{ik}^+. \tag{4.2.5}$$

This model (4.2.5) obviously contains the simple linear model $a + bx_i$ as a special case (when $b_1 = \cdots = b_k = 0$) and it thereby provides a way of testing the fit of the linear model. Also, the parameters have a rather simple interpretation in that a is the value of the linear predictor when $x = 0$, b is the slope of the linear predictor for $x \leq r_1$, that is, in the first interval, and $b_j, j = 1, \ldots, k$, is the change of slope of the linear predictor when x "passes" r_j. (The slope is b in the reference interval, $b + b_1$ in the next, $b + b_1 + b_2$ in the next, etc.)

For the PBC3 example we get the estimates $\widehat{b} = -0.245(0.182)$, $\widehat{b}_1 = 0.460(0.309)$, $\widehat{b}_2 = -0.122(0.185)$, $\widehat{b}_3 = -0.0592(0.0654)$, $\widehat{b}_4 = -0.0278(0.0174)$, and the resulting linear spline function (set to be 0 for bilirubin= 7.66) is shown (as the dashed line) in Figure 4.2.5. For bilirubin values above 10.3 the curve is concave. The likelihood ratio test for linearity is 39.13 which, evaluated in the $\chi^2(4)$-distribution gives $P<0.001$.

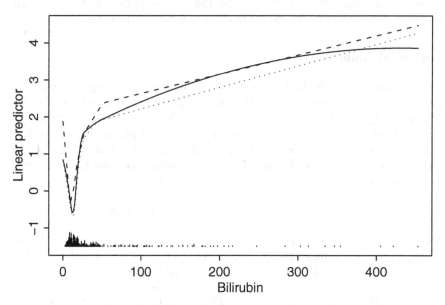

Fig. 4.2.5. Estimated linear predictor for the PBC3 study assuming an effect of serum bilirubin modeled as a linear spline (dashed), an unrestricted quadratic spline (solid), or a quadratic spline restricted to be linear for bilirubin values above 51.4 (dotted). The distribution of bilirubin is shown on the horizontal axis.

Although the linear predictor for model (4.2.5), as mentioned, is continuous and, therefore, more plausible than a model with jumps at the interval end points it is still not a smooth function of x: it has a break at each r_j. A smooth regression spline curve may be obtained using "splines of higher order," for example, quadratic or cubic splines. Such a model may also be seen as an extension of *polynomial* models discussed in the next section but we prefer to discuss these models now as they do rely on a choice of intervals .

For simplicity, attention is restricted to a model with quadratic regression splines. This model is easily defined based on the explanatory variables introduced in (4.2.4) by having the linear predictor

$$\mathrm{LP}_i = a + b_1 x_i + b_2 x_i^2 + b_{1,1}(x_{i1}^+)^2 + \cdots + b_{1,k}(x_{ik}^+)^2. \tag{4.2.6}$$

It can be shown that this is a smooth function of x_i (even at the interval endpoints $r_1, \ldots, r_k$) and furthermore (4.2.6) contains both the linear model $a + b_1 x_i$ and the quadratic model $a + b_1 x_i + b_2 x_i^2$ (discussed in the next section) as special cases (corresponding to $b_2 = b_{1,1} = \cdots = b_{1,k} = 0$ and $b_{1,1} = \cdots = b_{1,k} = 0$, respectively).

For the PBC3 example the resulting quadratic spline is also shown in Figure 4.2.5 (as a solid line). This curve corresponds to the lower-right panel in the earlier Figure 4.2.1. In this model, the likelihood ratio test statistic for linearity is 40.97 on five degrees-of-freedom, again highly significant.

Restricted splines

As further discussed in the next section, the model (4.2.6) may give extreme values of the linear predictor for the last interval ($x > r_k$) and also for the first interval if the range of x is unrestricted. A slightly modified model is, therefore, frequently considered, in which the linear predictor is assumed to be linear in x for large or for small values of x (or both). Restricting LP_i to be linear for small values of x is obtained by deleting the term $b_2 x_i^2$ from the model; that is,

$$\mathrm{LP}_i = a + b_1 x_i + b_{1,1}(x_{i1}^+)^2 + \cdots + b_{1,k}(x_{ik}^+)^2.$$

A model restricted to be linear in x for large values is obtained by deleting $b_{1,k}(x_{ik}^+)^2$ and replacing x_i^2 by $x_i^2 - (x_{ik}^+)^2$ and $(x_{ij}^+)^2$ in (4.2.6) by $(x_{ij}^+)^2 - (x_{ik}^+)^2$ for $j = 1, \ldots, k - 1$. Thereby, the linear predictor becomes

$$\mathrm{LP}_i = a + b_1 x_i + b_2 \left(x_i^2 - (x_{ik}^+)^2 \right) + b_{1,1} \left((x_{i1}^+)^2 - (x_{ik}^+)^2 \right)$$
$$+ \cdots + b_{1,k-1} \left((x_{ik-1}^+)^2 - (x_{ik}^+)^2 \right).$$

To obtain linearity for both small and large values of x we do both to obtain the linear predictor

$$\mathrm{LP}_i = a + b_1 x_i + b_{1,1} \left((x_{i1}^+)^2 - (x_{ik}^+)^2 \right) + \cdots + b_{1,k-1} \left((x_{ik-1}^+)^2 - (x_{ik}^+)^2 \right).$$

For the PBC3 example the quadratic spline restricted to be linear only for large values of bilirubin (above 51.4) is also shown in Figure 4.2.5 (as a dotted line) not changing the shape of the curve dramatically.

The cubic model is dealt with analogously and the two models are likely to provide quite similar results, particularly if the linear restrictions for both small and large x are imposed. Although these models have the advantage of providing a linear predictor that is a smooth function of x, a drawback is that the coefficients in (4.2.6) no longer have simple interpretations. Rather, it is the shape of the whole function LP_i which is of interest and therefore such models are most suited for descriptive purposes.

4.2.2 Polynomials

This section deals with models where the linear predictor, as was the case for the higher-order spline models in the previous section, is a smooth function of x. The models we study all contain the simple linear model as a special case and they are not based on any selection of intervals covering the range of x. More specifically, we consider models where the linear predictor is a *polynomial* in x.

One of the simplest mathematical extensions of the linear model $LP_i = a + bx_i$ is the *quadratic* model

$$LP_i = a + b_1 x_i + b_2 x_i^2, \tag{4.2.7}$$

where the linear predictor is a second-order polynomial ("a parabola"). This model provides a simple alternative to the linear model and testing the hypothesis $b_2 = 0$ gives a test for linearity. Because of its simplicity the model (4.2.7) has been much used, although it certainly has a number of disadvantages. Thus, the coefficients b_1, b_2 have no simple interpretation and numerically large values of x may have a large influence of the estimates. Note that when $b_2 > 0$, (4.2.7) is a convex function (a "happy parabola") with minimum at $x = -\frac{b_1}{2b_2}$ whereas the situation $b_2 < 0$ corresponds to a concave function (a "bad-tempered parabola") with maximum at $x = -b_1/(2b_2)$. In both cases the curve is symmetric around $x = -b_1/(2b_2)$.

For the PBC3 example, with x representing (untransformed) bilirubin, the estimates in model (4.2.7) are $\widehat{b}_1 = 0.0227$ (0.0031), $\widehat{b}_2 = -0.0000369$ (0.00000871), and the likelihood ratio test statistic for linearity is 20.82 which evaluated in a $\chi^2(1)$-distribution gives $P < 0.0001$. The significantly negative sign of $\widehat{b}_2$ again signals a concave relationship between bilirubin and LP. The curve has a maximum point at bilirubin$= 0.0227/(2 \times 0.0000369) = 307.6$. The values of the regression coefficients would change if x were centered by subtracting a suitable reference value, whereas the model as such would not change.

Figure 4.2.6 shows Cook's distance based on $dev_i(b_1)$ and $dev_i(b_2)$ plotted against bilirubin and against time. The most influential points correspond to three censorings among patients with a large value of bilirubin (Cook's distance above 0.12). These are the same three observations that were seen to be mostly influential in Figure 4.1.24 where the covariate was log(bilirubin).

Fractional polynomials

Much more flexibility (however, with some of the same disadvantages as just mentioned for (4.2.7)) is obtained by introducing more powers q of x than just $q = 2$. In particular the use of the function class called *fractional polynomials* (e.g., Royston and Altman, 1994; Royston and Sauerbrei, 2008) provides flexible models. With fractional polynomials, powers of x are usually chosen

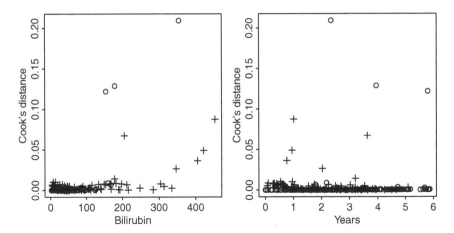

Fig. 4.2.6. Cook's distance for the model with a quadratic effect of bilirubin plotted against bilirubin and time: +: observed failure times, o: censored observations.

from the limited set $q = 0, \pm0.5, \pm1, \pm2, \pm3$ where $q = 0$ is taken to mean the natural logarithm $\log(x)$. Note that this power and $q = \pm0.5$ (i.e., $\sqrt{x}$ and $1/\sqrt{x}$) are only valid for positive x and, therefore, the method of fractional polynomials is most often used in this situation, inasmuch as then, the whole range of powers is available. For similar reasons, centering of covariates by subtracting a suitable reference value is usually not considered for the class of models based on fractional polynomials.

Models with fractional polynomials are purely descriptive with no simple parameter interpretation, thus one often simply seeks the best fitting model with a given number of terms. As becomes apparent in the next chapter on multiple regression (see also the discussion in Section 6.1.3), the method is most useful when the desire is to obtain an effective adjustment for a confounder variable when studying the effect on an exposure of primary interest. We exemplify fractional polynomials using the PBC3 example and fit models that extend the simple linear one corresponding to $q = 1$. Thus, we fit all eight 2-term models and all 28 3-term models including a linear term plus one or two more terms chosen from the set of eight additional powers mentioned above. The results in terms of likelihood ratio tests compared with the simple linear model are found in Table 4.2.1.

It is seen from Table 4.2.1 that, according to the one-degree-of-freedom test statistics, the "best fitting model" with one additional term (i.e., the one with the largest test statistic, marked in bold in the table) is the one including $\log(\text{bilirubin})$. This model has estimates -0.000723 (0.00222) for the linear term and 1.0661 (0.202) for the log term ($q_1 = 0$). Thus, in this model the linear effect is insignificant and the log term highly significant. The resulting linear predictor is shown in Figure 4.2.7 (as a dashed line) and is seen to be concave in the entire range considered. In a similar vein, the best fitting

Table 4.2.1. Likelihood ratio tests comparing fractional polynomial models for the effect of bilirubin in the PBC3 study to a model with a linear effect. First column: one additional term in the model; next columns two additional terms in the model.

		q_2						
q_1	—	–3	–2	–1	–0.5	0	0.5	2
–3	4.29							
–2	12.10	19.10						
–1	25.51	29.32	32.38					
–0.5	30.69	32.75	**34.12**	34.09				
0	**32.32**	33.10	33.24	32.57	32.35			
0.5	30.56	30.68	30.57	31.08	31.77	32.42		
2	20.82	21.47	23.65	28.69	31.17	32.50	32.44	
3	16.59	17.88	21.19	28.00	31.06	32.46	32.00	26.59

model with two additional terms corresponds to $q_1 = -0.5, q_2 = -2$ (also marked with bold in the table). In this model the linear term is insignificant with an estimated coefficient of 0.00242 (0.00165) whereas both the term for the power –0.5 and that for –2 are significant. The estimated coefficients are 40.301 (13.889) and –12.575 (2.372), respectively. The estimated linear predictor is also shown in Figure 4.2.7 (as a solid line) and it is seen that this estimate, like those based on the quintile division of bilirubin, has a minimum around a bilirubin value of 5 whereas for larger values it has a concave shape. The two models that are highlighted in Table 4.2.1 are not nested so they cannot be compared using, for example, the likelihood ratio test statistic. However, they are both nested in the model with the four terms corresponding to $q \in \{0, 1, -0.5, -2\}$ and the likelihood ratio tests for the reduction from this model to $q \in \{0, 1\}$ or $q \in \{1, -0.5, -2\}$ are 1.81 (2 d.f., $P = 0.40$) and 0.01 (1 d.f., $P = 0.92$), respectively. Hence, both models are clearly acceptable compared to the extended 4-term model, however, based on P-values the model corresponding to $q \in \{1, -0.5, -2\}$ may be preferable.

4.2.3 Other nonlinear models with a linear predictor

In this section we leave the general theme of studying alternatives to models with a simple linear effect of a quantitative explanatory variable. We study two special situations where the effect of a quantitative covariate x can be expected to have a particular nonlinear effect on the linear predictor: first when x has a particular value (or a certain interval) corresponding to "nonexposed individuals" and, second, when the effect of x may be periodic, that is, repeat itself in certain intervals, for example, calendar time periods.

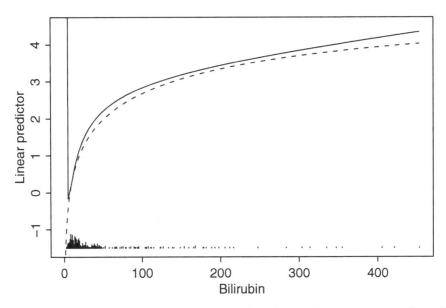

Fig. 4.2.7. Estimated linear predictor for the PBC study assuming an effect of serum bilirubin which is modeled either as a fractional polynomial with powers 1 and 0 (dashed) or with powers 1, –0.5, and –2 (solid). The distribution of bilirubin is shown on the horizontal axis.

Models with a zero exposure category

In this section, x is a quantitative explanatory variable and we study models for the effect of x on an outcome variable y where one particular value (or perhaps an interval) of x is considered special and therefore treated separately. For simplicity we assume that x is nonnegative although similar models may be considered for any quantitative x.

Motivation comes from epidemiological studies where x is an "exposure" and where, among the exposed, a dose–response relationship may be expected but where the nonexposed may fall outside this dose–response relationship. We again for the sake of simplicity, restrict attention to linear dose–response relationships although models with nonlinear effects of positive xs (cf. Sections 4.2.1–4.2.2) may also be of interest in some situations. Let $x = 0$ indicate no exposure and consider the dummy variable for being exposed: $I(x_i > 0)$. We then look at models where the linear predictor for individual i is given by

$$\text{LP}_i = a + b_1 x_i + b_0 I(x_i > 0). \tag{4.2.8}$$

In (4.2.8), a is the value of the linear predictor when $x = 0$, b_1 is the slope of the linear dose–response relationship for positive xs (i.e., the difference between values of LP for groups with positive exposure differing one unit in x), and b_0 is the difference between the LP-value for $x = 0$ and the extrapolation into

$x = 0$ of the line for the exposed. The test for the hypothesis $b_1 = 0$ is a *trend test among exposed, only* .

As an example of this kind we once more consider the PBC3 trial and the explanatory variable $x_i = $ bilirubin for patient i. Bilirubin has an upper limit for "normal" values at 17.1 μmol/L and a model where the linear effect of log(bilirubin) only applies above the normal range may be of interest. Using a model like (4.2.8) we can estimate how the hazard function for values of bilirubin in the normal range are compared to the assumed linear function for values outside that range. To do this we consider the indicator for the abnormal range; that is $I(x_i > 17.1)$. We then study a model such as (4.2.8) with x_i replaced by $(\log(x_i) - \log(17.1)) \cdot I(x_i > 17.1) = (\log(x_i) - \log(17.1))^+$ (and where, as usual, a is the log(baseline hazard), $\log(h_0(t))$, here the log(hazard) for bilirubin values in the normal range, including 17.1). The estimates in this model are $\widehat{b}_1 = 0.858(0.129)$ and $\widehat{b}_0 = 1.296(0.397)$ (Table 4.2.2). Thus, for values above the normal range the linear predictor increases highly significantly with log(bilirubin) (Wald test for the hypothesis $b_1 = 0$ is $(0.858/0.129)^2 = 43.9$). Furthermore, the step of the linear predictor from the normal range to values above (i.e., at log(17.1); see Figure 4.2.8) is $\widehat{b}_0 = 1.296(0.397)$ and yields a significant Wald test statistic $(1.296/0.397)^2 = 10.65$.

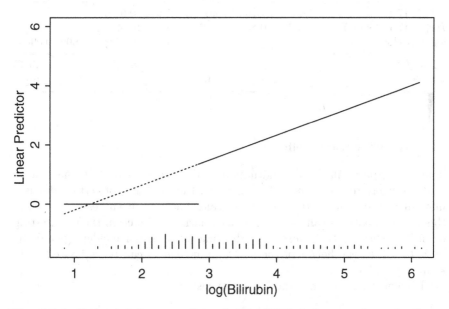

Fig. 4.2.8. Estimated linear predictor for the PBC study assuming a log-linear effect of serum bilirubin for values outside the normal range (>17.1 μmol/L) and constant within the normal range. The distribution of log(bilirubin) is shown on the horizontal axis.

Because the model (4.2.8) is not nested in the simple model with a linear effect of log(bilirubin), these two models cannot be formally compared using, for example, the likelihood ratio test statistic. However, both models can be nested in the three-parameter model allowing for a linear effect of $\log(x_i)$ also within the normal range but with a different slope than outside the normal range. This extended model may be obtained by adding the covariate $\log(x_i)$ (or preferably, $\log(x_i) - \log(17.1)$ to keep a reasonable interpretation of the baseline hazard as the hazard function, now as that for patients with a bilirubin value of 17.1) to (4.2.8). Note that the effect of $\log(x_i) - \log(17.1)$ determines the slope of the linear predictor within the normal range. The results from such an analysis are also shown in Table 4.2.2. Here it is seen that the extended model may be reduced to (4.2.8) (LR-test statistic is 1.66 with 1 d.f., $P = 0.20$) but not to the simple model containing only $\log(x_i)$ (LR-test statistic is 10.58 with 2 d.f., $P = 0.005$). We may thus conclude that the simple model including log(bilirubin) may be improved by considering different effects of bilirubin inside and outside the normal range.

Table 4.2.2. PBC3 study: analysis of the effect of bilirubin x_i within and outside the normal range ($<17.1 \ \mu$mol/L).

Covariate	Model (4.2.8)	Extended Model	Reduced Model
$I(x_i \geq 17.1)$	1.296 (0.397)	1.964 (0.699)	
$I(x_i \geq 17.1)(\log(x_i) - \log(17.1))$	0.858 (0.129)	1.930 (0.821)	
$\log(x_i) - \log(17.1)$		-1.073 (0.811)	1.009 (0.0985)
$-2\log(L)$	836.43	834.77	845.35
LR-test	1.66		10.58

Models with periodic effects

Sometimes, particularly in longitudinal studies, there may be (time) effects that are likely to be *periodic*. For example, the incidence of certain diseases may show the same pattern over the calendar year in successive years. If this periodic pattern can be modeled as a harmonic function then interesting quantities such as the *phase* (i.e., the time of maximal incidence) and the *amplitude* (i.e., the height of the maximal incidence) can be estimated quite simply, as follows.

The generic harmonic function is the cosine

$$\cos(x).$$

This function has a period of 2π and takes its maximal value at $x = 0$. Therefore, if x is in months and a yearly period (i.e., 12 months) is expected then the scaled cosine function

$$\cos(\frac{2\pi}{12}x)$$

may be used. This function still has maximum for $x = 0$ and to allow for an unknown phase f the translated cosine function

$$\cos(\frac{2\pi}{12}(x - f))$$

with maximum at $x = f$ is the choice. Finally, allowing for an unknown amplitude A a term like

$$A\cos(\frac{2\pi}{12}(x - f)) \tag{4.2.9}$$

can be added to the intercept a in the linear predictor. The trick is now to apply the formula for the cosine of a difference to get

$$A\cos(\frac{2\pi}{12}(x - f)) = A\cos(\frac{2\pi f}{12})\cos(\frac{2\pi x}{12}) + A\sin(\frac{2\pi f}{12})\sin(\frac{2\pi x}{12}). \tag{4.2.10}$$

Because x is the observed month of the year both $\cos(2\pi x/12)$ and $\sin(2\pi x/12)$ are observable explanatory variables and the corresponding regression coefficients $b_1 = A\cos(2\pi f/12)$ and $b_2 = A\sin(2\pi f/12)$ may be estimated because the linear predictor is linear in these two parameters. Because $\cos^2(t) + \sin^2(t) = 1$, we can then estimate the amplitude A by

$$\widehat{A} = \sqrt{\widehat{b}_1^2 + \widehat{b}_2^2}$$

and the phase f (because $\tan(t) = \sin(t)/\cos(t)$) can be estimated by

$$\widehat{f} = \frac{12}{2\pi}\tan^{-1}(\widehat{b}_2/\widehat{b}_1).$$

Digression. Standard deviations

Inference for b_1, b_2 also yields estimated standard deviations for $\widehat{b}_1$ and $\widehat{b}_2$ and an estimated correlation between $\widehat{b}_1$ and $\widehat{b}_2$. From these quantities standard deviations for $\widehat{A}$ and $\widehat{f}$ may be obtained using the "delta-method." This yields the following expressions:

$$(SD(\widehat{A}))^2 = \frac{\widehat{b}_1^2(SD(\widehat{b}_1))^2 + \widehat{b}_2^2(SD(\widehat{b}_2))^2 + 2\widehat{b}_1\widehat{b}_2 SD(\widehat{b}_1)SD(\widehat{b}_2)corr(\widehat{b}_1, \widehat{b}_2)}{\widehat{b}_1^2 + \widehat{b}_2^2}$$

and

$$(SD(\widehat{f}))^2 = \left(\frac{12}{2\pi}\right)^2 \frac{\widehat{b}_1^2(SD(\widehat{b}_1))^2 + \widehat{b}_2^2(SD(\widehat{b}_2))^2 - 2\widehat{b}_1\widehat{b}_2 SD(\widehat{b}_1)SD(\widehat{b}_2)corr(\widehat{b}_1, \widehat{b}_2)}{\widehat{b}_1^2 + \widehat{b}_2^2}.$$

◇

4.3 Exercises

Exercise 4.1. Use the tryptase dataset 3 from Example 1.12 for the following:

1. Perform an analysis relating baseline tryptase values to a linear predictor $LP_i = a + b \times$ age. Perform model checks to see whether age and/or baseline tryptase should be transformed in order to better meet the traditional assumptions of a simple linear regression.
2. Try a model where the effect of age is modeled by a linear spline with thresholds at the age of 60. Show that there is a significant change of slope at 60 years and describe the conclusion.
3. Do we see a change of slope already at the age of 40?

Exercise 4.2. Use the tryptase dataset 2 from Example 1.12 to investigate the relationship between baseline tryptase value and tryptase value in the allergic situation.

1. Make a scatterplot and comment on a reasonable model for describing reaction tryptase as a function of baseline tryptase.
2. Estimate the parameters in a linear relation between logarithmic values of reaction tryptase and logarithmic values of baseline tryptase. Transform back to original scale to get a power relation between the two. Does it fit well?

Exercise 4.3. Use the tryptase dataset 2 from Example 1.12 and look at the patients that have been subjected to a test for allergy following the surgery (tested = 1).

1. Relate the probability of a positive test result to the value of the reaction tryptase, using a logit link and a linear effect of tryptase value.
2. Show that the Wald test statistic for this relationship is 25.46 and state the conclusion.
3. Show that the odds ratio for a positive test is 2.66 for an increase of 10 units in reaction tryptase, and find the associated confidence interval for this quantity.
4. Do we see any signs of deviation from linearity in reaction tryptase? Try, for example, including a squared term in reaction tryptase.
5. Perform a model check by making a residual plot of Pearson residuals against reaction tryptase.

Exercise 4.4. Use the tryptase dataset 1 from Example 1.12 to compare the tryptase value before and after surgery.

1. Estimate a linear relationship between the tryptase value before (x) and after (y) surgery.
2. Compare with the line obtained by switching the roles of the outcome and the covariate.
3. Comment upon the fact that these two lines are not identical.

Exercise 4.5. The tryptase dataset 2 from Example 1.12 contains information on the type of allergic reaction, classified into four groups. Collapse these into a binary outcome by combining categories 1–2 and 3–4.

1. Perform a logistic regression relating the probability of a severe reaction to age.
2. Investigate whether the effect of age is linear by including a quadratic term and testing its significance.

Exercise 4.6. Use the tryptase dataset 2 from Example 1.12 for relating tryptase values during the allergic reaction (reaction tryptase values) to age.

1. Try the linear predictor $LP_i = a + b \times$ age as well as a linear spline with threshold in 60 years.
2. Show that at 60 years, the line bends in an upward direction, with an estimated change of slope of 0.16.
3. Is this change significant, or could we just as well use the simpler model with a linear effect of age?

Exercise 4.7. Baseline tryptase is considered "elevated" if it is above 11.4. Use the tryptase dataset 2 from Example 1.12 for investigating whether the probability of this event (during the suspected allergic reaction) depends on the age of the patient.

1. Calculate the confidence interval for the odds ratio for the occurrence, for a ten-year increase in age. Show that the confidence interval for this odds ratio is (1.2,1.7). Formulate an appropriate conclusion.
2. Make a residual plot (Pearson residuals) to investigate the appropriateness of the linearity in age.
3. Try including a quadratic term in age and test whether it improves the model significantly.

Exercise 4.8. Use the vitamin D dataset to investigate whether body mass index for girls is an important explanatory variable for vitamin D level.

1. Make a simple linear regression without transforming either of the two variables and perform model checks to investigate the appropriateness of this model.
2. Make a logarithmic transformation of the vitamin D concentration and perform the regression again. Compare with the above results and comment on which analysis to prefer.

Exercise 4.9. Use the surgery data from Example 1.4 to investigate whether age is an important predictor for the duration of anesthesia.

1. Estimate in the model relating mean duration to age through a linear predictor with age as a linear effect.
2. Perform model checks to investigate the appropriateness of the assumed linearity in age, graphically as well as numerically.

3. What could be a possible explanation for a poor model fit? See Exercise 5.6 from Chapter 5.

Exercise 4.10. Use data from the PBC-3 Example 1.3 to investigate the importance of aspartate transaminase for the survival after treatment of liver cirrhosis.

1. Estimate the hazard ratio corresponding to a doubling of aspartate transaminase, with 95% confidence limits.
2. Perform a model check for the linearity assumption corresponding to the chosen scale of aspartate transaminase, by categorization of the covariate into quintile groups.

Exercise 4.11. Use data from the PBC-3 Example 1.3 to investigate the effect of age on the survival after treatment of liver cirrhosis.

1. Choose a spline function with thresholds 50 and 60 years and investigate whether these thresholds give rise to significant changes in the effect of age on the logarithmic hazard rate.
2. Make a plot describing the estimated effect of age.

Exercise 4.12. Use the data from the study of malignant melanoma, Example 1.10, to study the effect of tumor thickness on the survival.

1. Categorize the tumor thickness into four categories of approximately the same size (quartiles), and compare the survival curves in these four groups. Do we see a trend?
2. Use the tumor thickness as a quantitative covariate with a linear effect on the log hazard rate. Is survival significantly related to tumor thickness in this model?
3. Perform a model check for the effect of tumor thickness.

Exercise 4.13. Use the data from the study of malignant melanoma, Example 1.10, to study the effect of age on the survival.

1. Choose a spline function with a single threshold at 60 years to investigate whether age has a linear effect on the logarithmic hazard rate.
2. Could the effect of age be due to other possible covariates, such as tumor thickness, as studied in Exercise 4.12? (See also Exercise 5.8 in Chapter 5.)

5

Multiple regression, the linear predictor

In the previous two chapters we studied regression models where the linear predictor depended on a single explanatory variable, x. In Chapter 3, x was categorical and for a *binary* variable (Section 3.1) with values g_0, g_1 we added

$$bI(x_i = g_1)$$

to the intercept a, whereas in general, for a variable with $k+1$ levels (Section 3.2) we added instead the expression

$$b_1I(x_i = g_1) + b_2I(x_i = g_2) + \cdots + b_kI(x_i = g_k),$$

with dummy variables for all categories except the reference category ($x_i = 0$). In Chapter 4, x was *quantitative* and we added a term (Section 4.1)

$$bx_i$$

to a if a *linear* effect was to be obtained or we could model nonlinear effects (Section 4.2) by adding instead terms of the form

$$b_1f_1(x_i) + b_2f_2(x_i) + \cdots + b_rf_r(x_i),$$

where $f_1(x), f_2(x), \ldots, f_r(x)$ are given functions of x (e.g., polynomials or dummy variables).

In some studies only one explanatory variable needs to be considered. Typical examples are randomized experiments with two or more treatment groups, such as a number of dose groups. In such situations relevant models for quantitative, binary, or survival time outcomes have been discussed in Chapters 3 and 4. However, more often several explanatory variables are required. In some experiments, subjects may be randomized to combinations of different treatments, or practical considerations may force researchers to randomize within a number of *blocks*, for example, hospitals, which need to be taken into account when analyzing effects of treatments. Furthermore (and this is in fact our main motivation), in observational studies conducted in, for example, epidemiology, some risk factors associated with the explanatory variable of primary interest (the exposure) must be considered in order to achieve a "fair comparison" between exposure groups. This may, in fact, also be relevant in randomized studies where, in spite of the randomization, important factors may not be quite balanced between the treatment groups.

In this chapter *multiple regression models* (i.e., regression models with several explanatory variables) are studied. We do this by adding the simple building blocks from the previous chapters to the model intercept. The *linear predictor* obtained in this way is then *linked* to the mean value, the failure probability, or to the hazard rate. That is, we focus on the linear predictor in general and exemplify using concrete types of outcome y.

Studying two or more explanatory variables in the same model has two important consequences. First of all, the interpretation of a regression parameter b_j is now the "effect" of the corresponding covariate "adjusted for" other covariates or "for any given values of" other covariates. This means that the effect of a particular explanatory variable describes the expected difference in outcome for groups of subjects differing one unit in this particular explanatory variable, when all other covariates are "held fixed." Note that (unless the link function is the identity function and covariates are independent) this interpretation is different from the *marginal interpretation* and an estimate of the effect of an explanatory variable should, therefore, always be accompanied by a list of the remaining explanatory variables in the model. For example, in an analysis of weight as outcome variable and gender as explanatory variable the effect of gender will depend strongly on whether adjustment for height is carried out. The phenomenon that adjusted and unadjusted effects may differ is the concept of *confounding*: if we want to study the effect of an explanatory variable x_1 on an outcome variable y and if x_1 is unevenly distributed in subgroups of another important covariate x_2, then the unadjusted effect of x_1 is confounded by x_2.

Second, the consequence of simply adding terms for the covariates to be included in the model is that the effect of each variable is assumed to be the same for all values of the other covariates: the assumption of *no interaction* between the covariates. This is a critical assumption which often requires careful examination as part of the statistical analysis and, obviously, more general regression models allowing for interaction are needed. Presence of interaction complicates the analysis and, for that reason, an attempt to eliminate interaction parameters from the model is often done. It should be noted, however, that interaction is not always just a nuisance for the researcher. In many cases it may be of considerable interest to study whether the effect of an explanatory variable differs, for example, between men and women, in which case the examination of a possible interaction is an important part of the scientific questions addressed. An alternative name for interaction, frequently used in epidemiology is "effect-modification". However, we have chosen to stick to the classical statistical phrase, "interaction."

Interaction and confounding have nothing in common as the following hypothetical example illustrates; see Figure 5.0.1. Here, the quantitative co-variate x_1 and the categorical variable x_2 are highly (positively) correlated. There is a negative x_1-effect *marginally* (see the dashed line in the figure); there is a marginal effect of x_2 (see the averages of y in x_2-groups indicated on the vertical axis). Adjusting for x_2 there is a positive effect of x_1 (see the four parallel solid lines corresponding to the four values of x_2) and a some-what increased effect of x_2 (vertical distance between the parallel lines, not shown in the figure). However, there is no interaction: for any given x_2-group the effect (slope) for x_1 is the same.

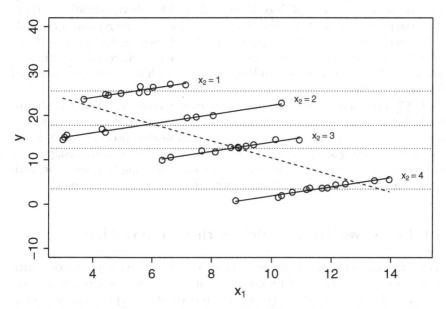

Fig. 5.0.1. Illustration of a confounding categorical variable x_2 when the effect of a quantitative variable x_1 on y is studied; see text.

Recall that, in spite of our use of the term "effect", we do not necessarily assume explanatory variables and outcome to be causally related.

The structure of this chapter is as follows. In Sections 5.1 and 5.2 we study models with only two explanatory variables: in Section 5.1 models without in-teraction and in Section 5.2 models with interaction. We consider the different combinations of covariate types: two categorical covariates in Section 5.1.1, one categorical and one quantitative with a linear or a nonlinear effect in Section 5.1.2, and two quantitative covariates (with linear or nonlinear ef-fects) in Section 5.1.3. In each section the model is exemplified using outcome variables of different types, with emphasis on parameter interpretation and signs of possible confounding. In Section 5.2 we return to all the examples from Section 5.1 and supplement with examination and discussion of interaction. For each combination of types of explanatory variables different ways of *parametrizing* the model are possible and may play various roles for *testing* the hypothesis of no interaction or for *presenting* the results from a model with interaction. Again, focus is on interpreting models and results. The reason why we concentrate on situations with only two covariates in Sections 5.1 and 5.2 is that this is, one the one hand, the simplest extension of the simple regression models considered in Chapters 3 and 4 and, at the same time, it still illustrates most of the new problems encountered in multiple regression models. Therefore, in Section 5.3 where we discuss general models including any number of explanatory variables, we emphasize that such models in many aspects are not more complicated than models with only two covariates. However, the problem of *higher-order interactions* does become relevant in models with several covariates. The chapter is concluded (Section 5.4) by a brief discussion of the situation where responses are paired or matched and where it is crucial, during the analysis, to keep track of which observations come from the same matched group.

In Chapters 3 and 4 we have been quite careful checking all model assumptions, however, in the present chapter less emphasis is put on that aspect of inference. This is of course not because we find model checking unimportant but only to save space and to concentrate on what is new in this chapter. In the discussion in Chapter 6 we return to model checking in connection with general model building procedures as well as in the worked examples.

5.1 Two covariates: Models without interaction

As mentioned in the introduction to this chapter, we first study models with only two explanatory variables and without interaction. In separate subsections we consider the different combinations of covariate types: two categorical covariates in Section 5.1.1, one categorical and one quantitative with a linear or nonlinear effect in Section 5.1.2, and two quantitative covariates (with linear or nonlinear effects) in Section 5.1.3. We concentrate on the situation with two covariates to keep the discussion as simple as possible while at the same time illustrating the consequences of adjusting the effect of one explanatory for that of another.

5.1.1 Two categorical covariates

This section deals with a regression model with two explanatory variables, both of which are categorical. As our primary example we return to the study of vitamin D status for women from different European countries (cf. Example 1.1), that is, the outcome variable is *quantitative*. Following the discussion in Section 3.1.1 we use the log-transformed values and define $y_i = \log_{10}(25\text{OHD}$ measurement for woman no. i). The main question addressed is how body mass index, denoted by $x_{i,1}$, dichotomized into overweight versus normal weight, is related to vitamin D status and it is of interest to see if this relation is stable over countries, denoted by $x_{i,2}$.

Two binary covariates

We first include only women from Ireland and Poland and study the two binary explanatory variables:

$$I(x_{i,1} \geq 25) \quad \text{and} \quad I(x_{i,2} = \text{Ireland}).$$

The model specifies the mean $E(y_i)$ of y_i to be

$$E(y_i) = LP_i = a + b_1 I(x_{i,1} \geq 25) + b_2 I(x_{i,2} = \text{Ireland}). \tag{5.1.1}$$

Note that the linear predictor in (5.1.1) is obtained by adding the terms, $b_1 I(x_{i,1} \geq 25)$ and $b_2 I(x_{i,2} = \text{Ireland})$ to the model intercept, a. Thereby the expected values, given in tabular form in Table 5.1.1 are obtained.

Table 5.1.1. Expected values in four groups according to model (5.1.1).

	Normal Weight	Overweight
Poland	a	$a + b_1$
Ireland	$a + b_2$	$a + b_1 + b_2$

These satisfy that:

1. The effect of body mass index for women from Ireland is the same as that for women from Poland. (The former is $(a + b_1 + b_2) - (a + b_2) = b_1$ and the latter is $(a + b_1) - a = b_1$.)
2. The difference between countries for overweight women is the same as that for normal weight women. (The former is $(a + b_1 + b_2) - (a + b_1) = b_2$ and the latter is $(a + b_2) - a = b_2$.)

We see that the interpretation of the regression coefficient b_1 for body mass index x_1 in the model which also includes country x_2 is an effect of body mass index for separate values of country and this effect is assumed to be the same for all values of x_2, that is, both for Ireland and for Poland. In a similar vein, the interpretation of the regression coefficient b_2 for country x_2 in the model that also includes body mass index x_1, is the effect of country, that is, the difference between countries, for separate values of body mass index and, again, this effect is assumed to be the same for all values of x_1, that is, for normal weight and for overweight women. We say that the effects of body mass index and country are *mutually adjusted* and that the model assumes there is *no interaction* between body mass index and country .

Table 5.1.2 shows the number of women and the average $\log_{10}(25\text{OHD}$ values) in each of the four country by BMI groups and Figure 5.1.1 shows these numbers graphically.

Table 5.1.2. Average $\log_{10}(25\text{OHD}$ values) (and numbers of women) in four country by BMI groups.

	Normal Weight	Overweight	Difference
Poland	1.598 (12)	1.443 (53)	−0.155
Ireland	1.720 (16)	1.593 (25)	−0.127
Difference	0.121 (28)	0.150 (78)	0.028

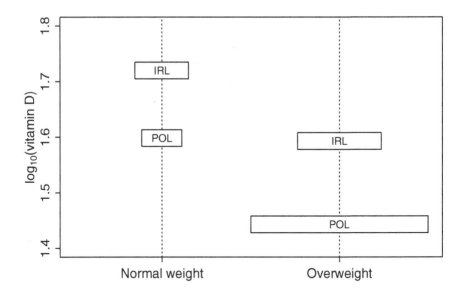

Fig. 5.1.1. Average $log_{10}(25\text{OHD}$ values) in four country by BMI groups. The size of a bar reflects the sample size.

Fitting the additive model (5.1.1) to the data we find the estimates: $\hat{a} = 1.587(0.043)$, $\hat{b}_1 = -0.141(0.044)$, and $\hat{b}_2 = 0.142(0.039)$. The interpretation of these estimates is that $\hat{a}$ is the expected $\log_{10}(25\text{OHD})$ value in the *combined* reference group for both covariates, that is, for Polish women with normal BMI. Furthermore, $\widehat{b}_1$ is the (assumed common) effect of BMI for both Polish and Irish women. It is an average of the two differences between averages for overweight and normal weight: $1.443 - 1.598 = -0.155$ in Poland and $1.593 - 1.720 = -0.127$ in Ireland (cf. Table 5.1.2 and Figure 5.1.1) *weighted according to group size*. Finally, $\widehat{b}_2$ is the (assumed common) effect of country for both normal weight and overweight women, and it is an average of the differences between averages for Ireland and Poland: $1.720 - 1.598 = 0.121$ among normal weight women and $1.593 - 1.443 = 0.150$ among overweight women, again weighted according to group size.

Table 5.1.3 shows the estimated expected $\log_{10}(25OHD)$ values according to the additive model. Note that, because by coincidence $\widehat{b}_1 + \widehat{b}_2 \approx 0$, two of these values are almost identical.

Table 5.1.3. Expected values in four groups after fitting model (5.1.1).

	Normal Weight	Overweight
Poland	1.587	1.446
Ireland	1.729	1.588

We say that the estimates $\widehat{b}_1$ and $\widehat{b}_2$ are *mutually adjusted* or that $\widehat{b}_1$ is the effect of BMI for *given values* of the other explanatory variables in the model, here for given country (and vice versa for $\widehat{b}_2$). We can compare these values with the *unadjusted* estimates for BMI and country. These are $-0.177(0.045)$ for BMI (overweight versus normal weight) and $0.171(0.040)$ for country (Ireland versus Poland). The difference between the adjusted and unadjusted estimates is due to *confounding*. The unadjusted effect of BMI does not provide a fair comparison between overweight and normal weight women because of the influence of country: the group of overweight women is dominated by the women from Poland (Polish women constitute $53/(53+25) = 68\%$ of the overweight women and only $12/(12+16) = 43\%$ of the normal weight women) and the Polish women tend to have lower y-values than the Irish. Therefore the adjusted BMI estimate is smaller than the unadjusted. We can interpret the difference between the estimated effects of country similarly, however, these are not great. From the standard deviations we can see that both covariates have highly significant effects on the outcome even after mutual adjustment: the Wald test for no effect of BMI is $(-0.141/0.044)^2 = 10.46$ and for country it is $(0.141/0.039)^2 = 12.88$ both providing small P-values when evaluated in the $F(1, 75)$ (or $\chi^2(1)$)-distribution. Alternatively, the square root of the statistic may be evaluated in the $t(75)$ (or the standard Normal) distribution.

The estimates presented all relate to the scale of $\log_{10}(25OHD)$. As discussed in Section 3.1.1, a simpler interpretation in terms of ratios of medians in the original (25OHD) scale is available if the distribution of the log-transformed values is roughly symmetric. These are simply

$$10^{\widehat{b_1}} = 0.72,\ 10^{\widehat{b_2}} = 1.39$$

with the interpretation that for given country, median 25OHD-values among overweight women are about 72% of those for normal weight women. Similarly, for a given BMI group. Irish women have median 25OHD values about 39% larger than Polish women. Confidence intervals with 95% coverage for such a transformed parameter are simply from

$$10^{\widehat{b}-1.96 \cdot \text{SD}} \quad \text{to} \quad 10^{\widehat{b}+1.96 \cdot \text{SD}}$$

and for the effect of BMI we get the interval (0.59,0.88). That is, the median 25OHD values for overweight women is between 59% and 88% of that for normal weight women. For country we get the interval (1.16,1.65) meaning that Irish women have median 25OHD values between 16 and 65% larger than Polish women. When calculating the confidence interval one could, alternatively, have replaced the Normal quantile 1.96 by the corresponding $t(75)$-quantile 1.99, or one could simply take the estimate plus or minus "about 2" standard deviations.

Interaction

Turning to the assumption of no interaction we can give an initial evaluation of this by calculating differences in rows and columns as we did above. These represent BMI effects for each country separately and country effects for each BMI group separately, respectively. The fact that these are not very different (row differences are: −0.155 for Poland and −0.127 for Ireland, column differences are 0.121 for normal weight women and 0.150 for overweight women) suggests that the *additive* model (5.1.1) provides a satisfactory fit to the data (cf. Table 5.1.2 and Figure 5.1.1). We return to a more careful evaluation of interaction in Section 5.2.

Two-way ANOVA

The model (5.1.1) with two categorical explanatory variables and a quantitative outcome, y, is known as the 2-way analysis of variance (ANOVA) model. This model is usually discussed for planned experiments with balanced data, for example, when the numbers of observations in all cells of a table like Table 5.1.2 are the same. In this case, estimators in the model can be presented as simple explicit expressions. However, we consider the model in generality as a special case of a regression model without paying specific attention to balanced data.

Normal distribution and variance homogeneity

The model only specifies how the *mean response* depends on the two categorical covariates, so for the model to make sense the mean value parameter should be a useful characteristic of the distribution. This is definitely the case if y_i follows a *Normal* distribution, but as discussed in, for example, Section 3.1.1, the model may be relevant without the assumption of normality . However, *variance homogeneity* should be reasonably fulfilled, an assumption that may be evaluated graphically using, for example, residual plots as exemplified in Chapters 3 and 4. In the present situation with relatively few (four) groups, variance homogeneity may also be checked simply by computing the empirical standard deviations in each group and applying formal test statistics such as Levene's test.

Figure 5.1.2 shows the residuals from the additive model plotted against the fitted values in the four groups and this figure does not speak strongly against variance homogeneity. (Note that, according to Table 5.1.3, two of the fitted values are almost identical.) Variance homogeneity is supported by Levene's test for comparison of the standard deviations in the four groups giving the P-value 0.37 for homogeneity. The four SDs are shown in Table 5.1.4.

It can be noticed that without the log-transformation of the 25OHD values, variance homogeneity is rejected using Levene's test with a P-value of 0.027.

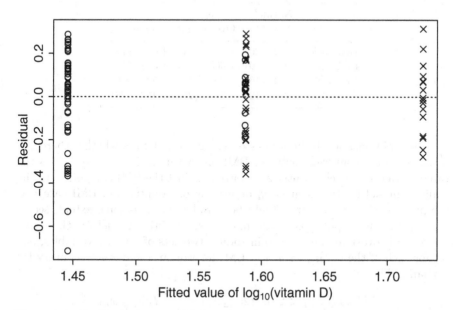

Fig. 5.1.2. Residuals from model (5.1.1) in four country by BMI groups plotted against fitted values: x: Ireland, o: Poland.

Table 5.1.4. SDs of $\log_{10}(25\text{OHD values})$ (and numbers of women) in four country by BMI groups.

	Normal Weight	Overweight
Poland	0.126 (12)	0.213 (53)
Ireland	0.164 (16)	0.192 (25)

General categorical covariates

To illustrate two-way analysis of variance with more than two levels of the two categorical explanatory variables we study a more complete version of the vitamin D dataset, that is, including women from all four countries (Denmark, Finland, Ireland, and Poland) and considering BMI in three categories: normal weight, slight overweight, and obese. Table 5.1.5 shows the average $\log_{10}(25\text{OHD})$ values and the numbers of women in these 12 categories. The general picture seems to be that, in all countries, normal weight women have higher values than those who are overweight or obese and that Polish women have lower values than what is seen in the other three countries.

Table 5.1.5. Average $\log_{10}(25\text{OHD})$ values (and numbers of women) in four countries and three BMI groups.

	Normal Weight	Slight Overweight	Obese
Denmark	1.692 (20)	1.545 (21)	1.603 (12)
Finland	1.664 (9)	1.665 (32)	1.562 (13)
Ireland	1.720 (16)	1.626 (16)	1.534 (9)
Poland	1.598 (12)	1.393 (25)	1.488 (28)

The main question to be addressed using these data is whether there is a relation, across countries, between BMI and vitamin D. In Figure 5.1.3 the three averages for each country are plotted against the BMI categories. In the additive model for the mean of y_i depending on country and BMI category, the profiles for each country should be parallel. This, to some extent, seems to be a tenable hypothesis. To formulate the additive model for these two categorical covariates we need to introduce two sets of dummy variables, one set for each of the covariates $x_{i,1} = $ BMI for woman i and $x_{i,2} = $ country for woman i. These are

$$I(18.5 \leq x_{i,1} < 25), I(25 \leq x_{i,1} < 30), I(30 \leq x_{i,1})$$

and

$$I(x_{i,2} = \text{Denmark}), I(x_{i,2} = \text{Finland}), I(x_{i,2} = \text{Ireland}), I(x_{i,2} = \text{Poland}),$$

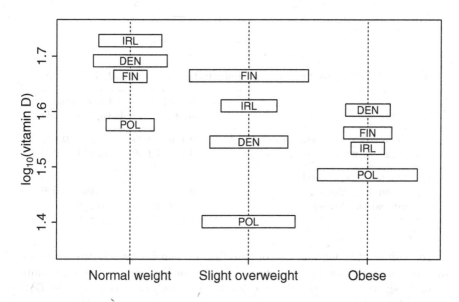

Fig. 5.1.3. Average OHD-values in four countries plotted against BMI group.

respectively. We then study the additive model

$$E(y_i) = a + b_{1,1}I(25 \le x_{i,1} < 30) + b_{1,2}I(30 \le x_{i,1}) \qquad (5.1.2)$$
$$+ b_{2,1}I(x_{i,2} = \text{Denmark}) + b_{2,2}I(x_{i,2} = \text{Finland}) + b_{2,3}I(x_{i,2} = \text{Ireland}).$$

Here the intercept a is the expected $\log_{10}(25\text{OHD})$ value for women in the combined reference category (normal weight women from Poland). Furthermore, $b_{1,1}$ is the difference in expected values between slight overweight and normal weight women *from the same country*, $b_{1,2}$ is the difference in expected values between obese and normal weight women *from the same country*, $b_{2,1}$ is the difference in expected values between women from Denmark and women from Poland *belonging to the same BMI category*, $b_{2,2}$ is the difference in expected values between women from Finland and women from Poland *belonging to the same BMI category*, and $b_{2,3}$ is the difference in expected values between women from Ireland and women from Poland *belonging to the same BMI category*.

The estimates from the model (5.1.2) are shown in Table 5.1.6 (left panel). We see that the expected $\log_{10}(25\text{OHD})$ values are largest for the normal weight women and that Poland seems to have values at a lower level than the other three countries. The likelihood ratio tests in this model are strongly significant for both explanatory variables: 11.67 which evaluated in the $\chi^2(2)$ distribution gives $P = 0.003$ for BMI and 21.78, $\sim \chi^2(3)$, $P < 0.0001$ for country. The corresponding F-statistics are 5.83 $\sim F(2, 207)$ for BMI and 7.43 $\sim F(3, 207)$ for country giving rise to similar P-values. The estimated intercept is $\hat{a} = 1.565(0.038)$.

Table 5.1.6. Adjusted and unadjusted effects of country and BMI group.

Parameter	Adjusted Estimate	SD	Unadjusted Estimate	SD
$b_{1,1}$: slight overweight vs. normal weight	−0.116	0.036	−0.116	0.037
$b_{1,2}$: obese vs. normal weight	−0.113	0.040	−0.143	0.040
$b_{2,1}$: Denmark vs. Poland	0.120	0.040	0.142	0.040
$b_{2,2}$: Finland vs. Poland	0.171	0.039	0.168	0.040
$b_{2,3}$: Ireland vs. Poland	0.147	0.043	0.171	0.043

To evaluate the amount of confounding we can study the estimates obtained by analyzing two models each with just one explanatory variable, country or BMI; see right part of Table 5.1.6. The unadjusted country and BMI effects tend to be numerically larger than those that are mutually adjusted, and so do the likelihood ratio tests for no effect of the covariates: 14.07 with 2 d.f., $P = 0.001$ for BMI and 24.18, 3 d.f., $P < 0.0001$ for country. The corresponding F-statistics are $7.17 \sim F(2, 210)$ for BMI and $8.38 \sim F(3, 209)$ for country. However, the confounding is not great because the distribution of BMI is fairly stable over countries. We return to a general discussion of confounding in Chapter 6.

Digression. Stratified "Mantel–Haenszel"-type analysis

For a binary outcome variable, a classical way of dealing with one binary "exposure" and one categorical "confounder" variable in epidemiology has been to conduct *stratified analysis* according to the "Mantel–Haenszel" approach. That is, to study the effect of the binary exposure $x_{i,1}$, adjusting for the confounder $x_{i,2}$, the association between the exposure and the binary outcome y_i is assessed, first by separate (2×2)-tables within strata defined by the values of the confounder and, next, results from the separate strata are summarized to obtain a single measure of the effect of the exposure on the outcome.

As an example we consider the fever in pregnancy study (Example 1.2). Recall that no association between fever in early pregnancy and fetal death was seen (OR= 0.996(0.620, 1.600)), however, this lack of association could be due to confounding by, for example, the women's alcohol consumption. Table 5.1.7 shows the basic two by two table of fever episodes versus fetal death together with the same data stratified by alcohol consumption. To avoid too "thin" strata, alcohol consumption has been divided into only three categories. It is seen that the odds ratios for the association between fever episodes and risk of fetal death do not vary systematically between the three alcohol strata (i.e., no interaction) and, furthermore, that the three separate odds ratios have wide confidence limits due to the rareness of the outcome, fetal death.

Table 5.1.7. Analysis of the effect of fever episodes on the odds of fetal death: marginally and stratified by alcohol assumption.

Drinks per Week	0		0.5–1		1.5+		Total	
Stratum	$s = 0$		$s = 1$		$s = 2$		All strata	
Fever episodes	No	Yes	No	Yes	No	Yes	No	Yes
No fetal deaths	5701	1253	2692	549	1201	262	9595	2064
Fetal deaths	56	12	29	5	13	4	98	21
Odds ratio	0.975		0.845		1.411		0.996	
95% CI	(0.521,1.824)		(0.326,2.194)		(0.456,4.360)		(0.620,1.600)	

Based on these observations, a common odds ratio across strata is not contra-indicated and the so-called "Mantel–Haenszel" estimator provides such an adjusted estimate which may be calculated by a simple, explicit expression:

$$\widehat{\text{OR}}_{\text{MH}} = \frac{\sum_s \frac{n_{as} n_{ds}}{n_s}}{\sum_s \frac{n_{bs} n_{cs}}{n_s}}. \tag{5.1.3}$$

In (5.1.3), $n_{as}, n_{bs}, n_{cs}, n_{ds}$, following the notation introduced in Section 3.1.2 are the cell counts in stratum $s = 0, 1, 2$ and n_s is the total count in that stratum. The estimator, a weighted average between the separate stratum-specific odds ratios, takes the value $\widehat{\text{OR}}_{\text{MH}} = 0.997$ not much different from the crude odds ratio without adjustment for alcohol consumption. An explicit significance test for no association between exposure and outcome adjusted for the potential confounder is also available, namely the "Mantel–Haenszel" test:

$$X^2_{\text{MH}} = \sum_s \frac{\left(n_{as} - \frac{(n_{as}+n_{bs})(n_{as}+n_{cs})}{n_s}\right)^2}{\frac{n_{as} n_{bs} n_{cs} n_{ds}}{n_s^2(n_s-1)}}.$$

The test statistic takes the value $X^2_{\text{MH}} = 0.0002$ which is highly nonsignificant when evaluated in the $\chi^2(1)$-distribution. Thus, there is absolutely no indication of an effect of fever episodes on the risk of fetal death even after adjustment for alcohol consumption, a fact which is further illustrated by the 95% confidence interval (0.621,1.601) for the commom odds ratio.

The Mantel–Haenszel technique is an old-fashioned method for assessment of the effect of a binary exposure on a binary outcome adjusting for a potential confounder which is categorical. It has the advantage that all computations are explicit (though this is of course of minor importance because computations are carried out using some computer package, anyway) but it also has the advantage that it "forces" the user to study the tabulated stratified data. This may be forgotten when the more obvious method, logistic regression, is used. However, our general recommendation is always to study tables such as those in Table 5.1.7 also when regression models are used. In the present example, results for the fever effect based on the relevant logistic model are very close to those reported above. This model is given by

$$\ell_i = a + b_1 I(x_{i,1} \geq 1) + b_{2,1} I(x_{i,2} = 0.5 \text{ or } x_{i,2} = 1) + b_{2,2} I(x_{i,2} \geq 1.5),$$

where ℓ_i is the log(odds) for fetal death for woman i and $x_{i,1}$ and $x_{i,2}$ are, respectively, her reported number of fever episodes and her reported number of drinks per week. The estimated odds ratio for fever is $\exp(\widehat{b}_1) = 0.997(0.621, 1.601)$; that is, with three decimal places the maximum likelihood estimate based on the logistic regression model as well as the associated 95% confidence interval is identical to the results from the Mantel–Haenszel analysis. In fact, it can be shown that the Mantel–Haenszel method is almost fully efficient for OR-values close to 1.

For a survival time outcome similar techniques, the "stratified Cox regression model" and the "stratified logrank test," are available. We explain these techniques in the context of the PBC3 study (Example 1.3) evaluating the treatment effect adjusting for bilirubin by stratification. We have seen previously (Section 3.1.3) that without adjustment for bilirubin the treatment effect is small and insignificant: estimated hazard ratio 0.943 (0.624,1.426). The analyses reported in Section 5.1.2 show that adjusting in various ways for bilirubin as a quantitative covariate will change this hazard ratio considerably, the magnitude of change depending on the exact way in which the effect of bilirubin is modeled.

To get a preliminary view of the data, Table 5.1.8 shows the number of treatment failures for CyA- and placebo-treated patients stratified by bilirubin quintiles. It is seen that the number of treatment failures increases dramatically with bilirubin and that, in the highest quintile group, the treatment allocation is somewhat uneven (42 out of 70 patients, 60%, were in the CyA group). That is, in spite of the randomization, bilirubin may confound the simple treatment comparison.

Table 5.1.8. Numbers of patients with or without treatment failure by treatment and bilirubin quintile group.

Bilirubin Stratum	≤ 10.3 $s = 0$		$(10.3,16]$ $s = 1$		$(16,26.7]$ $s = 2$		$(26.7,51.4]$ $s = 3$		> 51.4 $s = 4$	
Treatment group	Plac.	CyA	Plac.	CyA	Plac.	CyA	Plac.	CyA	Plac.	CyA
No treatment failure	33	31	37	33	24	29	25	22	8	17
Treatment failure	3	3	2	1	7	6	14	9	20	25
Hazard ratio	1.235		0.500		1.012		0.748		0.532	
95% CI	(0.249,6.129)		(0.045,5.524)		(0.325,3.144)		(0.321,1.743)		(0.291,0.973)	
"Expected" E^s_{tment}	3.3	2.7	1.5	1.5	7.0	6.0	12.4	10.6	13.7	31.3

In strata with many treatment failures, CyA treatment tends to be beneficial and in strata with few failures the stratum-specific treatment effect has wide confidence limits. Therefore, an evaluation of the effect adjusted for the bilirubin strata is likely to show a treatment effect that differs from the marginal insignificant effect quoted above. The significance of such an adjusted effect may be tested using the *stratified logrank test* based on observed and "expected" numbers of treatment failures (and variances) within strata (s) (cf. Section 3.1.3). The expected numbers of treatment failures by treatment group E^s_{tment} are also given in Table 5.1.8 and the version of the stratified logrank test statistic using a variance estimator (cf. (3.1.31) and (3.1.32)), is

$$X^2_{\text{lr,strat}} = \frac{\left(\sum_s (O^s_{\text{CyA}} - E^s_{\text{CyA}})\right)^2}{\sum_s V^s},$$

where O^s_{CyA} denotes the observed number of treatment failures in stratum s in the CyA group. An alternative version (see Section 3.1.3) uses only the observed and expected numbers of treatment failures. The first test statistic takes the value 3.24 which, evaluated in the $\chi^2(1)$-distribution gives $P = 0.07$. This test is the *score test* for the hypothesis $b_1 = 0$ in the *stratified Cox model*

$$l_i(t) = \log(h_{s0}(t)) + b_1 I(x_{i,1} = \text{CyA}), \tag{5.1.4}$$

where, as previously $l_i(t)$ is the log(hazard rate) for individual i belonging to stratum s. Note that in (5.1.4), the baseline hazards $h_{s0}(t)$ are allowed to vary between strata in an unspecified way, in particular, they are not assumed to be proportional. Such a model may be used for evaluating the proportional hazards assumption as we show in Section 6.2.3.

The estimated hazard ratio for treatment is $\exp(\widehat{b}_1) = 0.671(0.435, 1.036)$ with associated Wald and likelihood ratio tests both equal to $3.24(P = 0.07)$. ◇

Matched studies

A special situation arises when data are *matched* or *paired*, for example, when the same subject is observed both before and after an intervention. Such matched studies may be handled by including "subject" as a categorical covariate in the linear predictor as we show in Section 5.4.

5.1.2 One categorical and one quantitative covariate

In this section we study the situation with two explanatory variables one of which is categorical (in fact, binary) and the other is quantitative. We study both the situation where the effect of the latter is assumed to be linear and the situation where this assumption is not made.

Linear effect of the quantitative covariate: the vitamin D study

Our first illustrative example is a continuation of the vitamin D study (Example 1.1) with the quantitative outcome variable $y_i = \log_{10}(25\text{OHD}$ measurement for woman i). The quantitative covariate, the effect of which is assumed to be linear, is BMI $x_{i,1}$ measured in kg/m^2 and the binary covariate is country $x_{i,2}$ (Ireland versus Poland). The questions addressed include a comparison of the vitamin D status in these two countries taking potential differences in BMI into account and a study of the relationship between BMI and vitamin D status and its stability over countries.

The simple additive model for these two explanatory variables then states the mean of y_i to have the form

$$E(y_i) = a + b_1 x_{i,1} + b_2 I(x_{i,2} = \text{Ireland}). \tag{5.1.5}$$

Model (5.1.5) is obtained, in the now usual way, by adding the linear effect, $b_1 x_{i,1}$ of BMI, and that of country, $b_2 I(x_{i,2} = \text{Ireland})$ to the intercept a. The interpretation of the parameters in the model are as follows: a is the expected $\log_{10}(25\text{OHD})$ value for individuals with both covariates equal to 0; that is, Polish women with BMI= 0, b_1, the effect of BMI, is the expected difference in $\log_{10}(25\text{OHD})$ values for women from the same country differing 1 kg/m^2 in BMI, and b_2, the effect of country, is the expected difference in $\log_{10}(25\text{OHD})$ values between women from Ireland and women from Poland with the same BMI. Because of the awkward interpretation of the intercept, the model is often reparametrized by replacing $x_{i,1}$ by, for example, $x_{i,1}-25$. In the reparametrized model, the intercept is the expected $\log_{10}(25\text{OHD})$ value for Polish women with BMI= 25 and interpretations (and estimates) of b_1, b_2 are unchanged. In short, model (5.1.5) states that the relationship between BMI and y_i is linear within both countries, with the same slope b_1 and with the distance b_2 between the two parallel lines.

The estimates in model (5.1.5) (with BMI centered around 25) are $\widehat{b_1} = -0.0152(0.0045)$, $\widehat{b_2} = 0.131(0.040)$, $\widehat{a} = 1.532(0.030)$. The estimated mean values (regression lines) are shown, together with the scatterplot of y_i versus BMI, in Figure 5.1.4. That is, the lines here have the common slope -0.0152 and their vertical distance is 0.131. The value of the line for Poland at BMI= 25 is 1.532. Apart from some outliers for the Polish data the figure does not speak strongly against the model.

We can compare these *mutually adjusted* estimates $\widehat{b_1}, \widehat{b_2}$ with the unadjusted estimates to evaluate the amount of confounding. The unadjusted estimate for country is $\widehat{b_2} = 0.171(0.040)$ whereas that for BMI is $\widehat{b_1} = -0.0195(0.0045)$; that is, adjustment has changed both estimates towards 0 due to the fact that Polish women have lower y-values than those from Ireland while, at the same time, they tend to have higher BMI $(\bar{x}_{1,\text{Irl}} = 26.36, \bar{x}_{1,\text{Pol}} = 28.94)$. The unadjusted estimate for country is simply the difference between average y-values:

$$\bar{y}_{\text{Irl}} - \bar{y}_{\text{Pol}} = 1.643 - 1.472 = 0.171.$$

The BMI-adjusted estimate is the difference between *adjusted* average y-values:

$$\bar{y}_{\text{Irl}}^{\text{adj}} = 1.643 - (-0.0152)(26.36 - 27.94) = 1.618$$

and

$$\bar{y}_{\text{Pol}}^{\text{adj}} = 1.472 - (-0.0152)(28.94 - 27.94) = 1.487.$$

Here, the value 27.94 is the overall average BMI-value in Ireland and Poland and the numbers 1.618 and 1.487 have, therefore, been adjusted to that value

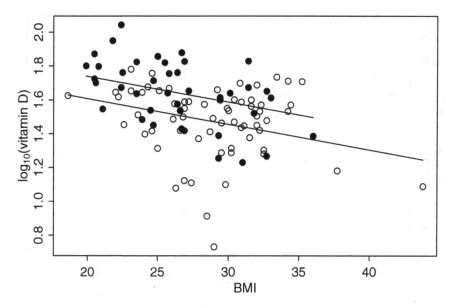

Fig. 5.1.4. Scatterplot of $\log_{10}(25OHD$ values) by BMI for women from Ireland (dots) or Poland (circles). Fitted parallel regression lines are added.

of BMI. However, because the adjusted estimate for country is simply the (vertical) difference between the two regression lines, adjustment to any other value for BMI would have resulted in the same difference. Thus, adjustment to BMI= 25 would give adjusted averages 1.664 for Poland and 1.532 for Ireland, respectively. The discrepancy between adjusted and unadjusted average values is illustrated in Figure 5.1.5. The procedure by which we compare countries after adjustment for the quantitative covariate BMI is known as *analysis of covariance* (ANCOVA) but as we have seen this is simply a regression model for parallel regression lines .

It is important to note that if the true model is (5.1.5) then the "marginal" model only studying the relationship between y_i and BMI need not be linear. Linearity of the marginal model will depend on the relationship between country and BMI. It will hold if the distribution of BMI is the same in both countries, however, even without this assumption being formally fulfilled, the marginal linear relationship with BMI may provide a satisfactory approximation for practical purposes.

As in the previous section, estimates with simpler interpretations than $\widehat{b}_1, \widehat{b}_2$ can be obtained by back-transformation with antilog$_{10}$. Thus, the adjusted ratio between medians for Irish and Polish women with the same BMI is $10^{0.131} = 1.35$ with 95% confidence limits from $10^{0.131-1.96\cdot0.040} = 1.13$ to $10^{0.131+1.96\cdot0.040} = 1.62$. Similarly, the ratio between medians for women from

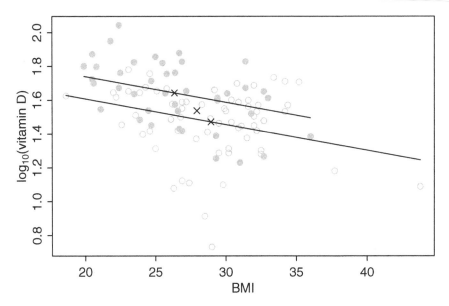

Fig. 5.1.5. Illustration of adjusted country effect (vertical difference between regression lines for Ireland and Poland) and unadjusted country effect (difference between marginal averages, that is, vertical distance between the left (26.36,1.643) and the right (28.94,1.472) "x"). The middle "x" (27.94,1.538) indicates overall averages for BMI and $\log_{10}$(vitamin D).

the same country differing, for example, 5 kg/m^2 in BMI, is $10^{-0.0152 \cdot 5} = 0.84$ with 95% confidence interval (0.76,0.93).

Model assumptions

The results presented rely on a number of model assumptions:

- Linear effect of BMI on $\log_{10}$(25OHD)
- No interaction between BMI and country (i.e., parallel regression lines)
- Variance homogeneity
- Symmetric distributions of residuals

To investigate some of these model assumptions, Figure 5.1.6 shows the scatterplot of y_i versus BMI for both countries with separate regression lines for Ireland and Poland added and Figure 5.1.7 shows the same scatterplot, now with separate smoothers for Ireland and Poland added. In Section 5.2.2 we return to formal tests of no interaction. Here we just notice that the assumption of parallel curves is not strongly contraindicated. The assumption of linearity may be formally tested as described in Section 4.2, for example, by adding linear splines to the model. We have done that using the cutpoints

25 and 30 corresponding to the categories previously used. Table 5.1.9 shows the results. There is no evidence against linearity in either country.

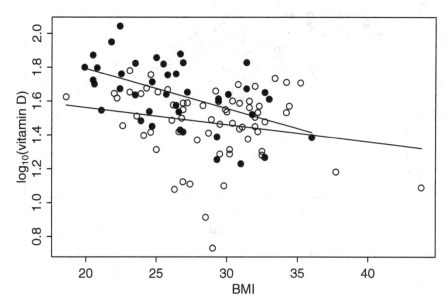

Fig. 5.1.6. Scatterplot of $\log_{10}(25\text{OHD}$ values) by BMI for women from Ireland (dots) and Poland (circles). Fitted regression lines are added separately for the two countries.

Table 5.1.9. Tests for linearity (i.e., estimates in both columns 3 and 4 equal to 0), separately in the two countries, based on linear splines.

Country	BMI	(BMI-25)I(BMI$\geq$ 25)	(BMI-30)I(BMI$\geq$ 30)	P for linearity
Poland	−0.0422 (0.0301)	0.0393 (0.0412)	−0.0033 (0.0248)	0.53
Ireland	−0.0221 (0.0201)	−0.0084 (0.0348)	0.0203 (0.0430)	0.89

Figure 5.1.8, showing residuals plotted against fitted values, also suggests a reasonable fit of the model with residuals being symmetrically distributed around 0. The variation for Polish and Irish data seems to be of the same order of magnitude, a fact which is also illustrated by a formal test for variance homogeneity:

$$F = \frac{s_{\text{Pol}}^2}{s_{\text{Irl}}^2} = \frac{0.205^2}{0.166^2} = 1.53.$$

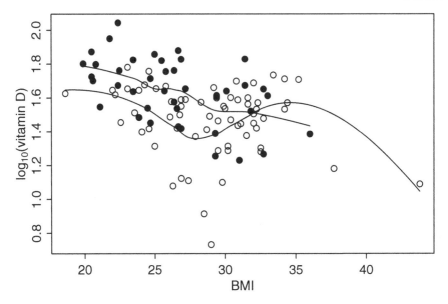

Fig. 5.1.7. Scatterplot of $\log_{10}(25\text{OHD values})$ by BMI for women from Ireland (dots) and Poland (circles). Scatterplot smoothers are added separately for the two countries.

When evaluated in the $F(63, 39)$ distribution this gives a P-value of 0.16 and the common estimate for the residual standard deviation is 0.192.

Nonlinear effect of the quantitative covariate: The PBC3 trial

This section, thus far, has dealt with the situation where the effect of the quantitative covariate x_1 was assumed to be linear, whereby it is described by a single-slope parameter b_1. In our example, the vitamin D study, this assumption was examined and it was found to provide a reasonable data description. In the remaining part of the section we briefly discuss the situation with one categorical covariate and one quantitative covariate whose effect cannot be assumed to be linear. Our example is the PBC3 liver cirrhosis trial with the binary covariate treatment $x_{i,2}$ and the quantitative covariate bilirubin $x_{i,1}$. The analyses in Section 4.2 showed that the effect of the latter could not reasonably be described as a linear function and a number of models with transformations of bilirubin were studied. The question addressed in the following is how the treatment groups differ when adjusting for bilirubin and in Section 5.2.2 we continue this example with an evaluation of a possible interaction between treatment and bilirubin.

In spite of the randomization, the distributions of bilirubin differ somewhat between the two treatment groups. Table 5.1.10 presents average values and SD for both bilirubin and $\log_{10}(\text{bilirubin})$ for placebo- and CyA-treated

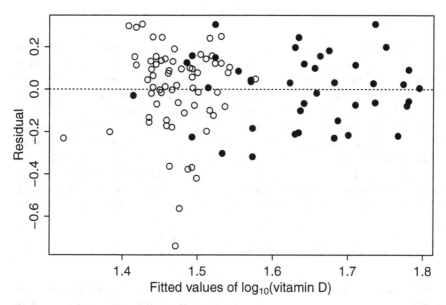

Fig. 5.1.8. Scatterplot of residuals by fitted values for women from Ireland (dots) and Poland (circles).

patients. It is seen that CyA-treated patients tend to have higher bilirubin values than those from the placebo group. Note the large standard deviations compared to the averages for the untransformed values indicating a strongly right-skewed distribution, that is, with a heavy right-hand tail. Because of the strong association between bilirubin and survival this difference may confound the treatment comparison. Note that a significance test for comparing the mean values makes no sense. Such a test would examine whether the differences are larger than explained by chance; however, if randomization is performed properly, chance is in fact the only possible explanation for the differences. What matters is not statistical significance of the difference but rather the size of the difference in absolute terms combined with the prognostic influence of bilirubin.

Table 5.1.10. PBC3: distribution of bilirubin in the CyA and placebo treatment groups.

Treatment	Bilirubin (SD)	$\log_{10}$(Bilirubin) (SD)
CyA	48.56 (69.38)	3.26 (1.05)
Placebo	42.34 (65.90)	3.14 (0.99)

Recall from Section 3.1.3 that unadjusted for bilirubin, that is, in the model

$$\log(h_i(t)) = \log(h_0(t)) + b_2 x_{i,2},$$

the estimated log(hazard ratio) for treatment was $\widehat{b}_2 = -0.0585(0.210)$ leading to a 95% confidence interval for the hazard ratio $\exp(b_2)$ from 0.624 to 1.426 ($P = 0.78$); see first row of Table 5.1.11. We now assess the treatment effect using three different ways of adjustment for bilirubin, all of which were discussed in Section 4.2. The simplest adjustment considered a linear effect of the single transformed covariate $\log(x_{i,1})$. Alternatives were based on the fractional polynomials $x_{i,1}^{-0.5}$ and $x_{i,1}^{-2}$ and a third way of adjustment (Section 4.2.3) involved the range of normal values $(0,17.1)$ μmol/L by including the two covariates $I(x_{i,1} > 17.1)$ and $I(x_{i,1} > 17.1)(\log(x_{i,1}) - \log(17.1))$. The latter covariate may also be written as $I(x_{i,1} > 17.1)\log(x_{i,1}/17.1)$. Table 5.1.11 also shows the results of fitting these models which all have the form

$$\log(h_i(t)) = \log(h_0(t)) + b_2 x_{i,2} + \sum_{j=1}^{r} b_{1,j} f_j(x_{i,1}). \qquad (5.1.6)$$

That is, in (5.1.6) the effect of bilirubin $x_{i,1}$ is modeled by including r nonlinear functions, $f_1, f_2, \ldots, f_r$ of $x_{i,1}$ and the model is obtained in the usual way by adding the treatment effect $b_2 x_{i,2}$ to the effect, $\sum_j b_{1,j} f_j(x_{i,1})$ of bilirubin. In the first model, we have $r = 1$ and $f_1(x) = \log(x)$, in the second, $r = 2$ and $f_1(x) = x^{-0.5}, f_2(x) = x^{-2}$, whereas in the third, $r = 2$ and $f_1(x) = I(x > 17.1), f_2(x) = I(x > 17.1)\log(x/17.1)$.

Table 5.1.11. PBC3: treatment effects: unadjusted and from models (5.1.6) with nonlinear adjustment for bilirubin. Effects of bilirubin are also shown.

Adjustment for Bilirubin		Effect of Bilirubin		Effect of Treatment	
$f_1(x_{i,1})$	$f_2(x_{i,1})$	$\widehat{b}_{1,1}$	$\widehat{b}_{1,2}$	$\widehat{b}_2$	P for $b_2 = 0$
—	—	—	—	-0.0585 (0.210)	0.78
$\log(x_{i,1})$	—	1.040 (0.210)	—	-0.399 (0.215)	0.064
$x_{i,1}^{-0.5}$	$x_{i,1}^{-2}$	-15.705 (1.689)	50.829 (11.265)	-0.424 (0.217)	0.050
$I(x_{i,1} > 17.1)$	$I(x_{i,1} > 17.1)$ $\cdot \log(x_{i,1}/17.1)$	1.292 (0.396)	0.896 (0.130)	-0.387 (0.216)	0.073

It is seen that the adjustment in all cases has a considerable influence on the treatment effect which changes from a marginal hazard ratio of $\exp(-0.0585) = 0.94$ to hazard ratios in the neighborhood of $\exp(-0.4) = 0.67$

indicating a beneficial effect of treatment for a given value of bilirubin. Also, in all adjusted models, the effect is borderline significant.

As discussed in Chapter 4, the parameters for bilirubin are not all easy to interpret. What matters is the shape of the relationship between bilirubin and the linear predictor; see Figures 5.1.9 and 5.1.10 which show the linear predictors ("parallel response curves"; i.e., the linear predictor as a function of log(bilirubin)), for the fractional polynomial model and for that based on the normal range. It is seen that the difference between the two types of models has to do with the effect of low values of bilirubin where the model using fractional polynomials predicts a higher mortality. However, for very low values of bilirubin this high mortality may be implausible as it has the same order of magnitude as that for the highest bilirubin values. Note that, for the model in the second row of Table 5.1.11, the linear predictor is simply two parallel lines (as in Figure 5.1.4) when plotted against log(bilirubin).

All (adjusted) treatment and bilirubin effects in Table 5.1.11 rely on the assumption of no interaction between the two covariates. In Section 5.2.2 we return to an evaluation of this hypothesis.

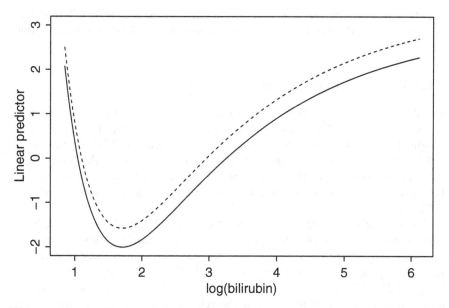

Fig. 5.1.9. The PBC study: parallel linear predictors as a function of bilirubin in treatment groups (CyA: solid line, placebo: dashed line) modeled as fractional polynomials with powers –0.5 and –2.

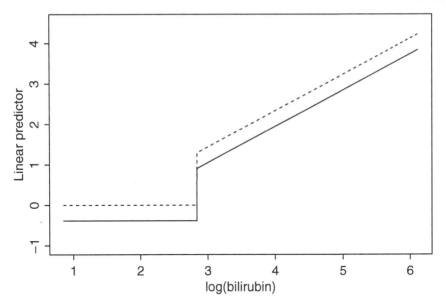

Fig. 5.1.10. The PBC study: parallel linear predictors as a function of bilirubin in treatment groups (CyA: solid line, placebo: dashed line) modeled as constant within the normal range (0,17.1).

5.1.3 Two quantitative covariates

Finally, we turn to the situation with two quantitative explanatory variables, $x_{i,1}$ and $x_{i,2}$. An example is the birthweight study, Example 1.8 of the birthweight (BW) for 107 babies for whom both the abdominal (AD) and biparietal (BPD) diameters were measured shortly before birth using ultrasound. Recall that the purpose of this study was to describe the relationship between birthweight and these two ultrasound measurements and thereby to predict birthweight.

Because of the "geometry" of the problem, AD and BPD are likely to affect birthweight *multiplicatively* and in order to prepare for a linear model we therefore define both the response variable and the two explanatory variables in terms of log-transformations: $y_i = \log_{10}(BW_i), x_{i,1} = \log_{10}(AD_i), x_{i,2} = \log_{10}(BPD_i)$. Figures 5.1.11 and 5.1.12 show the scatterplots of y_i versus $x_{i,1}$ and $x_{i,2}$, respectively. It is seen that the relationship with $x_{i,1}$ seems roughly linear whereas that with $x_{i,2}$ may have some deviation from linearity, however, mostly owing to the relatively high value of y_i for the observation with the lowest value of $x_{i,1}$. The fitted straight lines are

$$E(y_i) = -1.062 + 2.237x_{i,1}$$

and

$$E(y_i) = -3.077 + 3.332x_{i,2},$$

respectively, the standard deviation of the coefficient for $\log_{10}(AD)$ is 0.111, that for $\log_{10}(BPD)$ is 0.202, and the residual standard deviations in the two models are 0.0554 and 0.0646.

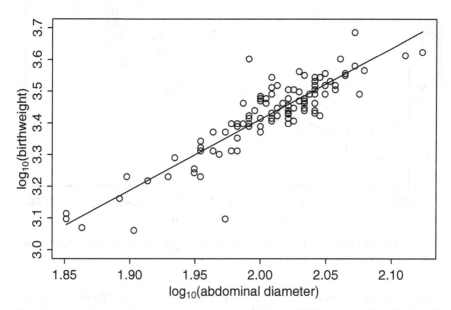

Fig. 5.1.11. Birthweight study: scatterplot of $\log_{10}(BW)$ versus $\log_{10}(AD)$ with estimated regression line.

Two linear effects

The simplest case with two quantitative explanatory variables is when both can be assumed to have a linear effect. In this case the linear predictor can be written in the form

$$LP_i = a + b_1 x_{i,1} + b_2 x_{i,2}, \tag{5.1.7}$$

where, again, the linear effects of $x_{i,1}$ and $x_{i,2}$ are simply added. Figure 5.1.13 shows the three-dimensional scatterplot where y_i is plotted against both $x_{i,1}$ and $x_{i,2}$ and, graphically, the linear predictor can be represented as a plane in the three-dimensional space. The estimated parameters in (5.1.7) then characterize the plane that fits the scatterplot best. For a quantitative outcome variable, as in the current example, the parameters for the best fitting plane minimize the residual sum of squares

$$\sum_i (y_i - (a + b_1 x_{i,1} + b_2 x_{i,2}))^2$$

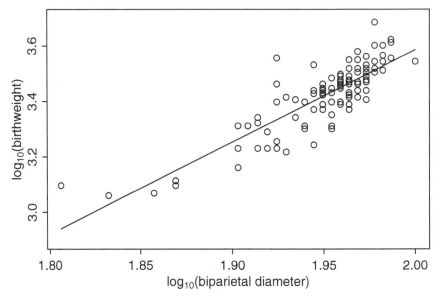

Fig. 5.1.12. Birthweight study: scatterplot of $\log_{10}(\text{BW})$ versus $\log_{10}(\text{BPD})$ with estimated regression line.

and, in general, parameter estimates are obtained using the likelihood principle. For the birthweight example the fitted plane is

$$\widehat{\text{LP}}_i = -2.546 + 1.467x_{i,1} + 1.552x_{i,2}$$

with a residual standard deviation of 0.0464. The standard deviations of the parameter estimates are $\text{SD}(\widehat{b}_1) = 0.147, \text{SD}(\widehat{b}_2) = 0.229$. Results are summarized in Table 5.1.12.

Table 5.1.12. Birthweight study: adjusted and unadjusted effects of $\log_{10}(AD)$ and $\log_{10}(BPD)$ on $\log_{10}(BW)$.

Model	$\log_{10}(AD)$		$\log_{10}(BPD)$		Residual SD
	$\widehat{b}$	SD	$\widehat{b}$	SD	
Mutually adjusted	1.467	0.147	1.552	0.229	0.0464
Unadjusted	2.237	0.111	3.332	0.202	0.0554, resp. 0.0646

The fitted plane has the property that for fixed value, say $x_{0,1}$, for the first covariate (i.e., when intersecting the plane for the linear predictor with a vertical plane at $x_{0,1}$ in the direction of the second covariate) we obtain a straight line with slope $\widehat{b}_2 = 1.552$ (and intercept $\widehat{a} + \widehat{b}_1x_{0,1} = -2.546 + 1.467x_{0,1}$) (Figure 5.1.14). Thus, the slope b_2 represents the effect of $x_{i,2}$ for

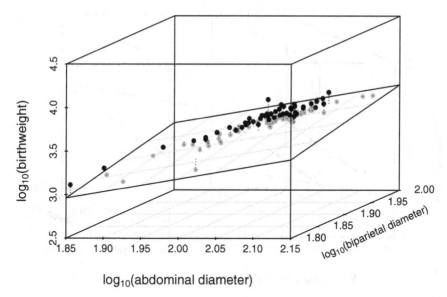

Fig. 5.1.13. Birthweight study: scatterplot of $\log_{10}(\mathrm{BW})$ versus $\log_{10}(\mathrm{BPD})$ and $\log_{10}(\mathrm{AD})$ with fitted plane and "residual needles" added.

any given value of $x_{i,1}$ showing once more that a consequence of adding the effects of the two explanatory variables to the intercept a is an assumption of no interaction between $x_{i,1}$ and $x_{i,2}$: the effect of one covariate is the same for all values of the other. A consequence of Equation (5.1.7) is, therefore, that for a given value of one covariate the effect of the other is linear. It is important to notice that it does *not* follow from (5.1.7) that the ("marginal") relation between the linear predictor and just one of the covariates is linear. The structure of this marginal relationship depends on the structure of the relation between $x_{i,1}$ and $x_{i,2}$.

Figure 5.1.15 shows the scatterplot of $\log_{10}(\mathrm{BPD})$ versus $\log_{10}(\mathrm{AD})$ and because this is roughly linear and we are studying a linear model for the mean of a quantitative outcome, the scatterplots of $\log_{10}(\mathrm{BW})$ versus either of the two explanatory variables should also be roughly linear as seen in Figures 5.1.11 and 5.1.12.

Confounding in this example is quite obvious. The two explanatory variables are strongly interrelated and also both strongly related to the outcome. Therefore, the effect of, say $x_{i,1}$, depends on whether we adjust for $x_{i,2}$: the unadjusted coefficient is 2.237 (0.111) and the adjusted coefficient is 1.467 (0.147) (Table 5.1.12). The inadequacy of a model including only $\log_{10}(\mathrm{BPD})$ may be seen by plotting the residuals from this model against $\log_{10}(\mathrm{AD})$; see Figure 5.1.16. A scatterplot smoother has been added that clearly shows a tendency to large residuals for large values of $\log_{10}(\mathrm{AD})$. However, residual

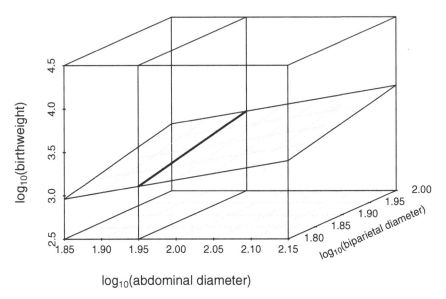

Fig. 5.1.14. Birthweight study: fitted plane for the linear predictor and its intersection with a vertical plane through $x_{0,1} = 1.95$ in the direction of $x_{i,2} = \log_{10}(BPD_i)$.

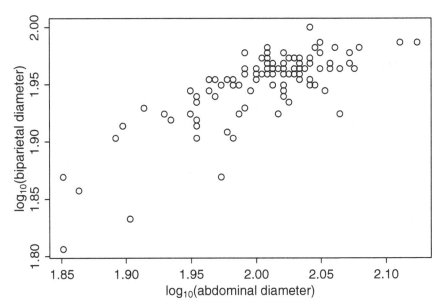

Fig. 5.1.15. Birthweight study: scatterplot of $\log_{10}(\text{BPD})$ versus $\log_{10}(\text{AD})$.

plots from model (5.1.7) including both covariates (see Figure 5.1.17) show no clear systematic pattern. The strong reduction in residual standard deviation when adding $\log_{10}(AD)$ to the model including only $\log_{10}(BPD)$ should also be noted. In the one-covariate model this is 0.0646 whereas after adjustment it reduces to 0.0464 (Table 5.1.12). The interpretation is that inclusion of $\log_{10}(AD)$ has explained some of the residual variation (Figure 5.1.16) when only taking $\log_{10}(BPD)$ into account. Note, however, that the standard deviation of the estimated effect $\widehat{b}_2$ of $\log_{10}(BPD)$ does not decrease. This is because the SD of the estimated effect not only depends on the residual SD but also on the joint distribution of the explanatory variables. In this case, adjustment for a covariate $\log_{10}(AD)$ which is rather strongly correlated with $\log_{10}(BPD)$ (Figure 5.1.15), increases $SD(\widehat{b}_2)$ in spite of the fact that the residual SD decreases. We return to a more general discussion of this phenomenon in Section 6.1.

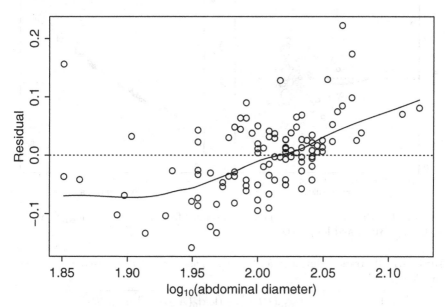

Fig. 5.1.16. Birthweight study: scatterplot of residuals (with smoother) from regression of $\log_{10}(BW)$ on $\log_{10}(BPD)$ plotted against $\log_{10}(AD)$.

The assumptions of linearity for both covariates can be examined as explained in Section 4.2 by adding nonlinear functions of $x_{i,1}$ and $x_{i,2}$ to the linear predictor, for example $(\log_{10}(AD))^2$ or $(\log_{10}(BPD))^2$. The results obtained by doing this are shown in Table 5.1.13 which also repeats the estimates from the model (5.1.7) with two linear effects.

The (Wald) P-value for linearity is 0.16 for $\log_{10}(AD)$, however, it is 0.04 for $\log_{10}(BPD)$ suggesting some deviations as also indicated in Figure 5.1.17

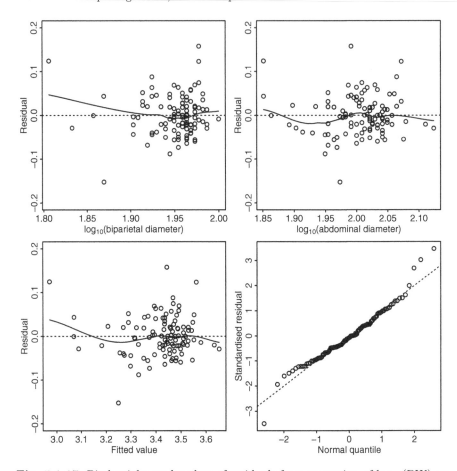

Fig. 5.1.17. Birthweight study: plots of residuals from regression of $\log_{10}(BW)$ on both $\log_{10}(BPD)$ and $\log_{10}(AD)$.

Table 5.1.13. Tests for linearity for $\log_{10}(AD)$ and $\log_{10}(BPD)$ based on quadratic functions.

$\log_{10}(AD)$	$\log_{10}(BPD)$	$(\log_{10}(AD))^2$	$(\log_{10}(BPD))^2$
1.467 (0.147)	1.552 (0.229)		
−5.688 (5.098)	1.699 (0.251)	1.785 (1.271)	
1.418 (0.146)	−18.933 (9.852)		5.354 (2.574)

via the relatively high birthweight for the baby with the lowest observed BPD. However, looking at Cook's distance (Section 4.1.1) for the model including $(\log_{10}(BPD))^2$, Figure 5.1.18, it is seen that this observation has by far the largest influence on the estimates. If we leave out this observation from the dataset and refit the model with linear effects of both covariates as well as that with a quadratic effect of $\log_{10}(BPD)$ the results are as follows. The estimates in the linear model do not change dramatically $\hat{b}_1 = 1.432, \hat{b}_2 = 1.818$ whereas, in the latter model, the quadratic term completely loses its significance, $P = 0.96$. Thus, the evidence against linearity is not strong because it seems to come from a single observation, and a larger study including more small fetuses would be useful to shed further light on this question.

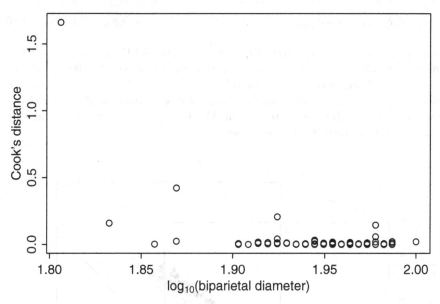

Fig. 5.1.18. Birthweight study: Cook's distance for the model with quadratic effect of $\log_{10}(BPD)$ plotted against $\log_{10}(BPD)$.

Nonlinear efects

When one covariate has a nonlinear effect, say $x_{i,2}$ with an effect of $\sum_j b_{2,j} f_j(x_{i,2})$, the situation is to some extent similar. The linear predictor

$$LP_i = a + b_1 x_{i,1} + \sum_j b_{2,j} f_j(x_{i,2})$$

is now a surface in the three-dimensional space with the property that its intersection with a vertical plane at a fixed value $x_{0,2}$ of the second covariate

$x_{0,2}$ in the direction of the first covariate is a straight line with slope b_1 (and intercept $a + \sum_j b_{2,j} f_j(x_{0,2})$); that is, all such lines are parallel. On the other hand, the intersection of the surface of the linear predictor with a vertical plane at $x_{0,1}$ in the direction of the second covariate is a curve of the form $a + b_1 x_{0,1} + \sum_j b_{2,j} f_j(x_{i,2})$; that is, all such curves are also parallel. This, again, signals no interaction as a consequence of adding the terms for the two covariates in the linear predictor.

As an illustration, we fit a model for the entire birthweight dataset (i.e., including the observation with the lowest BPD) where the effect of $x_{i,1}$ is kept linear and that of $x_{i,2}$ is described as a quadratic spline with knots at 85, 90, and 95 mm. That is, the linear predictor is now

$$\text{LP}_i = a + b_1 x_{i,1} + b_{2,1} x_{i,2} + b_{2,2} x_{i,2}^2 + b_{2,3}(x_{i,2} - \log_{10}(85))^2 I(x_{i,2} \geq 85)$$
$$+ b_{2,4}(x_{i,2} - \log_{10}(90))^2 I(x_{i,2} \geq 90) + b_{2,5}(x_{i,2} - \log_{10}(95))^2 I(x_{i,2} \geq 95).$$

In this model, the linear effect of $x_{i,1}$ is $\widehat{b}_1 = 1.384(0.145)$ whereas, as noted in Section 4.2, the $b_{2,j}$-coefficients are difficult to interpret directly. What matters is the shape of the estimated linear predictor. This is shown as a 3D plot in Figure 5.1.19 and Figure 5.1.20 shows it as a function of $x_{i,2}$ for three fixed values (90, 100, and 110 mm) of AD. It is seen, as expected, that the deviations from linearity are not great.

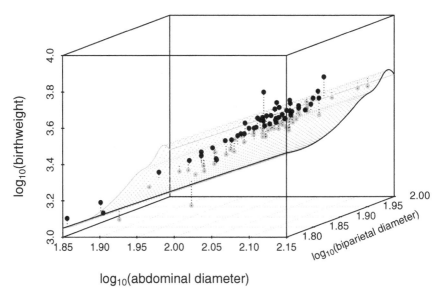

Fig. 5.1.19. Birthweight study: 3D plot of the linear predictor (when the effect of $\log_{10}(\text{BPD})$ is a quadratic spline) against $\log_{10}(\text{AD})$ and $\log_{10}(\text{BPD})$.

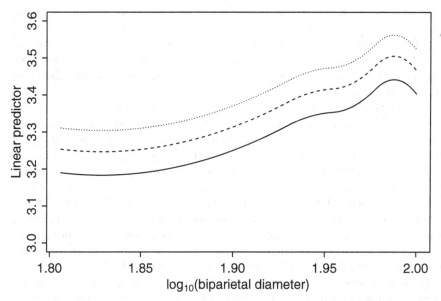

Fig. 5.1.20. Birthweight study: the linear predictor when the effect of $\log_{10}$(BPD) is a quadratic spline plotted against $\log_{10}$(BPD) for values 90, 100, 110 mm of AD.

5.2 Two covariates: Models with interaction

In the previous Section 5.1 a number of regression models with two explanatory variables were discussed. Situations with different types of covariates were studied: two categorical ones (Section 5.1.1), one categorical and one quantitative (Section 5.1.2), and two quantitative (Section 5.1.3). Common to all these situations was the assumption of *no interaction* between the two explanatory variables: the effect of one variable was constant over all values of the other. This assumption was imposed when simply adding the terms for the two covariates in the linear predictor. We did some preliminary examinations of that assumption, and in the present section we conduct careful studies of interaction in all these examples. We discuss in each situation how interaction is interpreted as well as ways of parametrizing models with interaction. It is important to note that some parametrizations may be useful for testing for no interaction and others more useful for reporting estimates when interaction is present. Reparametrizations do not change the model, only the way in which the results appear.

It is also important to note that interaction is a symmetrical concept: if the effect of x_1 depends on the level of x_2 then, also, the effect of x_2 will depend on x_1. How to report the results from a model with interaction will depend on the scientific purpose of the analysis and the status of x_1 and x_2. Furthermore, interaction is scale-dependent: for a quantitative outcome interaction may be quite apparent when data are analyzed in the original scale whereas it may disappear after a log transformation. For binary outcomes, a logistic regression model may show no interaction but for a model with another link function (studied in Section 7.4.1), adding interaction terms may improve the fit. Our general attitude is that identifying a scale with no interaction gives interpretative advantages due to increased simplicity; see also the discussion in Section 2.3.3.

Interaction means that the effect of x_1 depends on the level of x_2, therefore an obvious introductory approach to studying interaction is *subgroup analysis*. Here, after *stratification* on x_2, separate models for the effect of x_1 are fitted within strata. However, in spite of the simplicity, we do not, in general, recommend such an approach, for several reasons. First of all, for models with other explanatory variables, $x_3, x_4, \ldots$, stratification on x_2 will not only provide the desired interaction with x_1 but also different effects of $x_3, x_4, \ldots$ in the different strata. Second, after stratification on x_2, separate x_1-effects will be estimated in strata and, therefore, it is possible to perform as many tests for the effect of x_1 as there are strata, which will considerably inflate the type I error risk. Our recommendation is not to overemphasize that x_1-effects may be significant for some values of x_2 and insignificant for others, unless rejection of an overall test for no interaction or, more important, a careful evaluation of confidence intervals has signaled that the separate x_1-effects do, indeed, seem to be different.

A final remark is that, in general, it makes no sense to interpret a main effect, or to test for such an effect when interaction is present. We discuss all these aspects of interaction in connection with the concrete examples in the following sections.

5.2.1 Two categorical covariates

In Section 5.1.1 we discussed the vitamin D study, Example 1.1. Focus was on the relation between $\log_{10}(25\text{OHD})$ measurements of vitamin D, y_i, in women and groups of BMI, $x_{i,1}$ (normal weight, $18.5 \leq x_{i,1} < 25$, versus overweight, $x_{i,1} \geq 25$) and country, $x_{i,2}$ (Ireland or Poland). The model (5.1.1) which we studied specified the mean $\text{E}(y_i)$ of y_i to be

$$\text{E}(y_i) = a + b_1 I(x_{i,1} \geq 25) + b_2 I(x_{i,2} = \text{Ireland}).$$

In this model the effect b_1 of body mass index for women from Ireland is the same as that for women from Poland and the effect b_2 of country for overweight women is the same as that for normal weight women. The average values in the four groups are shown in Table 5.2.1 and the estimates in the additive model are: $\widehat{a} = 1.587(0.043), \widehat{b}_1 = -0.141(0.044), \widehat{b}_2 = 0.142(0.039)$.

To evaluate the assumption of no interaction we computed differences in rows and columns and noted that these were not very different: row differences are –0.155 for Poland and –0.127 for Ireland, and column differences are 0.121 for normal weight women and 0.150 for overweight women; see the graphical illustration in Figure 5.1.1.

Table 5.2.1. Average 25OHD values (number of women) in four country by BMI groups.

	Normal Weight	Overweight	Difference
Poland	1.598 (12)	1.443 (53)	−0.155
Ireland	1.720 (16)	1.593 (25)	−0.127
Difference	0.121 (28)	0.150 (78)	0.028

Testing for no interaction

As an alternative to the additive model (5.1.1) we now introduce the corresponding model *with interaction* between BMI and country, that is, a model where BMI effects are, indeed, different in the two countries and where differences between countries depend on BMI group.

Let us first recall that in the model without interaction the expected values in the four groups were as presented in Table 5.2.2.

Table 5.2.2. Expected values in four groups according to model (5.1.1).

	Normal Weight	Overweight
Poland	a	$a + b_1$
Ireland	$a + b_2$	$a + b_1 + b_2$

One way of parametrizing the model with interaction is shown in Table 5.2.3. Here, the effect of BMI (overweight versus normal weight) for Polish women (the reference group for country), is still $(a + b_1) - a = b_1$ whereas, in Ireland the BMI effect is now $(a+b_1+b_2+b_{1,1})-(a+b_2) = b_1+b_{1,1}$. Similarly, the effect of country (Ireland versus Poland) for normal weight women (the reference group for BMI), is still $(a + b_2) - a = b_2$ whereas for overweight women it is now $(a + b_1 + b_2 + b_{1,1}) - (a + b_1) = b_2 + b_{1,1}$. Thus, the new parameter $b_{1,1}$ is the difference between the BMI effects for Ireland and for Poland (the reference group for country) and, at the same time, $b_{1,1}$ is the difference between the country effects for overweight women and for normal weight women (the reference group for BMI).

Table 5.2.3. Expected values in four groups according to model (5.2.2).

	Normal Weight	Overweight
Poland	a	$a + b_1$
Ireland	$a + b_2$	$a + b_1 + b_2 + b_{1,1}$

Note the symmetry: when the effect of country depends on BMI then, at the same time, the effect of BMI depends on country. From both points of view the magnitude of the interaction is described by the *interaction parameter*, $b_{1,1}$. With this parametrization the model with interaction is

$$E(y_i) = a + b_1 I(x_{i,1} \geq 25) + b_2 I(x_{i,2} = \text{Ireland}) \qquad (5.2.1)$$
$$+ b_{1,1} I(x_{i,1} \geq 25 \text{ and } x_{i,2} = \text{Ireland}).$$

Note that the added dummy variable is simply the product of the two separate dummy variables

$$I(x_{i,1} \geq 25 \text{ and } x_{i,2} = \text{Ireland}) = I(x_{i,1} \geq 25) \cdot I(x_{i,2} = \text{Ireland})$$

and that the hypothesis of no interaction can be formulated simply as

$$H_0 : b_{1,1} = 0.$$

That is, with this parametrization *testing* for no interaction is simple, whereas the interpretation of the parameter $b_{1,1}$, is less direct: it is a "difference between differences." In fact, in this simple situation with no other covariates in the model the maximum likelihood estimates of the regression parameters $b_1, b_2, b_{1,1}$ are obtained simply as differences that may be computed directly from Table 5.2.1.

- Intercept, level of $\log_{10}(25\text{OHD})$ in "combined reference group" (normal weight women from Poland): $\widehat{a} = 1.598$ (0.056).
- Effect of BMI in the reference group for country: $\widehat{b}_1 = 1.443 - 1.598 = -0.155$ (0.062).
- Effect of country (i.e., difference between countries) in the reference group for BMI: $\widehat{b}_2 = 1.720 - 1.598 = 0.121$ (0.074).
- Interaction parameter, difference between BMI effects in Poland and in Ireland = difference between country effects among overweight and normal weight women: $\widehat{b}_{1,1} = (1.593 - 1.720) - (1.443 - 1.598) = (1.593 - 1.443) - (1.720 - 1.598) = 0.028$ (0.088).

In general, neither the estimates nor the standard deviations can be calculated explicitly but will be part of the regression output. The Wald test statistic for no interaction, $b_{1,1} = 0$, takes the value $(0.028/0.088)^2 = 0.11$ which, evaluated in the $\chi^2(1)$-distribution gives the P-value of 0.75. Thus, in this example there is no indication of different effects of BMI in Ireland and in Poland. The test for no interaction has one degree-of-freedom because it deals with a single parameter $b_{1,1}$. In general, for two categorical variables with, say $k_1 + 1$ and $k_2 + 1$ categories, respectively, the number of degrees-of-freedom for the no interaction test is $k_1 \cdot k_2$. Examples are provided later in this section.

Note that in this model one can also test the hypotheses $b_1 = 0$ or $b_2 = 0$. These hypotheses, however, no longer correspond to tests for no overall effects of BMI and country, respectively, but relate to effects of one covariate only in the reference group for the other.

Also note that the discussion of a possible interaction between the two explanatory variables has nothing to do with the fact that the effect of one of them may be confounded by the other. In fact, *the concepts of confounding and interaction have nothing in common* (although they are often mixed up); see also Figure 5.0.1.

Presenting estimates in models with interaction

If there is indication of an interaction between two explanatory variables then alternative parametrizations to (5.2.2) are advantageous. Recall that presence of interaction means that the effect of one covariate depends on the value of another, so to report a model with interaction an obvious possibility is to present these different effects. To exemplify, we first study presentation of BMI effects separately for women from Ireland and from Poland and parametrize the model with interaction between BMI and country as:

$$
\begin{aligned}
\mathrm{E}(y_i) = a &+ b_2 I(x_{i,2} = \text{Ireland}) \\
&+ b_{1,0} I(x_{i,1} \geq 25 \text{ and } x_{i,2} = \text{Poland}) \qquad (5.2.2) \\
&+ b_{1,1} I(x_{i,1} \geq 25 \text{ and } x_{i,2} = \text{Ireland}).
\end{aligned}
$$

The expected values from model (5.2.2) are shown in Table 5.2.4. Here, a is still the expected $\log_{10}(25\text{OHD})$ level in the combined reference group (normal weight Polish women), b_2 is again the effect of country (Ireland versus Poland) in the reference group (normal weight) for BMI, and $b_{1,0}$ and $b_{1,1}$, respectively, are the effects of BMI for Poland and for Ireland. With this parametrization, the hypothesis of no interaction is:

$$
H_0 : b_{1,0} = b_{1,1}.
$$

Note that the interpretation of $b_{1,1}$ has changed from (5.2.2) to (5.2.2). This illustrates the important fact in multiple regression models that *the interpretation of the parameter corresponding to any explanatory variable depends on which other covariates are included in the model* (even though, in this case, we do not even change the model as such).

Note that the added dummy variable may, again, be computed simply as a product of two dummy variables

$$
\begin{aligned}
I(x_{i,1} \geq 25 \text{ and } x_{i,2} = \text{Poland}) &= I(x_{i,1} \geq 25) \cdot I(x_{i,2} = \text{Poland}) \\
&= I(x_{i,1} \geq 25) \cdot (1 - I(x_{i,2} = \text{Ireland})).
\end{aligned}
$$

The maximum likelihood estimates may again be computed directly from Table 5.2.1:

- Intercept, level of $\log_{10}(25\text{OHD})$ in "combined reference group" (normal weight women from Poland): $\widehat{a} = 1.598 \ (0.056)$.

- Effect of country in the reference group for BMI: $\widehat{b}_2 = 1.720 - 1.598 = 0.121$ (0.074).
- Effect of BMI for women from Poland: $\widehat{b}_{1,0} = 1.443 - 1.598 = -0.155$ (0.062).
- Effect of BMI for women from Ireland $\widehat{b}_{1,1} = 1.593 - 1.720 = -0.127$ (0.062),

where $\widehat{a}$ and $\widehat{b}_2$ are unchanged compared to the previous parametrization. Note that in the model with interaction, the estimates corresponding to one particular parametrization can always be computed directly from the estimates in another parametrization of the same model. However, this is not the case for their standard deviations.

Table 5.2.4. Expected values in four groups according to model (5.2.2).

	Normal Weight	Overweight
Poland	a	$a + b_{1,0}$
Ireland	$a + b_2$	$a + b_2 + b_{1,1}$

Because, as mentioned previously, interaction is a symmetric concept the model may also be reparametrized to focus on effects of country within BMI categories. To this end the model is written as

$$\begin{aligned}
E(y_i) = a &+ b_1 I(x_{i,1} \geq 25) \\
&+ b_{0,1} I(x_{i,1} < 25 \text{ and } x_{i,2} = \text{Ireland}) \\
&+ b_{1,1} I(x_{i,1} \geq 25 \text{ and } x_{i,2} = \text{Ireland})
\end{aligned} \tag{5.2.3}$$

and the expected values are shown in Table 5.2.5. Here a is still the expected $\log_{10}(25\text{OHD})$ level in the combined reference group (normal weight Polish women), b_1 is again the effect of BMI (overweight versus normal weight) in the reference group for country, Poland, whereas $b_{0,1}$ and $b_{1,1}$, respectively, are the effects of country (Ireland versus Poland) for normal weight and for overweight women. With this parametrization, the hypothesis of no interaction is:

$$H_0 : b_{0,1} = b_{1,1}$$

and once more the interpretation of $b_{1,1}$ has changed. Note that again the new dummy variable may be computed simply as a product of two other dummy variables

$$I(x_{i,1} < 25 \text{ and } x_{i,2} = \text{Ireland}) = I(x_{i,1} < 25) \cdot I(x_{i,2} = \text{Ireland}).$$

The maximum likelihood estimates in (5.2.3) are obtained from Table 5.2.1:

- Intercept, level of $\log_{10}(25\text{OHD})$ in "combined reference group" (normal weight women from Poland): $\widehat{a} = 1.598$ (0.056).

- Effect of BMI in the reference group for country: $\widehat{b}_1 = 1.443 - 1.598 = -0.155$ (0.062).
- Effect of country for normal weight women: $\widehat{b}_{0,1} = 1.720 - 1.598 = 0.121$ (0.074).
- Effect of country for overweight women: $\widehat{b}_{1,1} = 1.593 - 1.443 = 0.150$ (0.047).

Table 5.2.5. Expected values in four groups according to model (5.2.3).

	Normal Weight	Overweight
Poland	a	$a + b_1$
Ireland	$a + b_{0,1}$	$a + b_1 + b_{1,1}$

Alternative parametrizations of model with interaction

One final way of parametrizing the model with interaction treats the four combinations of BMI group and country as levels of a new categorical covariate. Here, the model is specified as

$$\begin{aligned}
E(y_i) = {} & a + b_{1,0}I(x_{i,1} \geq 25 \text{ and } x_{i,2} = \text{Poland}) \\
& + b_{0,1}I(x_{i,1} < 25 \text{ and } x_{i,2} = \text{Ireland}) \quad\quad (5.2.4) \\
& + b_{1,1}I(x_{i,1} \geq 25 \text{ and } x_{i,2} = \text{Ireland})
\end{aligned}$$

giving expected values as presented in Table 5.2.6. The regression parameters now give differences between three of the categories for the combined variable and the reference category $(0,0)$ (normal weight Polish women), as follows: $b_{1,0}$ for the category $(1,0)$, overweight Polish women, $b_{0,1}$ for the category $(0,1)$, normal weight Irish women, and $b_{1,1}$ for the category $(1,1)$, overweight Irish women.

Table 5.2.6. Expected values in four groups according to model (5.2.4).

	Normal Weight	Overweight
Poland	a	$a + b_{1,0}$
Ireland	$a + b_{0,1}$	$a + b_{1,1}$

The maximum likelihood estimates in (5.2.4) are, again, obtained from Table 5.2.1.

- Intercept, level of $\log_{10}(25\text{OHD})$ in "combined reference group" (normal weight women from Poland): $\widehat{a} = 1.598$ (0.056).

- Effect of BMI in the reference group for country, that is, difference between averages for overweight Polish women and normal weight Polish women: $\widehat{b}_{1,0} = 1.443 - 1.598 = -0.155$ (0.062).
- Effect of country for normal weight women, that is, difference between averages for normal weight Irish women and normal weight Polish women: $\widehat{b}_{0,1} = 1.720 - 1.598 = 0.121$ (0.074).
- Difference between averages for overweight Irish women and normal weight Polish women: $\widehat{b}_{1,1} = 1.593 - 1.598 = -0.005$ (0.068).

With this parametrization the hypothesis of no interaction is not so simple:

$$H_0 : b_{1,1} = b_{0,1} + b_{1,0}$$

and in many situations this "corner parametrization" may not be very useful. However, if both x_1 and x_2 are treatment or exposure variables, and if they do exhibit an interaction then it may be advantageous to consider their combination as a single treatment or exposure variable and study the outcome for its various categories compared to a chosen reference category.

In this section we have presented models with interaction between two categorical explanatory variables using *dummy variables*. This is a very flexible approach that can be applied in all computer programs for multiple regression. However, specific programs frequently offer possibilities for specifying model formulas using a notation such as "$x_1 * x_2$" or "$x_1 . x_2$" for interaction terms and the user then has to determine which parametrization was actually applied. We have chosen the dummy variable approach because of its generality.

Stratification

As mentioned in the introduction to Section 5.2, interaction can be handled by stratifying the data, for example by analyzing data from Ireland and from Poland separately, thereby automatically getting stratum- (country) specific effects of BMI. In the simple model with no other covariates included, this would correspond closely to the analysis presented above (except for also getting separate SD estimates in the two strata). However, with more covariates in the model, as we study in Section 5.3, the difference between stratifying and introducing interaction terms in the model becomes more prominent. This is, as already noted in the introduction to Section 5.2, because stratifying on one covariate because of its potential interaction with another will introduce not only the desired interaction but at the same time interactions among the stratification variable and all other covariates in the model. Because of this, and even though stratification is an intuitively simple approach, we recommend studying interactions as exemplified above, and as we further demonstrate in the next sections (i.e., by adding interaction terms to the model).

Another difference between stratification and modeling using interaction terms has to do with the type of hypotheses that are typically tested and the order in which this is done. When stratifying on country in the vitamin D example one would test for no effect of BMI in Poland and Ireland separately. Such a test could lead to the conclusion that BMI is of importance in only one of the countries, typically that with the largest sample or the smallest SD, whereas no difference may be identified in the other group. However, by first testing for no interaction and thereby "borrowing strength from one group when analyzing the other," the conclusion could rather be that there is no interaction and that BMI thus might affect vitamin D in both groups. We show an example of this phenomenon in the next Section 5.2.2.

The CSL1 liver cirrhosis trial

Recall from Section 1.5 that CSL1 was a randomized clinical trial where 488 patients with liver cirrhosis were treated with either the active drug prednisone (251 patients) or placebo (237 patients). The outcome of interest was death, whereas patients who dropped out or were alive at the closing day of the study were censored: 142 prednisone patients and 150 placebo patients were observed to die. An important prognostic factor for these patients is ascites, that is, excess fluid in the abdomen, categorized as: no, slight, or moderate/marked. The numbers of patients and deaths classified by treatment and ascites are given in Table 1.5.2.

The survival data from the trial were analyzed using Cox regression models with treatment and ascites as categorical explanatory variables. Table 5.2.7 shows estimated log(hazard ratios), both marginally and mutually adjusted in a model with no interaction. It is seen that there is no effect of treatment, whereas the hazard rate increases with amount of ascites. There is not much confounding: marginal estimates and adjusted estimates are almost identical. This is no surprise because of the randomization that should result in similar distributions of ascites in both treatment groups (although this did not quite happen for bilirubin in the PBC3 trial, Example 1.3); see Section 5.1.2.

Table 5.2.7. CSL1 trial: unadjusted and adjusted log(hazard ratios) of treatment and ascites.

	Unadjusted b	Adjusted b
Treatment: prednisone vs. placebo	−0.010 (0.117)	−0.034 (0.118)
Ascites: slight vs. no	0.584 (0.175)	0.583 (0.175)
Ascites: moderate/marked vs. no	1.301 (0.171)	1.296 (0.172)

However, the insignificant treatment effect conceals that there is an *interaction* between treatment and ascites; see Table 5.2.8. Patients without ascites seem to benefit significantly from prednisone treatment whereas the very same treatment seems to be harmful for patients with ascites. The table shows the parametrization where the treatment effects in subgroups of ascites are seen directly; see also Table 5.2.4. With this parametrization, the effects of ascites are those in the reference group (placebo) for treatment. To obtain those for the prednisone group, the treatment effects in the upper panel of the table should be added in the appropriate way. Table 5.2.9 shows the parametrization using the parameters useful for testing; see also Table 5.2.3. Note that the new parameters (but not their SD) can be calculated from Table 5.2.8: $0.875 = 0.560 - (-0.315)$ and $1.171 = 0.856 - (-0.315)$. Also note that $2 = (3 - 1)(2 - 1)$ interaction parameters are needed because ascites has three categories and treatment has two.

Table 5.2.8. CSL1 trial: log(hazard ratios) for treatment and ascites in model with interaction.

	b
Treatment: prednisone vs. placebo, patients with no ascites	−0.315 (0.139)
Treatment: prednisone vs. placebo, patients with slight ascites	0.560 (0.330)
Treatment: prednisone vs. placebo, patients with moderate/marked ascites	0.856 (0.314)
Ascites: slight vs. no placebo-treated patients	0.129 (0.275)
Ascites: moderate/marked vs. no placebo-treated patients	0.764 (0.254)

Table 5.2.9. CSL1 trial: model with interaction between treatment and ascites, interaction parameters.

	b
Treatment: prednisone vs. placebo in reference group, (i.e., patients with no ascites)	-0.315 (0.139)
Treatment: prednisone vs. placebo, difference between effects for patients with slight ascites and for reference group	0.875 (0.359)
Treatment: prednisone vs. placebo, difference between effects for patients with moderate/marked ascites and reference group	1.171 (0.344)
Ascites: slight vs. no placebo-treated patients	0.129 (0.275)
Ascites: moderate/marked vs. no placebo-treated patients	0.764 (0.254)

Table 5.2.10 presents likelihood ratio test statistics. It is seen that in models without interaction, ascites is highly significant (model 2 versus 0 or model 3 versus 1) whereas treatment is not (model 1 versus 0 or 3 versus 2). These test statistics, however, are not relevant to quote because of the highly significant interaction between treatment and ascites (model 4 versus 3). Thus the best way to summarize the results of the analyses is provided by the parameters in Table 5.2.8, in particular, when transforming to the hazard ratio scale. Thus the hazard ratios for treatment (prednisone versus placebo) are (with 95% confidence intervals): 0.73 (0.56,0.96) for patients without ascites, 1.75 (0.92,3.34) for patients with slight ascites, and 2.35 (1.27,4.36) for patients with moderate/marked ascites.

Table 5.2.10. CSL1 trial: LR tests for treatment, ascites and interaction.

Model	$-2\log L$	Test	LR Test	df	P
0: no covariates	3178.11				
1: only treatment	3177.38	1 vs. 0	0.73	1	0.39
2: only ascites	3128.48	2 vs. 0	49.63	2	<0.0001
3: treatment and ascites	3128.40	3 vs. 1	48.98	2	<0.0001
		3 vs. 2	0.08	1	0.78
4 interaction	3112.93	4 vs. 3	15.47	2	0.0004

5.2.2 One categorical and one quantitative covariate

Linear effect of the quantitative covariate: The vitamin D study

In Section 5.1.2 we discussed the vitamin D study, Example 1.1. Focus was on the relation between $\log_{10}(25OHD)$ measurements of vitamin D, y_i, and the quantitative covariate $x_{i,1}(= BMI - 25)$ and country $x_{i,2}$ (Ireland or Poland). The model (5.1.5), that we studied specifies the mean $E(y_i)$ of y_i to be

$$E(y_i) = a + b_1 x_{i,1} + b_2 I(x_{i,2} = \text{Ireland}).$$

In model (5.1.5) the linear effect (slope) b_1 of body mass index for women from Ireland is the same as that for women from Poland and the effect b_2 of country is the same for all values of BMI. The estimates in this *additive model* are: $\widehat{a} = 1.532(0.030), \widehat{b}_1 = -0.0152(0.0045), \widehat{b}_2 = 0.131(0.040)$.

To evaluate the assumption of no interaction we studied the scatterplot of y_i versus BMI, Figure 5.1.6, with separate regression lines for Poland and Ireland added. We now evaluate the hypothesis of no interaction more carefully. As in the previous subsection we show that different parametrizations of the model with interaction are useful for testing the hypothesis and for presenting results allowing for interaction, respectively.

Testing for no interaction

As an alternative to the additive model (5.1.5) we now introduce the corresponding model *with interaction* between BMI and country. One way of parametrizing this model is:

$$E(y_i) = a + b_1 x_{i,1} + b_2 I(x_{i,2} = \text{Ireland}) + b_{1,1} x_{i,1} \cdot I(x_{i,2} = \text{Ireland}), \quad (5.2.5)$$

where $x_{i,1}$ is now BMI-25 for the ith woman. In (5.2.5), the intercept a is then the expected $\log_{10}(25\text{OHD})$-value for Polish women with BMI= 25, b_2 the expected difference between $\log_{10}(25\text{OHD})$ values in Ireland and Poland when BMI= 25, b_1 is the slope of the regression line for Polish women, and $b_{1,1}$ the difference between the slopes of the regression lines for Ireland and Poland. Thus, the effect of BMI for Polish women is b_1 and for Irish women it is $b_1 + b_{1,1}$. The effect of country (Ireland versus Poland) is $b_2 + b_{1,1}(BMI - 25)$ for a woman with a given BMI. Note that the added covariate is the product of the two covariates from the additive model and that the hypothesis of no interaction can be formulated simply as no effect of this covariate:

$$H_0 : b_{1,1} = 0.$$

With this parametrization, testing for no interaction is simple, whereas the interpretation of the parameter, $b_{1,1}$, is less direct: it is a "difference between slopes." The maximum likelihood estimates of the regression parameters, $b_1, b_2, b_{1,1}$, are:

- Intercept, level of $\log_{10}(25\text{OHD})$ in the reference group for country (Poland) when BMI= 25: $\hat{a} = 1.512 \ (0.033)$
- Effect of BMI in the reference group for country (Poland): $\hat{b}_1 = -0.0101$ (0.0057)
- Effect of country (i.e., difference between countries) for BMI= 25: $\hat{b}_2 = 0.163 \ (0.045)$
- Interaction parameter, difference between BMI effects (slopes) in Ireland and in Poland: $\hat{b}_{1,1} = -0.0135 \ (0.0093)$

The Wald test statistic for no interaction, $b_{1,1} = 0$, takes the value $(-0.0135/0.0093)^2 = 2.10$ which, evaluated in the $\chi^2(1)$-distribution (or the $F(1, 102)$-distribution) gives a P-value of 0.15. Thus in this example there is no indication of different effects of BMI in Ireland and in Poland. The test for no interaction has one degree-of-freedom because it deals with a single parameter $b_{1,1}$. In general, for the test for no interaction between a categorical variable with, say $k + 1$ categories, and a quantitative covariate with a linear effect, the number of degrees of freedom is k.

Note that, in this model one can also test the hypotheses $b_1 = 0$ or $b_2 = 0$. These hypotheses, however, no longer correspond to tests for no overall effects of BMI and country, respectively, but relate to effects of one covariate only for a particular value for the other. In particular, the parameter b_2 for country relates to the value 25 for BMI and for other ways of centering BMI; that is, by subtracting values other than 25, this parameter would have been different. For example, without centering, the country effect (now for BMI= 0) would be 0.500 (0.257). Note that the standard deviation is considerably increased due to the fact that the parameter now corresponds to a heavy extrapolation outside the BMI range observed in the data. The test for no interaction, however, is not dependent on possible centering of BMI.

Presenting estimates in models with interaction

If there is indication of an interaction between the two explanatory variables then an alternative parametrization to (5.2.6) is to be preferred. Presence of interaction means that the effect of one covariate depends on the value of another, so, to report a model with interaction an obvious possibility is to present these different effects. In the previous Section 5.2.1 several such possibilities were available. With a binary and a quantitative covariate the relevant parametrization of the model with interaction, for the purpose of presenting estimates, is:

$$E(y_i) = a + b_2 I(x_{i,2} = \text{Ireland}) \qquad (5.2.6)$$
$$+ b_{1,0} x_{i,1} I(x_{i,2} = \text{Poland}) + b_{1,1} x_{i,1} I(x_{i,2} = \text{Ireland}).$$

In (5.2.6), a is still the expected $\log_{10}(25\text{OHD})$ level for BMI= 25 in the reference group for country (Poland), b_2 is again the effect of country (Ireland versus Poland) for BMI= 25, and $b_{1,0}$ and $b_{1,1}$, respectively, are the effects of BMI for Poland and for Ireland. With this parametrization, the hypothesis of no interaction is:

$$H_0 : b_{1,0} = b_{1,1}.$$

The maximum likelihood estimates in this parametrization may be computed directly from the previous ones:

- Intercept, level of $\log_{10}(25\text{OHD})$ in the reference group for country (Poland) when BMI=25: $\widehat{a} = 1.512 \ (0.033)$
- Effect of BMI for Poland: $\widehat{b}_{1,0} = -0.0101 \ (0.0057)$
- Effect of BMI for Ireland: $\widehat{b}_{1,1} = -0.0101 - 0.0135 = -0.0236 \ (0.0074)$
- Effect of country for BMI=25: $\widehat{b}_2 = 0.163 \ (0.045)$

Note that $\widehat{a}$ and $\widehat{b}_2$ are unchanged compared to the previous parametrization, that the new $\widehat{b}_{1,0}$ is identical to the old $\widehat{b}_1$, and that the interpretation (and value) of $\widehat{b}_{1,1}$ has changed.

Even though interaction is a symmetric concept, a reparametrization with focus on effects of country for different values of BMI is less appealing because there are, in fact, infinitely many country effects $b_2 + (b_{1,1} - b_{1,0})(BMI - 25)$. However, the estimated country effect as a function of BMI can be shown graphically; see Figure 5.2.1 where this straight line is shown with 95% confidence limits. The horizontal line in the figure represents the (constant) effect of country, 0.131, from the model with no interaction.

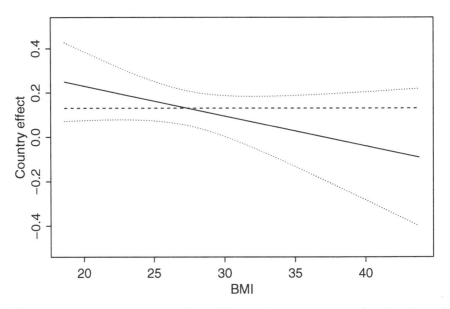

Fig. 5.2.1. Estimated country effect (difference between countries) as function of BMI.

In Section 5.1.2 we noticed that the log-transformation simplified the analysis in the sense that variance homogeneity was not rejected. Similarly, the transformation has simplified the model in the sense that the model with no interaction gave an adequate description of the data. Indeed, with the original 25OHD-values as outcome variable estimates in the model (5.2.5) with interaction are:

- Intercept, level of 25OHD in the reference group for country (Poland) when BMI= 25: $\widehat{a} = 35.115$ (2.508)
- Effect of BMI in the reference group for country (Poland): $\widehat{b}_1 = -0.647$ (0.437)
- Effect of country (difference between countries) for BMI= 25: $\widehat{b}_2 = 16.131$ (3.483)
- Interaction parameter, difference between BMI effects (slopes) in Ireland and in Poland: $\widehat{b}_{1,1} = -1.741$ (0.715)

On this scale the Wald test statistic for no interaction, $b_{1,1} = 0$, takes the significant value $(-1.741/0.715)^2 = 5.93$ ($P = 0.017$).

Stratification

We now illustrate how interaction can be handled by stratifying the data, that is, by analyzing data from Ireland and from Poland separately. Hereby, we automatically get country-specific effects of BMI whereas country effects are not presented explicitly. Thereby, an asymmetry between the two covariates is introduced. Note that stratification only works for a categorical covariate. As mentioned in the introduction to Section 5.2, in the simple model with no other covariates included this corresponds closely to the analysis presented above. The estimates are presented in Table 5.2.11. It is seen from the Wald tests that one could now conclude that the effect of BMI is only important in Ireland and not in Poland. However, our recommendation would be first to examine a possible interaction and next, if interaction does not seem important, to estimate the BMI effect jointly based on data from both countries, thereby obtaining a more precise estimate. With such an approach, simpler models are usually obtained and our recommendation, therefore, closely follows the principles discussed in Section 2.3.3.

Table 5.2.11. Vitamin D study: Estimates in country-specific models for BMI.

Country	Intercept	BMI-25	Wald (P)	Residual SD
Poland	1.511 (0.035)	−0.0101 (0.0061)	2.76 (0.10)	0.205
Ireland	1.675 (0.027)	−0.0236 (0.0064)	13.66 (0.0007)	0.166

Nonlinear effect of the quantitative covariate: the PBC3 trial

In Section 5.1.2 we studied the effect of treatment x_2, CyA versus placebo, in the PBC3 liver cirrhosis trial after adjustment for the effect of bilirubin x_1. We saw that, in spite of the randomization, bilirubin confounded the simple marginal comparison of the treatment groups because CyA-treated patients tended to have a somewhat higher bilirubin value than patients from the control group and because of the overwhelming effect of bilirubin. Previous analyses had shown that the effect of bilirubin was not linear thus we studied a hazard model of the form

$$\log(h_i(t)) = \log(h_0(t)) + b_2 x_{i,2} + \sum_{j=1}^{r} b_{1,j} f_j(x_{i,1})$$

(cf. (5.1.6)). Here, we used a number of different functions of x_1. In the simplest adjustment we considered the single transformed covariate $f_1(x_{i,1}) = \log(x_{i,1})$ and alternatives were based on the fractional polynomials $f_1(x_{i,1}) = x_{i,1}^{-0.5}$ and $f_2(x_{i,1}) = x_{i,1}^{-2}$. A third way of adjustment involved the range of normal bilirubin values by including the two covariates $f_1(x_{i,1}) = I(x_{i,1} > 17.1)$

and $f_2(x_{i,1}) = I(x_{i,1} > 17.1) \log(x_{i,1}/17.1)$. The adjusted treatment effects obtained from these models were all hazard ratios on the order of magnitude of $\exp(\widehat{b}_2) \approx 0.67$ and relied on the assumption of no interaction between treatment and bilirubin imposed by simply adding the terms for the two variables. In what follows we evaluate this assumption more systematically by extending model (5.1.6) with interaction terms. The simplest way of doing that (although notation is a bit involved, anyway) is to add covariates of the form $f_j(x_{i,1})x_{i,2}$, that is, product terms for the covariates from the additive model:

$$\log(h_i(t)) = \log(h_0(t)) + b_2 x_{i,2} + \sum_{j=1}^{r} (b_{1,j} f_j(x_{i,1}) + b_{1,j,1} f_j(x_{i,1}) x_{i,2}). \quad (5.2.7)$$

In (5.2.7) the hypothesis of no interaction is

$$H_0 : b_{1,1,1} = \cdots = b_{1,r,1} = 0$$

and $b_{1,j,1}$ is the difference between the effect of $f_j(x_{i,1})$ for CyA patients ($x_{i,2} = 1$) and placebo patients ($x_{i,2} = 0$). Test statistics for H_0 have r degrees-of-freedom. The treatment effect b_2 is the log(hazard ratio) when all $f_j(x_{i,1}) = 0$ and $b_{1,j}$ is the effect of $f_j(x_{i,1})$ for placebo-treated patients.

Table 5.2.12 shows the results from fitting these models and it is seen that the tests for no interaction are nowhere near significance. The coefficients $b_{1,j}$ and $b_{1,j,1}, j = 1, \ldots, r$ are hard to interpret but Figures 5.2.2 and 5.2.3 show the fitted linear predictors as a function of bilirubin, that is, $\sum_j \widehat{b}_{1,j} f_j(x_{i,1})$ for placebo and $\widehat{b}_2 + \sum_j (\widehat{b}_{1,j} + \widehat{b}_{1,j,1}) f_j(x_{i,1})$ for CyA. The figure for $f_1(x_{i,1}) = \log(x_{i,1})$ is omitted because this is just (much like Figure 5.1.6) two straight lines when plotted against log(bilirubin). Figures 5.2.2 and 5.2.3 show the nonparallel linear predictors ("response curves") and can be compared to the parallel curves in Figures 5.1.9 and 5.1.10. Although the tests for no interaction show that the extra flexibility in Figures 5.2.2 and 5.2.3 is not really needed, Figures 5.2.4 and 5.2.5 present the estimated treatment effects $\widehat{b}_2 + \sum_j \widehat{b}_{1,j,1} f_j(x_{i,1})$ as functions of bilirubin ($x_{i,1}$) with 95% confidence limits. These figures also show the (constant) treatment effect estimated from the corresponding models with parallel "response curves," that is, without interaction. For both sets of curves the difference lies in the predicted effect of treatment for low values of bilirubin (cf. the discussion in Section 5.1.2 where we concluded that the predictions from the model using fractional polynomials might be implausible for low values of bilirubin). Therefore, this model is included here only for purely illustrative purposes.

5.2.3 Two quantitative covariates

Two linear effects

In Section 5.1.3 we studied the data regarding birthweight (BW) and its relation to ultrasound measurements of abdominal diameter (AD) and biparietal diameter (BPD). We saw that, assuming no interaction between the

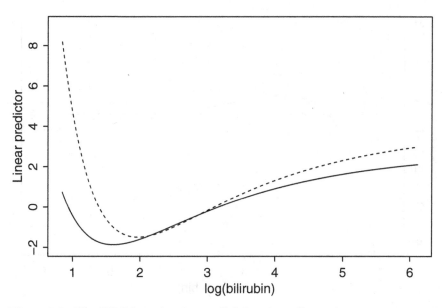

Fig. 5.2.2. The PBC-3 study: nonparallel linear predictors in treatment groups modeled using fractional polynomials.

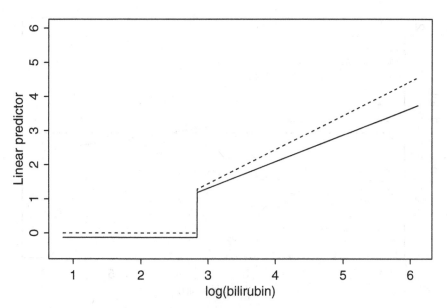

Fig. 5.2.3. The PBC-3 study: nonparallel linear predictors in treatment groups modeled as constant within the normal range (0,17.1).

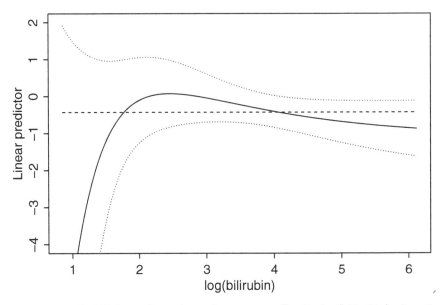

Fig. 5.2.4. The PBC3 study: estimated treatment effect by log(bilirubin) when the effect of bilirubin is modeled using fractional polynomials.

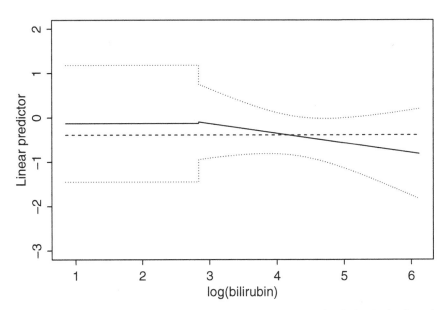

Fig. 5.2.5. The PBC3 study: estimated treatment effect by log(bilirubin) when the effect of bilirubin is modeled as constant within the normal range (0,17.1)

Table 5.2.12. PBC3: treatment effects and effects of bilirubin in models with interaction and nonlinear effects of bilirubin.

	Bilirubin			Interaction		Treatment	
$f_1(x_{i,1})$	$f_2(x_{i,1})$	$\widehat{b}_{1,1}$ (SD)	$\widehat{b}_{1,2}$ (SD)	$\widehat{b}_{1,1,1}$ (SD)	$\widehat{b}_{1,1,2}$ (SD)	$\widehat{b}_2$ (SD)	LR Test (P)
$\log(x_{i,1})$		1.111 (0.134)		−0.154 (0.193)		−0.209 (0.320)	0.63 (0.43)
$x_{i,1}^{-0.5}$	$x_{i,1}^{-2}$	−19.160 (2.623)	91.748 (24.742)	5.443 (3.537)	−53.794 (32.138)	−1.124 (0.528)	3.13 (0.21)
$I(x_{i,1} > 17.1)$	$I(x_{i,1} > 17.1)$ $\cdot \log(x_{i,1}/17.1)$	1.281 (0.428)	0.996 (0.171)	0.036 (0.799)	−0.220 (0.255)	−0.131 (0.671)	0.89 (0.64)

two covariates, the mean value of $y_i = \log_{10}(BW_i)$ could reasonably be described as increasing linearly with $x_{i,1} = \log_{10}(AD_i)$ for any fixed value of $x_{i,2} = \log_{10}(BPD_i)$ and, at the same time, it could be assumed to increase linearly with $\log_{10}(BPD)$ for any fixed value of $\log_{10}(AD)$. In this additive model

$$\text{LP}_i = \text{E}(y_i) = a + b_1 x_{i,1} + b_2 x_{i,2}$$

the estimates were $\widehat{b}_1 = 1.467, \widehat{b}_2 = 1.552$. A single strongly influential point with a low value of BPD was, however, discovered.

To examine a possible interaction between the two covariates a model describing departures from additivity is needed. In Section 5.1.3 we noted the geometric interpretation of additivity: the linear predictor described a plane in the three-dimensional space and for any fixed value, $x_{0,1}$, of the first covariate the intersection of that plane with one in the x_2-direction which is vertical and passes through $x_{0,1}$ is a line with slope b_2. If, more generally, the second covariate had a nonlinear effect then such an intersection would always provide a curve with the same shape. To model interaction between x_1 and x_2 corresponds to modeling how, for example, the effect of x_2 for given $x_1 = x_{0,1}$ varies among different choices of $x_{0,1}$ or, stated geometrically, to describing how such intersections vary from plane to plane.

Returning to the case with linear effects of both covariates and borrowing ideas from previous sections, a model allowing for interaction could be obtained by simply adding a product term to the linear predictor

$$\text{LP}_i = a + b_1 x_{i,1} + b_2 x_{i,2} + b_{1,1} x_{i,1} x_{i,2}. \tag{5.2.8}$$

In (5.2.8), the hypothesis

$$b_{1,1} = 0$$

corresponds to no interaction, so, testing for no interaction in this model is quite simple. The interpretation of the interaction parameter $b_{1,1}$ is, however, less intuitive. The effect of $x_{i,2}$ for given value, $x_{0,1}$, of the first covariate is

$$(b_2 + b_{1,1}x_{0,1})x_{i,2};$$

that is, for given value $(x_{0,1})$ of the first covariate, the effect of the second is linear with a slope that varies smoothly (in fact, linearly) with $x_{0,1}$.

For the birthweight data estimates from model (5.2.8) are: $\widehat{b}_1 = -7.119$ (4.052), $\widehat{b}_2 = -6.963(4.025)$, $\widehat{b}_{1,1} = 4.400(2.077)$; that is, the Wald test for no interaction is $(4.400/2.077)^2 = 4.49$ which, evaluated in the $\chi^2(1)$- (or $F(1, 103)$-) distribution gives $P = 0.037$ indicating a significant interaction between $\log_{10}(AD)$ and $\log_{10}(BPD)$ on the effect of $\log_{10}(BW)$. Table 5.2.13 presents the coefficients for the fitted lines giving the dependence of the linear predictor on $\log_{10}(BPD)$ for fixed values of AD= 90, 100, 110 mm, respectively. Figure 5.2.6 presents the results graphically. It is seen that the slope for $\log_{10}(BPD)$ increases with AD.

Table 5.2.13. Fitted linear effects of $x_2 = \log_{10}(BPD)$ for given values of $x_1 = \log_{10}(AD)$ according to model (5.2.8).

AD	$\log_{10}(AD)$	Intercept $\widehat{a} + \widehat{b}_1 \log_{10}(AD)$	Slope $\widehat{b}_1 + \widehat{b}_{1,1} \log_{10}(AD)$
90 mm	1.954	0.151	1.637
100 mm	2.000	−0.175	1.838
110 mm	2.041	−0.470	2.020

We see that, inasmuch as the interpretation of the interaction parameter $b_{1,1}$ is not very intuitive, it is not quite obvious how to present the results from a model including the product term $x_{i,1}x_{i,2}$ of two quantitative explanatory variables. Ease of interpretation may be obtained by *categorizing*, for example, $x_{i,1}$, and fitting separate linear effects for $x_{i,2}$ in each category (cf. Section 5.2.2). We did this using the cutpoints 95 and 105 mm for AD; that is, we fitted the model with the linear predictor

$$
\begin{aligned}
LP_i = a &+ b_{1,1}I(95 \leq AD < 105) + b_{1,2}I(105 \leq AD) \\
&+ b_{2,1}x_{i,2}I(AD < 95) + b_{2,2}x_{i,2}I(95 \leq AD < 105) \quad (5.2.9) \\
&+ b_{2,3}x_{i,2}I(105 \leq AD).
\end{aligned}
$$

In (5.2.9), the parameters $b_{2,1}, b_{2,2}$, and $b_{2,3}$ are the slopes for $\log_{10}(BPD)$ in each of the three intervals for AD and a is the intercept for the line for the first AD-interval (< 95 mm), $b_{1,1}$ the difference between intercepts for the second (95 to 105 mm) and the first AD-intervals, and $b_{1,2}$ the difference between intercepts for the third ($\geq$ 105 mm) and the first AD-intervals. The estimated slopes: 2.113 (0.273), 1.940 (0.477), 2.436 (0.510) are not significantly different ($P = 0.77$) and the estimated lines are shown in Figure 5.2.7. With this approach, estimates in the model with interaction are easier to interpret, however, the approach has a number of drawbacks. First, the choice

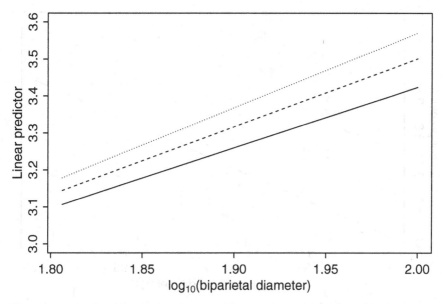

Fig. 5.2.6. Birthweight study: estimated linear effect of $\log_{10}$(BPD) for three different values of AD (90, 100, 110 mm).

of cutpoints for $x_{i,1}$ is not obvious: we chose "nice" values of AD close to tertiles in the distribution; second, the estimated linear predictor (5.2.9) is not a smooth function of $x_{i,1}$ which makes it less biologically plausible and, third, the test for no interaction is likely to be less powerful than when using $x_{i,1}$ as a quantitative variable.

All in all, the evidence against a model without interaction between $x_{i,1}$ and $x_{i,2}$ is not strong and, in fact, when studying Cook's distance for the model including the product term (Figure 5.2.8) it is seen that the same single observation which strongly affected the linearity of $\log_{10}$(BPD) (Section 5.1.3) is responsible for the significance of the product term. When removing this observation from the dataset, the product term is no longer significant ($P = 0.64$).

Nonlinear effects

In models where, for example, $x_{i,1}$ has a linear and $x_{i,2}$ a nonlinear effect, similar techniques for examining interaction may be applied. Thus, for a model with an effect

$$\sum_{j=1}^{r} b_{2,j} f_j(x_{i,2}) \tag{5.2.10}$$

of the second covariate one may add a product term between $x_{i,1}$ and (5.2.10), thereby obtaining a test for no interaction with as many degrees of freedom

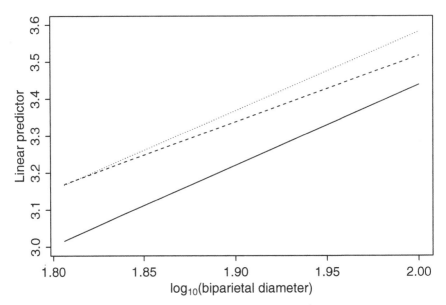

Fig. 5.2.7. Birthweight study: linear effects of $\log_{10}(\text{BPD})$ fitted separately for three different intervals of AD ($< 95, 95 - 105, \geq 105$ mm).

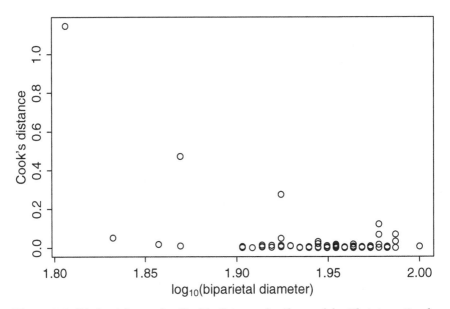

Fig. 5.2.8. Birthweight study: Cook's distance for the model with interaction between $\log_{10}(\text{AD})$ and $\log_{10}(\text{BPD})$ plotted against $\log_{10}(\text{BPD})$.

(r) as there are terms in the sum. Alternatively, one may categorize the first covariate and fit separate functions of the form (5.2.10) for the second covariate for each category. With, say k, categories for $x_{i,1}$ the resulting test for no interaction will have $r(k-1)$ degrees of freedom. Arguments for or against such approaches follow those for the situation with two linear effects closely.

5.2.4 Saving degrees-of-freedom

When examining interactions between two categorical explanatory variables, x_1, x_2, with k_1+1 and k_2+1 categories, respectively, we saw in Section 5.2.1 that the number of degrees-of-freedom in the test for the hypothesis of no interaction between x_1 and x_2 is $k_1 k_2$. Furthermore, in Section 5.2.2 we saw that the number of degrees-of-freedom when testing for no interaction between a categorical covariate x_1 with k_1+1 categories and a quantitative covariate x_2 with an effect modeled using k_2 functions was also $k_1 k_2$. Thus, when k_1 and k_2 are not small such tests will have many degrees-of-freedom .

Tests with many degrees-of-freedom tend to lack power (Section 2.3.3) because deviations from the hypothesis to be tested (here: the hypothesis of no interaction between x_1 and x_2) can be "in many directions." It is, therefore, of interest to reduce this number of degrees-of-freedom. That is the topic for the current section.

To illustrate ideas we continue the discussion of the CSL1 example (Example 1.7) from Section 5.2.1. We do this in spite of the fact that, in that example, the number of degrees-of-freedom when testing for no interaction between treatment (prednisone versus placebo) and ascites (no, slight, moderate/marked) was only two. However, the CSL1 example has already been introduced and the interaction is quite easy to understand. One way of presenting these two degrees-of-freedom is via parameters describing differences between the treatment effect for patients with slight ascites and for patients with no ascites and, on the other hand, the treatment effect for patients with moderate/marked ascites and for patients with no ascites. The estimates (on the log(hazard ratio) scale) for these two interaction parameters (Table 5.2.9) are 0.875 (0.359) and 1.171 (0.344), respectively, and the LR test for no interaction (Table 5.2.10) is 15.47 with two degrees-of-freedom ($P = 0.0004$).

One way of reducing the number of degrees-of-freedom (from 2 to 1) is to replace the categorical covariate ascites with a cruder version with only two categories: ascites absent versus ascites present, when describing the interaction while keeping the original covariate with three categories when describing the "main effect." That is, the model without interaction (Table 5.2.7) includes the same three indicator covariates as before: I(prednisone treatment), I(slight ascites), I(moderate/marked ascites), and the model with interaction is obtained by adding the single indicator variable I(prednisone, ascites present). Note that this variable can be obtained as

I(prednisone, ascites present)

$= I$(prednisone)$(I$(slight ascites) $+ I$(moderate/marked ascites))$.

The results from fitting the model with only one interaction parameter are found in Table 5.2.14. Minor changes are seen for the estimated main effects of ascites and the new interaction parameter 1.033, as expected, is between those quoted above (0.875 and 1.171) with a smaller SD signaling the gain in power. The LR test for no interaction is 15.05 with one degree-of-freedom ($P = 0.0001$).

Table 5.2.14. CSL1 trial: model with interaction between treatment and ascites including only one interaction parameter.

	b
Treatment: prednisone vs. placebo in reference group, (i.e., patients with no ascites)	-0.315 (0.139)
Treatment: prednisone vs. placebo, difference between effects for patients with ascites and for reference group	1.033 (0.269)
Ascites: slight vs. no placebo-treated patients	0.0292 (0.237)
Ascites: moderate/marked vs. no placebo-treated patients	0.840 (0.218)

Although the technique of reducing the number of degrees-of-freedom when testing the hypothesis of no interaction between two categorical covariates was not really needed in the CSL1 example, the idea can be used quite generally: keep the "detailed" covariates with "many" categories for modeling the main effects but use cruder versions with some categories collapsed for describing the interaction. For example, in the vitamin D study (Example 1.1), when testing for no interaction between the four countries and BMI in three categories, the test would have six degrees-of-freedom. This number could be reduced to three if two BMI categories were collapsed (e.g., those slightly overweight and those who are obese). Thereby the test would only examine whether the difference between vitamin D levels for women with or without a normal BMI differs between countries (assuming that the difference between the levels for obese and slightly overweight women was the same in all countries).

However, for the vitamin D study a more natural way of saving degrees-of-freedom would be to treat BMI as a quantitative covariate when testing for no interaction. This would also reduce the number of degrees-of-freedom to three. This idea seems most obvious to use when the main effect of BMI is also quantitative but it can, in fact, also be used when the main effect is categorical.

Let us finally study the situation with a categorical covariate (e.g., treatment: CyA versus placebo in the PBC-3 study, Example 1.3) and a quantitative covariate with a nonlinear effect (e.g., bilirubin in the PBC-3 study modeled using quadratic splines, Equation (4.2.6)). Here, the effect of bilirubin is modeled using six terms: a linear effect, a quadratic effect, and four quadratic splines, one for each quintile. Modeling interaction as described in Equation (5.2.7) would require another six parameters and the number of degrees-of-freedom for the test for no interaction is six. This number could be reduced to one if attention for the interaction were restricted to the linear term. That is, the main effect of bilirubin is then still modeled "detailed" using the six-parameter spline function but only a simplified version of this, the linear term, is allowed to interact with treatment, the idea being that this single degree-of-freedom may catch major deviations from parallel linear predictors.

5.3 Several covariates

In Section 5.1 we showed how to take the step from a model with a linear predictor with just one explanatory variable (as discussed in Chapters 3 and 4) to models with two. The basic idea consists of adding the building blocks for the two covariates. This results in a model without interaction between the two covariates and in Section 5.2 the discussion was extended to cover the situation where the study of such an interaction is in focus.

In this section, models with any number of explanatory variables are introduced. A main conclusion is that the step of extending the model from two to more covariates is as simple as the step of going from one to two. Therefore, this section is rather brief with many references to the two previous sections, however, as we show, a new concept of *higher-order interactions* (in particular, *three-factor interactions*) becomes relevant . To set ideas, we take as our starting point, a model with two covariates as discussed in Sections 5.1 and 5.2 and add further covariates (in fact, most often one covariate!) to this basic model. However, we emphasize that this is just to set the ideas and, in general, we do not recommend this kind of "forward selection" of variables into the models. In Chapter 6, we return to a more detailed discussion on when and why to include more covariates as well as to the interpretation of results from models with several covariates (Sections 6.1 and 6.2). We first, in Section 5.3.1, look at the situation where, in the initial model, the two covariates do not interact and study the consequences of adding further covariates to the linear predictor. In Section 5.3.2 we study the much more complex situation where the initial model contains an interaction.

5.3.1 Models without higher-order interactions

Let us, as our starting point, take the model for the vitamin D study (Example 1.1) considered in Section 5.1.2 where the outcome y_i is the $\log_{10}(25\text{OHD}$ for woman $i)$ and where two covariates were included: $x_{i,1}$ is

BMI (measured in kg/m^2) minus 25, and $x_{i,2}$ is country (Ireland versus Poland). We studied the additive model (cf. Equation (5.1.5)),

$$E(y_i) = a + b_1 x_{i,1} + b_2 I(x_{i,2} = \text{Ireland})$$

and obtained the estimates $\widehat{a} = 1.532$, $\widehat{b}_1 = -0.0152$, and $\widehat{b}_2 = 0.131$. That is, for given BMI, women from Ireland have on average a value of the outcome that is 0.131 larger than in Poland. Let us pose the question of how much this difference between countries is affected by also adjusting for age. We introduce the covariate $x_{i,3}$ defined as the age (in years) of woman i minus 70 years. Women from both countries are between 69 and 76 years old and they have similar average values (72.2 in Ireland and 71.6 in Poland). Furthermore, the distribution of BMI is not much related to age (see Figure 5.3.1) and therefore when adding age to the model, that is, studying the model

$$E(y_i) = a + b_1 x_{i,1} + b_2 I(x_{i,2} = \text{Ireland}) + b_3 x_{i,3}, \qquad (5.3.1)$$

we do not expect large changes in estimated values of b_1, b_2.

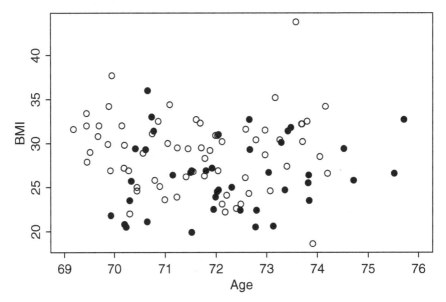

Fig. 5.3.1. Vitamin D study: BMI plotted against age for women from Ireland (circles) or Poland (dots).

This is, indeed, what we see when fitting (5.3.1) where the estimates are $\widehat{a} = 2.310(0.539)$, $\widehat{b}_1 = -0.0149(0.0045)$, $\widehat{b}_2 = 0.143(0.041)$, and $\widehat{b}_3 = -0.0187(0.0130)$. The interpretation of these values are as follows. The average value of the outcome for women from Poland, aged 70 years and with a

BMI of 25 is $\hat{a} = 2.310$; comparing women from the same country and with the same age and with body mass indices that differ by 1 kg/m^2 the average difference for the outcome is $\hat{b}_1 = -0.0149$; for women with the same BMI and same age, those from Ireland have average y-values that are $\hat{b}_2 = 0.143$ larger than for those from Poland and, finally, comparing women from the same country and with the same BMI and with ages that differ by 1 year the average difference for the outcome is $\hat{b}_3 = -0.0187$. Thus, the intercept is still the value of the linear predictor in (5.3.1) when all covariates are equal to 0, and regression coefficients are effects of the corresponding explanatory variables for given fixed values of all other covariates. In that respect, nothing is new here! Note, however, the new assumptions for the model.

- The effect of age is linear (when adjusting for country and BMI).
- There is no interaction between age and BMI (when adjusting for country).
- There is no interaction between age and country (when adjusting for BMI).

Also, the previous assumptions of no interaction between country and BMI and linear effect of BMI for given country should now be qualified as

- The effect of BMI is linear (when adjusting for country and age).
- There is no interaction between BMI and country (when adjusting for age)

The new assumptions (and the modifications of the old ones) can be examined using the type of methods that we have described previously. Thus, adding a quadratic term in age gives an $F(1, 101)$ distributed Wald test for linearity of $(-0.00446/0.00774)^2 = 0.34$ ($P = 0.57$). Furthermore, following the approach of Section 5.2.2, the test for no interaction between country and age gives $P = 0.55$, whereas that for no interaction between age and BMI (using a "linear-by-linear" interaction term, Section 5.2.3) gives $P = 0.72$. Thus, assumptions behind (5.3.1) seem not to be violated. This may be further illustrated via residual plots as exemplified in previous sections. The conclusion is that, for given age and BMI, Irish women have average $\log_{10}(25OHD)$ values which are 0.143 higher than Polish women. This value is close to what we saw without age adjustment and, in fact, age is insignificant in (5.3.1): Wald test for no age effect is $(-0.0187/0.0130)^2 = 2.07, P = 0.15$. The simplest interpretation of $\hat{b}_2 = 0.143$ is that $10^{\hat{b}_2} = 1.39$ is the ratio between median 25OHD values for women from Ireland compared to those from Poland for given values of BMI and age.

5.3.2 Models with higher-order interactions

Following the approach of the previous section one could add further covariates in the vitamin D example and study how the effect of country is affected. However, the situation is more complicated when the starting model contains interaction terms.

To illustrate this we study the CSL1 trial in liver cirrhosis (Example 1.7) discussed in Section 5.2.1. There we demonstrated that the effect of treatment (prednisone versus placebo) on survival depends on the level of ascites; see Tables 5.2.8 and 5.2.9. In the present section, for the sake of simplicity, we study a simpler version of the ascites variable with only two levels: absent versus present. To do this we define two explanatory variables:

$$x_{i,1} = I(\text{patient } i \text{ is treated with prednisone}),$$
$$x_{i,2} = I(\text{patient } i \text{ has ascites})$$

and consider the following model for the log(hazard) for patient i:

$$l_i(t) = l_0(t) + b_{1,0}x_{i,1}(1 - x_{i,2}) + b_{1,1}x_{i,1}x_{i,2} + b_2x_{i,2}.$$

Fitting this model we get $\widehat{b}_{1,0} = -0.313(0.139)$ as the estimated log(hazard ratio) for treatment (prednisone versus placebo) for patients without ascites, $\widehat{b}_{1,1} = 0.616(0.227)$ as the estimated log(hazard ratio) for treatment (prednisone versus placebo) for patients with ascites, and $\widehat{b}_2 = 0.425(0.197)$ as the estimated log(hazard ratio) for ascites (present versus absent) for patients treated with placebo. Wald tests for all three parameters are significant; that is, prednisone significantly reduces the hazard for patients without ascites and prednisone is significantly harmful for patients with ascites. Finally, presence of ascites increases the hazard for placebo-treated patients. The likelihood ratio test for no interaction between $x_{i,1}$ and $x_{i,2}$ is 12.33 which evaluated in the $\chi^2(1)$ distribution gives $P < 0.0001$.

   With this model as our starting point, we now study the effect of also including the covariate gender

$$x_{i,3} = I(\text{patient } i \text{ is a man}).$$

Simply adding $b_3x_{i,3}$ to the linear predictor gives estimates similar to those above: $\widehat{b}_{1,0} = -0.302(0.139)$, $\widehat{b}_{1,1} = 0.612(0.228)$, and $\widehat{b}_2 = 0.437(0.197)$, and the effect of gender (male versus female) is $\widehat{b}_3 = 0.223(0.121)$ with a Wald test of 3.40 (1 degree-of-freedom, $P = 0.07$). When adding this covariate, however, its potential interaction with both treatment and ascites should be considered. This leads to a number of different questions involving either "higher- (third) order interactions" or several two-factor interactions.

   We discuss these issues by focusing on the effect of treatment and start by considering the most general model where this effect is allowed to differ among all four combinations of ascites and gender. This corresponds to treating these four combinations as the values of a single categorical explanatory variable, as discussed in Section 5.2.1, and allow an interaction between this covariate and treatment. The parametrization of the resulting model is shown in Table 5.3.1. In the "overall reference group," placebo-treated women without ascites ($x_{i,1} = x_{i,2} = x_{i,3} = 0$), the log(hazard) is the baseline, $\log(h_0(t))$ and for other combinations of the three covariates, the parameters shown in the table should be added to the log(baseline hazard). For men, b_3 is added, for women with ascites, $b_{2,0}$ is added, for men with ascites, $b_{2,1}$ is added, and finally, for prednisone-treated patients, the relevant "b_{1,j_1,j_2}"-parameter is added when ascites, $x_{i,2} = j_1$ and gender, $x_{i,3} = j_2$, for $j_1, j_2 = 0$ or 1.

Table 5.3.1. CSL1 trial: parameters in model with interaction between treatment and combinations of gender and ascites.

| | Placebo: $x_{i,1} = 0$ | | Prednisone: $x_{i,1} = 1$ | |
Gender	No Ascites: $x_{i,2} = 0$	Ascites: $x_{i,2} = 1$	No Ascites: $x_{i,2} = 0$	Ascites: $x_{i,2} = 1$
Women: $x_{i,3} = 0$	Reference	$b_{2,0}$	$b_{1,0,0}$	$b_{2,0} + b_{1,1,0}$
Men: $x_{i,3} = 1$	b_3	$b_3 + b_{2,1}$	$b_3 + b_{1,0,1}$	$b_3 + b_{2,1} + b_{1,1,1}$

Table 5.3.2 shows the explanatory variables one needs to include to fit this model. The table also shows estimates and SD. These estimates have the following interpretations.

- b_3: The hazard ratio between placebo-treated men and women without ascites is $\exp(-0.017) = 0.983$.
- $b_{2,0}$: The hazard ratio between placebo-treated women with and without ascites is $\exp(0.335) = 1.397$.
- $b_{2,1}$: The hazard ratio between placebo-treated men with and without ascites is $\exp(0.495) = 1.640$.
- $b_{1,0,0}$: The hazard ratio between prednisone- and placebo-treated women without ascites is $\exp(-0.594) = 0.552$.
- $b_{1,1,0}$: The hazard ratio between prednisone- and placebo-treated women with ascites is $\exp(0.439) = 1.551$.
- $b_{1,0,1}$: The hazard ratio between prednisone- and placebo-treated men without ascites is $\exp(-0.123) = 0.884$.
- $b_{1,1,1}$: The hazard ratio between prednisone- and placebo-treated men with ascites is $\exp(0.719) = 2.052$.

It is seen that there is one effect of gender in the combined reference group for ascites and treatment, there are two effects of ascites, for women and men, respectively, in the reference group for treatment, and as discusssed above, there are four effects of treatment, one for each combination of gender and ascites. It should be emphasized that this is only one out of several possible ways of parametrizing the model with a three-factor interaction. It focuses on the treatment effect because this is the covariate of primary interest in the CSL1 study. For placebo-treated patients, there is an interaction between ascites and gender parametrized as separate ascites effects for women and men. For this interaction other parametrizations (as discussed in Section 5.2.1)

Table 5.3.2. CSL1 trial: covariates and estimates in model with interaction between treatment and combinations of gender and ascites.

Parameter	Covariate	Estimate, $\widehat{b}$	SD
b_3	$x_{i,3}$	−0.017	0.188
$b_{2,0}$	$x_{i,2}(1 - x_{i,3})$	0.335	0.304
$b_{2,1}$	$x_{i,2}x_{i,3}$	0.495	0.259
$b_{1,0,0}$	$x_{i,1}(1 - x_{i,2})(1 - x_{i,3})$	−0.594	0.227
$b_{1,1,0}$	$x_{i,1}x_{i,2}(1 - x_{i,3})$	0.439	0.367
$b_{1,0,1}$	$x_{i,1}(1 - x_{i,2})x_{i,3}$	−0.123	0.176
$b_{1,1,1}$	$x_{i,1}x_{i,2}x_{i,3}$	0.719	0.291

could have been studied. The interaction between gender and ascites in the placebo group is far from significant (the LR test statistic for no interaction is 0.17 with 1 d.f., $P = 0.68$) and the two covariates $x_{i,2}(1 - x_{i,3})$ and $x_{i,2}x_{i,3}$ could be replaced by ascites $x_{i,2}$ without changing the results for the treatment presented in the following. However, we have chosen to keep the interaction in the model.

To study the structure of the four treatment effects, a number of model reductions can be considered. Treatment effects in these reduced models are all shown in Table 5.3.3. First, one could ask whether the four treatment effects can be replaced by one common effect, that is, replacing the last four covariates in Table 5.3.2 by $x_{i,1}$. In this reduced model the treatment effect (log(hazard ratio) for prednisone versus placebo) is $\widehat{b}_1 = -0.052(0.118)$ (see lower-right corner of the table) but, as expected because of the interaction between treatment and ascites, the test for this model reduction is highly significant: LR test 15.0, 3 d.f., $P = 0.002$. Two alternative and "smaller" model reductions to study are those where either the treatment effect only depends on ascites or it only depends on gender. To fit the former, the last four covariates in Table 5.3.2 are replaced by $x_{i,1}(1 - x_{i,2})$ and $x_{i,1}x_{i,2}$, whereas, to fit the latter, they are replaced by $x_{i,1}(1 - x_{i,3})$ and $x_{i,1}x_{i,3}$. The estimated treatment effects for both submodels are shown in Table 5.3.3 (bottom line and rightmost column, respectively). When removing the interaction between treatment and gender, the estimated hazard ratios for treatment are $\exp(-0.303) = 0.738$ and $\exp(0.610) = 1.841$ for patients without and with ascites, respectively. The test for reducing to this model is insignificant: LR test 3.08, 2 d.f., $P = 0.21$. The test for reducing to the model where treatment only interacts with gender (i.e., no interaction between treatment and ascites) is, however, highly significant as expected: LR test 11.97, 2 d.f., $P = 0.003$.

Let us, finally, mention that still another reduction of the model may be studied, namely one where the four treatment effects for the ascites by gender combinations are additive in ascites and gender. The test for this reduction is insignificant: LR test 0.13, 1 d.f., $P = 0.72$. However, the interpretation of the estimates in the resulting model is rather complicated and therefore is not presented.

Table 5.3.3. CSL1 trial: treatment effects (SD) depending on gender and/or ascites.

Gender	No Ascites $x_{i,2} = 0$	Ascites $x_{i,2} = 1$	Both Ascites and no Ascites	P for Model Reduction
Women: $x_{i,3} = 0$	−0.594 (0.227)	0.439 (0.367)	−0.315 (0.193)	
Men: $x_{i,3} = 1$	−0.123 (0.176)	0.719 (0.291)	0.108 (0.149)	0.002
Both sexes	−0.303 (0.139)	0.610 (0.227)	−0.052 (0.118)	
P for Model Reduction	0.21		0.002	

All in all, as illustrated by the CSL1 example, models with higher-order interactions are complex and, in general, we recommend not to focus too much on examining such interactions when analyzing regression models.

Digression. Using "interaction notation"

As mentioned in Section 5.2, a special notation for interactions is sometimes used both in textbooks discussing the topic (e.g., Clayton and Hills, 1993, Ch. 24). Thus, an interaction term between two (categorical) explanatory variables A (ascites) and T (treatment) is denoted $A.T$ (or $A * T$) and a three-factor interaction between A, G (gender) and T is $A.G.T$. Using this notation, we first fitted the seven-parameter model including the three-factor interaction:

$$A + G + T + A.G + A.T + G.T + A.G.T$$

whereas the model excluding the interaction between ascites and gender for placebo-treated patients is the six-parameter model

$$A + G + T + A.T + G.T + A.G.T.$$

Furthermore, the reduced model taking the interaction between treatment and gender out is the five-parameter model

$$A + G + T + A.G + A.T$$

and allowing for no ascites–gender interaction it is the four-parameter model

$$A + G + T + A.T.$$

Leaving instead the interaction between ascites and treatment out, the five-parameter model becomes

$$A + G + T + A.G + G.T,$$

or, when also the ascites–gender interaction is eliminated, it is

$$A + G + T + G.T.$$

The final model where the gender–ascites interaction with treatment is additive is the six-parameter model

$$A + G + T + A.G + A.T + G.T$$

and, again, the ascites–gender interaction may be eliminated leading to

$$A + G + T + A.T + G.T.$$

However, as also discussed in Section 5.2, we have chosen not to highlight this notation because we believe that using indicator variables is a more direct way to set up the models parametrized in the most convenient way both when discussing them in mathematical terms and when implementing them in computer programs. Furthermore, different computer programs may use the interaction notation differently. ◇

This section and the previous one have shown that including more explanatory variables than two in multiple regression models is quite simple as long as no higher-order interactions are studied. This section has also shown how higher-order interactions may become relevant in such models but that this will complicate the models and their interpretation considerably. For this reason we believe that one should, in general, be reluctant to focus on higher-order interactions. In the next chapter (Section 6.1.7) as part of a discussion of general principles for model building, we also discuss principles more systematically for when to include interactions in models with a linear predictor.

5.4 Matched studies

Previously, we have studied the situation where only one response variable y_i was observed for the ith experimental unit (typically, the ith subject/patient). However, in many situations the same unit may provide several observations, often as a consequence of a *paired* or otherwise *matched* design. A special case of paired observations is one where the same response variable is recorded in the same subjects before and after an intervention or, more generally, several repeated measurements are taken over time in the same subjects. In such examples, independence between observations from the same subject or from the same matched set will most often be an unreasonable assumption.

In this section we discuss a simple approach to solve this problem, namely to include "subject" or "matched set" as a categorical covariate. We demonstrate how this works for both quantitative outcomes (the paired t-test), binary outcomes (conditional logistic regression, McNemar's test) as well as for survival times (the Cox regression model for survival in matched pairs). In Section 8.1, some more advanced techniques for how to address this problem are briefly introduced without going into details, as such details are beyond the scope of the book.

For notation, let $y_{i,j}, i = 1, \ldots, n, j = 1, \ldots, N_i$ be the observations of the response, where i refers to the subject (or matched set) and $j = 1, \ldots, N_i$ to the observations for the ith subject (or individuals in the ith matched set). We focus on paired data, that is, all $N_i = 2$, and for the three types of outcome variable we study the situation with a single binary covariate in detail and briefly discuss how to add more explanatory variables.

Quantitative outcomes

In Example 1.12 ("study 1"), 120 patients had their serum tryptase (in μ g/L) measured before and after orthopedic surgery and it is of interest to study whether the level of tryptase is affected by surgery. Thus, $n = 120$ patients provide $N = 2$ measurements each, $y_{i,1} =$"tryptase before surgery" and $y_{i,2} =$"tryptase after surgery" and we define the binary covariate $x_{i,1} = 0$ ($\sim$ "before") and $x_{i,1} = 1$ ($\sim$ "after"). The two repeated measurements from patient i cannot reasonably be considered independent but the deviations of the responses $y_{i,1}, y_{i,2}$ from a patient-specific level a_i may. We therefore consider the following model for the mean response

$$\mathrm{E}(y_{i,j}) = a_i + b_2 x_{i,j} \tag{5.4.1}$$

or written in a more familiar form, explicitly treating "patient" as a categorical covariate with reference level $i = 1$,

$$\mathrm{E}(y_{i,j}) = a + b_{1,i} I(\text{patient} = i) + b_2 x_{i,j},$$

where $a = a_1$ and $b_{1,i} = a_i - a_1, i = 2, \ldots, n$. That is, the a_i- (or $a, b_{1,i}$-) parameters describe the patient-specific tryptase levels and b_2 is the expected change in response from before to after surgery for any given patient. The assumption of no interaction between patient and covariate, that is, the same mean change in tryptase for all patients cannot be formally tested inasmuch as the model with interaction contains as many parameters as there are observations. However, it may be examined by plotting the "after" measurements $y_{i,2}$ against the "before" measurements $y_{i,1}$, or by plotting the within-patient differences against the patient averages (the "Bland–Altman plot"; see Altman and Bland, 1983); see Figure 5.4.1. In the figure, we have used the log-transformed tryptase measurements because the points on the after versus before plot seem to approximate a straight line with slope 1 closer when studying the log-transformed values than when using the raw data (Figure 1.5.6 in Section 1.5). We therefore restrict attention to the log-transformed values in the following and for those data the assumption of no interaction is not contraindicated.

The estimated effect of x is $\widehat{b_2} = -0.0953(0.0195)$ and the Wald test for no effect is $(-0.0953/0.0195)^2 = 23.80$ giving a P-value less than 0.0001. This shows that the level of tryptase decreases highly significantly (by about 9.5%) during surgery, likely owing to the fact that fluid is given to patients during

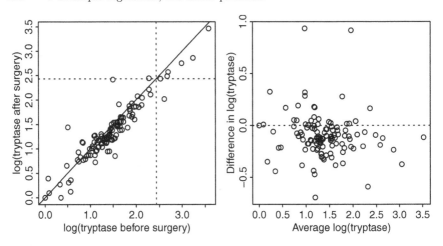

Fig. 5.4.1. Tryptase data, log scale. Left: measurements after surgery plotted against measurements before; the line is the identity line. A threshold at 11.4 μ g/L has been indicated. Right: difference between measurements after surgery and measurements before plotted against patient averages.

anesthesia. The intercept and the effects of "patient" are usually not given because there is one parameter estimate for each of the $n = 120$ subjects and, therefore, these estimates are of no interest, so-called "nuisance" parameters.

These results correspond to the *paired t*-test. The estimate is simply the mean difference between after and before measurements

$$\widehat{b}_2 = \frac{1}{n} \sum_{i=1}^{n} (y_{i,2} - y_{i,1})$$

and $\mathrm{SD}(\widehat{b}_2)$ the empirical standard deviation of this mean

$$\mathrm{SD}(\widehat{b}_2)^2 = \frac{1}{n-1} \sum_{i=1}^{n} (y_{i,2} - y_{i,1})^2.$$

If the differences are Normally distributed with a common SD the signed square root of the Wald test statistic follows a t-distribution with $n-1$ degrees of freedom when there is no effect of the covariate.

Writing the model as the linear model (5.4.1), it is simple to adjust the comparison between means of before and after measurements for other co-variates by adding more terms to the linear predictor. Note, however, that the effect of covariates which are constant within pairs cannot be estimated when, as in (5.4.1) each pair has its own fixed, unknown level, a_i. To estimate such effects, "random effects models," studied in Section 8.1.1, may be applied. Also, note that the model formulation (5.4.1) immediately generalizes to more than two measurements per subject by including a_i in the linear predictor for all measurements from subject i. The inference, however, becomes more complicated and can no longer be based on a single set of differences. In fact, when several measurements are taken over time, it is crucial to take the temporal aspects of the data into account and allow for a possible *autocorrelation* between repeated measurements; see Section 8.1.3 .

Binary outcomes

A completely analogous situation occurs for binary outcome data. We first study the situation with paired data; that is, $y_{i,1}$ and $y_{i,2}$ are now binary outcomes observed before ($x_{i,1} = 0$) or after ($x_{i,2} = 1$) intervention. In Example 1.12 we could have $y_{i,j} = 1$ if the tryptase measurement for patient i taken at occasion j (before or after surgery) were above the threshold for normal values, 11.4 μg/L; see Figure 5.4.1 where this threshold has been indicated. (Note that y now denotes this binary outcome and the y above was the tryptase measurement, possibly log-transformed.) We can then study the "standard" logistic regression model including the covariates x and the categorical covariate "patient":

$$\text{logit}(\text{pr}(y_{i,j} = 1)) = a_i + b_2 x_{i,j}. \tag{5.4.2}$$

Here, $\exp(b_2)$ is the ratio for any given patient between the odds of having tryptase above normal after surgery compared to before. However, inference for (5.4.2) turns out (e.g., Clayton and Hills, 1993, Ch. 29) to be complicated by the presence of the many nuisance parameters (one a_i parameter for each of the n patients), and maximum likelihood estimates based on this model are not consistent: even for large n, the parameter estimates do not get close to the true population values. Instead, *conditional logistic regression* may be used. Intuitively, pairs where either $y_{i,1} = y_{i,2} = 0$ or $y_{i,1} = y_{i,2} = 1$ do not provide any information on how x affects the outcome as long as the probability in (5.4.2) has an arbitrary level given by the parameter a_i. This means only pairs that are *discordant* with respect to the outcome contribute to the inference. Conditional logistic regression then amounts to studying the conditional likelihood where the contribution from such a discordant pair is the conditional probability of observing the configuration of outcomes seen in the data (either $y_{i,1} = 0, y_{i,2} = 1$ or $y_{i,1} = 1, y_{i,2} = 0$) given that one response was 0 and the other was 1. It turns out that this conditional probability does not depend on a_i and, thereby, "the nuisance parameters $a_1, \dots, a_n$ have been eliminated by conditioning."

Digression. Conditioning

Note that the problem of inconsistency of $\widehat{b}_2$ in the presence of n nuisance parameters did not occur for quantitative outcomes. However, conditioning on the sum $y_{i,1} + y_{i,2}$, as we just did for binary outcome data, would also lead to the paired t-test for quantitative data. ◇

For the tryptase data little information is left when dichotomizing the outcome as seen in Table 5.4.1 that includes only three pairs which are discordant on the outcome. The following analyses are, therefore, included only as an illustration and should not be taken as a serious analysis of these data.

Table 5.4.1. Tryptase data: numbers of patients according to normal ($\leq 11.4\,\mu$ g/L) or increased ($> 11.4\,\mu$ g/L) tryptase level before and after surgery.

	After		
Before	≤ 11.4	> 11.4	Total
≤ 11.4	$n_{0,0} = 112$	$n_{1,0} = 1$	113
> 11.4	$n_{0,1} = 2$	$n_{1,1} = 5$	7
Total	114	6	$n = 120$

In Table 5.4.1, the following notation is introduced: $n_{0,1} = 2$ is the number of discordant pairs of observations where $y_{i,1} = 1$, that is, tryptase was raised before surgery but not after, and $n_{1,0} = 1$ is the number of discordant pairs of observations where $y_{i,2} = 1$, that is, tryptase was raised after surgery but not before. The conditional maximum likelihood estimator for the odds ratio $\exp(b_2)$ is extremely simple in this two sample situation

$$\exp(\widehat{b_2}) = \frac{n_{1,0}}{n_{0,1}} = \frac{1}{2} = 0.5$$

and so is the score test for the hypothesis $b_2 = 0$

$$\frac{(n_{1,0} - n_{0,1})^2}{n_{1,0} + n_{0,1}} = \frac{1}{3} = 0.33.$$

This test is known as *McNemar's* test for paired binary data and has in large samples (which is hardly the situation here) an approximate Chi-squared distribution with one degree-of-freedom. The standard deviation of $\widehat{b_2}$ is

$$\text{SD}(\widehat{b_2}) = \sqrt{\frac{1}{n_{0,1}} + \frac{1}{n_{1,0}}} = \sqrt{1.5} = 1.22.$$

In particular in small samples, the hypothesis $b_2 = 0$ may be more reliably examined using a test for a probability of 0.5 based on observing $n_{0,1}$ (or $n_{1,0}$) in the Binomial distribution with count parameter $c = n_{0,1} + n_{1,0}$ (Section 2.3.3). However, for the tryptase example where $c = 3$ it makes no sense to present the details.

As for quantitative responses, adjustment for other covariates is possible simply by adding the appropriate terms to the linear predictor in (5.4.2). Note, however, that the conditional inference prevents estimation of effects of covariates which are constant within pairs. This is similar to the case of quantitative data and, as for those, estimation of such effects may be performed using random effects models (Section 8.1.1). Finally, again similarly to the case of quantitative responses, more than two binary responses may be handled using (5.4.2), although the contributions to the conditional likelihood become more complicated in that case.

Another example of paired binary responses appears in an individually matched case-control study (introduced in Section 7.4.2).

Survival time outcomes

For survival data, a model for matched pairs similar to (5.4.1) and (5.4.2) is the highly stratified Cox model for the log(hazard rate)

$$l_{i,j}(t) = \log(h_{0,i}(t)) + b_2 x_{i,j} \qquad (5.4.3)$$

(Holt and Prentice, 1974) where we first study the case where the covariate x is a binary exposure. Note that (5.4.3) is simply (5.1.4) but now, each matched pair i has a separate completely unspecified baseline hazard $h_{0,i}(t)$ and, obviously, it is impossible to estimate this based on only two possibly censored, survival times $y_{i,1}, y_{i,2}$. However, the effect of x is estimable using methods similar to what we saw above for binary responses based on a so-called "partial likelihood". Note that $\exp(b_2)$ is the ratio between the hazard rates for the two subjects from the same matched pair where one has $x = 1$ and the other has $x = 0$. Only pairs where the smaller of $y_{i,1}, y_{i,2}$ is an uncensored failure time provide information on b_2 because otherwise we have no information on the order in which the two subjects in a pair fail. Furthermore, among such pairs, only those that are *discordant on exposure* contribute. The estimator is $\exp(\widehat{b_2}) = n_{1,0}/n_{0,1}$, the score test for no effect of x is $(n_{1,0} - n_{0,1})^2/(n_{1,0} + n_{0,1})$, and $\text{SD}(\widehat{b_2}) = \sqrt{1/n_{1,0} + 1/n_{0,1}}$ just as for binary outcomes where now

$n_{1,0}$ = number of pairs, discordant on exposure, where the smaller of
$\qquad y_{i,1}, y_{i,2}$ is a failure time for an exposed subject,

and

$n_{0,1}$ = number of pairs, discordant on exposure, where the smaller of
$\qquad y_{i,1}, y_{i,2}$ is a failure time for an unexposed subject.

Digression. Partial likelihood

The arguments leading to the estimate for b_2 in (5.4.3) requires the concept of a "partial likelihood". This concept can also lead to the estimating equations for the standard Cox regression model that we have seen in previous chapters (e.g. (3.1.28) and (4.1.18)). However, as those equations also have more traditional likelihood interpretations (e.g., Andersen et al., 1993, Ch. 7) we have chosen not to introduce partial likelihood earlier. ◇

As for quantitative and binary responses adjustment for covariates that are not constant within pairs is performed by adding the proper terms to the linear predictor in (5.4.3). Also, extension to the case of more than two subjects per matched set is obvious. However, the fact that few out of the n matched sets contribute to the inference for b_2 (as a consequence of the completely unspecified baseline hazard) somewhat reduces the usefulness of (5.4.3) and, more often, random effects (or "frailty") models, briefly introduced in Section 8.1.1, are applied.

5.5 Exercises

Exercise 5.1. Use the tryptase data set 3 from Example 1.12 for identifying explanatory variables for baseline tryptase.

1. Include age as a linear spline with thresholds at 40 and 60, and with an interaction with gender.
2. Make model checks and consider the possibility of a logarithmic transformation of the baseline value.
3. Do we see a significant interaction between gender and age?
4. Is it necessary to include the bends in the effect of age, or can we reduce it to a linear effect?
5. Is the ASA classification significantly related to the baseline value?

Exercise 5.2. Use the tryptase data set 2 from Example 1.12 for identifying explanatory variables for reaction tryptase, on a logarithmic scale.

1. Include gender and ASA (categories 3 and 4 taken together) as categorical covariates and age as a linear effect.
2. What happens when we also include baseline tryptase (on a logarithmic scale) as an explanatory variable? Do we still see an effect of gender?
3. Does it make sense to include also the binary covariate "positive" that indicates whether the patient does in fact experience an allergic reaction? If it is included, what happens to the effects of age and gender? And why?

Exercise 5.3. The data set 2 from Example 1.12 contains information on the type of allergic reaction, classified into four groups. Collapse these into a binary outcome by joining categories 1–2 and 3–4.

1. Perform a logistic regression relating the probability of a severe reaction to age and gender.
2. Investigate whether the effect of age is linear, by including a quadratic term and testing its significance, and by using a linear spline with threshold in 60 years. Is the linearity a sufficiently good description?

3. Are baseline tryptase and/or reaction tryptase significant when entered into the model?

Exercise 5.4. Use the patients that have been subjected to a test for allergy following the surgery (tested= 1) in the tryptase data set 2 from Example 1.12.

1. Relate the probability of a positive test result to ASA class (three groups, combining class 3 and 4) and age, using a linear effect of age with a logit link.
2. Show that the interaction between ASA class and age is not significant.

Exercise 5.5. Use the tetrahymena data from Example 1.6 In Section 4.1.1 relating average cell diameter to cell concentration for the media without glucose. We now also include the media with glucose for comparison.

1. For the glucose media, make a logarithmic transformation of cell diameter and relate it to the logarithmic transformation of cell concentration through a simple linear regression.
2. Include both media in the model and compare the effect of cell concentration in the two media. Do we see the same effect?

Exercise 5.6. Use the surgery data from Example 1.4 for investigating the possible explanatory variables for the duration of anesthesia.

1. Include type of surgery and age as explanatory variables in a logistic regression.
2. Perform model checks for the assumption of a linear age effects, using residual plots as well as a numerical check by including a quadratic term in age.
3. Do we see any effect of the neuromuscular blocking agent?

Exercise 5.7. In Exercise 3.18 we used the surgery data from Example 1.4 for comparison of TOF-ratios for the three neuromuscular blocking agents. We now investigate this difference further.

1. Include blocking agent, type of surgery, and duration of anesthesia (linear effect) as explanatory variables in a logistic regression.
2. Perform model checks for the assumption of a linear effect of duration, using residual plots as well as a numerical check by including a quadratic term.
3. Do we see any effect of the neuromuscular blocking agent?

Exercise 5.8. Use the data from Example 1.10 to study possible covariates for the survival after malignant melanoma.

1. Include age and tumor thickness as quantitative covariates with linear effects in a Cox regression model.

2. How can we investigate a possible interaction between these two quantitative variables?

Exercise 5.9. Use data from the PBC-3 Example 1.3 to investigate the difference between the two treatments of liver cirrhosis.

1. Estimate the treatment effect, when adjusting for a linear effect of bilirubin, on a logarithmic scale and a linear effect of albumin on the untransformed scale.
2. Perform a model check for the linearity assumption corresponding to the untransformed albumin, by categorization of the covariate into quintile groups.

6

Model building: From purpose to conclusion

To investigate a scientific question, data are needed. Sometimes, data may already be available, but in many situations new data have to be collected because the question is concerned with a new procedure or treatment or requires new covariates to be considered for a previously studied phenomenon.

Careful planning before data collection may prevent a waste of time and money and help increase the probability that the investigation will be sufficiently informative to actually answer our questions. The first step after formulating the idea for the new scientific question is to study the literature to see if anything has been published regarding this matter. Previous studies related to the subject may help in developing your own idea into a plan for a new investigation that can provide the necessary information, for example, a list of outcome variables and explanatory variables that should be obtained in order to shed light on the problems at hand. Take care to think through the possible mechanisms involved in your problem in order to make sure that all relevant variables will be measured. Do not measure "everything" but at the same time, do not be too restrictive because obtaining information afterwards may be impossible or at least very cumbersome and perhaps expensive.

The design of a new investigation must be considered in combination with the available resources. For example, a prospective study will have a long time horizon before the study can be finished whereas a case-control study (see Section 7.4.2 for definition) may require data that can be hard to obtain. If possible (e.g., if comparing two treatments that are both considered adequate in a given situation), the investigation may be carried out as a randomized study, assigning the treatments randomly to each patient. In some situations, groups to be compared may be matched (so that two individuals who are identical on some prechosen characteristics such as gender and age are assigned to different treatment groups) or even paired (so that the same individual receives both treatments, separated adequately in time); see, for example, Section 5.4. For further discussion of such design questions, see standard text books such as Altman (1991, Ch. 5) or Senn (2002, Ch. 9).

If there exist known predictors for the outcome, you should consider making inclusion and/or exclusion criteria based on these variables. It is advantageous to choose subjects in such a way that the covariates of main interest show large variability, such as a large age range if you study the increase of blood pressure with age and both skinny and fat people when studying the relation between body mass index and vitamin D status. However, such a selection is of course only possible when the size of the explanatory variable is easily detectable, either by simple inspection (body mass index) or from previously registered data (age).

In the planning stage it is highly recommended to perform a power analysis, that is, to investigate the probability of getting an informative answer, as a function of the effect size and the sample size. From such an analysis a reasonable sample size can be determined before initiating the investigation, thereby avoiding a waste of time on an investigation that has a large risk of getting you nowhere. We deal with sample size determination in Section 6.3.

Before the collected data can be analyzed, it is necessary to have decided upon a reasonable initial model for the data, that is, which covariates first must be considered. In the previous chapters, we have seen examples where covariates have been combined into a linear predictor, which has subsequently been related to the outcome of interest through an appropriate link function, taking the nature of the outcome into account. This linear predictor and its relation to the outcome of interest are the basic ingredients of a regression model.

We believe model building to be a scientific process that is unique for each separate question. Hence, we do not advocate the use of expert systems or automatic model selection procedures. Instead, we summarize our own experiences into some general principles for the process, and these are collected in Section 6.1.

To illustrate the principles as well as the uniqueness of each new problem, Section 6.2 contains three detailed examples, the vitamin D Example 1.1, the surgery Example 1.4, and the PBC3 Example 1.3, all introduced in Chapter 1 and used as illustrations in various contexts in the previous chapters (as well as in the chapters to follow).

Finally, in Section 6.3 we look at an important part of the planning of a new investigation, namely the determination of an adequate sample size, that is, the necessary number of individuals to include in the study in order to have a good chance of providing a useful conclusion.

6.1 General principles for model selection

When data collection has been finalized and data have been made electronically available for statistical analysis, it is very tempting to start performing all kinds of analyses that apply to the kind of data obtained. At this stage, however, it is strongly advisable to initially stick to very simple explorative analyses such as illustrative figures and summary statistics as discussed in Section 2.2.

Before proceeding to proper analyses, it is necessary to go through a few steps in order to ensure the appropriateness of the scientific process. First, the problem needs to be defined precisely: what is already known and what would we like to know? It must be kept in mind that the more precisely the question is posed, the better are the chances of designing an investigation able to answer it. Also, the questions ought to be kept few, simple, and to the point (avoiding, if possible, comparison of several treatments in one single investigation).

The question that you want to address determines which variables you need to consider for each individual in your investigation. Each new question may require consideration of a different set of covariates and covariates may have different status as described in Section 6.1.1. A helpful graphical tool for determining a reasonable model for answering a specific problem is presented in Section 6.1.2.

Having decided upon the basic structure of the model (i.e. the outcome and the covariates) the next step is to build the linear predictor and choose an appropriate link function, that is, to build an initial model from which to start your analyses. This process is treated in Section 6.1.3, whereas Section 6.1.4 is concerned with the analysis of this initial model, leading up to final models on which to base your conclusion. Special topics in this analysis are treated in Sections 6.1.5 (model checks and diagnostics), Section 6.1.6 (how to detect and deal with collinearity), and Section 6.1.7 (how to deal with interactions between explanatory variables).

We emphasize that this chapter does not pretend to give an exhaustive account of the strategies and problems involved in the selection of an appropriate model. Our focus is to build models that facilitate the understanding of the relation between one or more explanatory variables of interest, and an outcome, rather than models that give accurate and precise predictions of the future or unmeasured variables. For an in-depth treatment of the latter approach, we refer to Harrell (2001).

6.1.1 Identification of covariates

As we have seen from previous chapters, an important part of model building is to identify possible explanatory variables for the outcome under study (i.e., the covariates of the problem). Some covariates may be known from previous studies (e.g., cigarette smoking when the outcome is lung function, age if the outcome is blood pressure, or gestational age if the outcome is birthweight), whereas others are the main focus of the current investigation. Furthermore, there may be potential covariates that are not considered of primary interest but which we may have to take into account to avoid confounding or to reduce standard deviation.

A very important exception from the general rules to follow in this section is the randomized clinical trial. When individuals have been randomized to treatment, the two (or perhaps more) treatment arms are by definition identical with respect to the distribution of all explanatory variables. This means that a simple comparison among the treatment groups creates valid conclusions, at least for large sample sizes. For small to moderate sample sizes there may, however, be chance differences among the distributions of some explanatory variables and if these have a strong effect, they should be taken into consideration in the models. Moreover, inclusion of explanatory variables in the model may in some situations (even for large randomized studies) provide more precise conclusions due to the elimination of random variation.

We may formulate the principles for inclusion of covariates as follows.

1. Variables in focus in the present investigation, such as a treatment, an exposure, or a new potential risk factor for development of some disease. These will typically have some theoretical justification but the form of their effect (if any) will usually not be known. The choice of how to include such covariates therefore involves careful considerations.
2. Variables known from previous investigations to have an effect on the outcome under study. As a basic principle, such covariates should be included in an initial model and should as a general rule also stay in the model, provided that their effect is not explained by some newly included covariates. However, there may be deviations from this principle according to the purpose of the investigation as explained in Section 6.1.2.
3. Very basic variables such as gender and age, which should almost always be considered for possible effect on any outcome.
4. A list of other potential explanatory variables. This list may be long and it will often not be reasonable, or even possible, to include all of these simultaneously in the model. However, a screening process may be undertaken, investigating each (or a few) of the variables in turn to get an idea of their possible importance. This activity is sometimes denoted a *fishing expedition*, and the results gathered in this fashion may need to be confirmed in future studies.   .

Note that covariates may also show interactions and we give some general advice on the inclusion of interactions in Section 6.1.7.

The decision on how many and which covariates to include in a model is not at all an easy one. It is important to stress that the interpretation of the effect of one covariate may depend strongly on which other covariates are included in the model. This is because the effect of a covariate is conditional upon all other covariates being held fixed, as explained in Chapter 5. For instance, an effect of body mass index on the level of vitamin D may change substantially if age is entered as another explanatory variable. This is because there may be some relation between age and body mass index (people tend to get a little heavier with age, although they do not grow in height) and also some connection between age and the level of vitamin D (e.g., due to different sun habits). This concept is known as *confounding* and is discussed further in Section 6.1.2.

The choice of covariates is also a choice of which scientific question to answer. This fact should be taken seriously although the order should be the reverse such that you include those covariates that are necessary for answering your question. Before you start your analyses, you should therefore carefully specify the question that you want to answer instead of performing any possible analysis and interpreting the results from these. A useful graphical tool in the process of determining a reasonable model for answering a specific problem is presented in Section 6.1.2.

In almost any investigation of a sufficient size, there will be missing values of one or more of the variables under study. We denote such subjects as *incomplete cases*. This is of course very annoying inasmuch as subjects with missing values on any one of the variables entering the model (be it the outcome or any one of the covariates) cannot be used in traditional analyses. Indeed, standard statistical software will automatically perform a *complete case analysis*, that is, leave out these subjects, hopefully making a note in the output that this has been done. Increasing the complexity of the models by adding more explanatory variables will increase the probability of encountering subjects with missing values and thus lead to loss of efficiency (power). Moreover, different models for the same data cannot be truly compared unless they are based on the same subjects.

Moreover, missingness may create bias problems because there may be a reason for their missingness that relates to the value that would have been seen if it had been measured. For instance, in an investigation of lung function, an observation may be missing because the patient was too ill to come to the hospital, or in an investigation involving questionnaires asking, for example, questions on alcohol consumption, subjects with a high consumption may tend to either lie about it (thus creating measurement error in a covariate, discussed in Section 8.2) or choose not to answer at all.

If missing values occur in the *outcome variable*, things may become critical. If the missing value occurs because somebody accidentally dropped a test tube, we should only be concerned with the loss of efficiency due to the smaller sample size. But if a selection takes place as a consequence of the way in which the measurement of the outcome variable is performed (such as in the above imaginary investigation involving patients coming to the hospital to have their lung function measured and where, for example, small values of the outcome may be systematically missing) a bias in the analysis will be the result. Typically, in such a situation, the estimated effect of a covariate will be biased towards zero.

If the missing values occur in one or more *covariates*, the situation need not be serious, even if we are dealing with selection that causes bias in the resulting distribution of the covariate. This is due to the fact that in regression models we are only concerned with the conditional distribution of the outcome given the values of all the covariates, not in the distribution of the covariates themselves.

The important consideration here is to make sure that the reason for the missingness is not related to the outcome. If this is the case, the consequence will be a bias, precisely as when the missing values occur in the outcome itself, simply because such incomplete cases will not be part of the analyses.

Digression. Imputation

An alternative to a complete case analysis is to perform *imputation* which means that values are filled in for the missing data. A simple approach is to fill in the appropriate sample average value instead of the missing value, but it is more common to impute by using the *conditional mean* of the variable given all the other variables in the problem. Note that this requires a model for the interdependencies among the covariates. After filling in the unobserved data, the analyses are carried on as if all data were observed, and this results in a downward bias of the standard deviations (because the data looks "nicer" than what would probably have been observed). Methods for correction of such a bias exist, but a safer approach is to perform instead "multiple imputation," which means that you create new datasets, each time imputing single values simulated from the conditional distribution (but not being identically equal to the conditional mean). The results from the analysis of all these different datasets are subsequently combined to obtain an appropriate measure of standard deviation (see, e.g. Harrell (2001, Ch. 3) or Rubin (1987). ◇

6.1.2 Model diagrams

As explained in Section 6.1.1, the interpretation of the effect of a covariate changes according to which other covariates are included in the model, because the effect of a covariate in a multiple regression model is conditional upon all other covariates being held fixed. The task of determining which covariates to include when answering a specific question should therefore not be taken lightly, and the purpose of the investigation should constantly be kept in mind. A useful tool may be to arrange the variables in a partially ordered (causal) chain (e.g., a chain referring to time), as explained below.

We consider a simple example involving a study of lung function, where we imagine that we want to compare two groups, say men and women. The outcome could be fev1 (forced expiratory volume in one second) and the covariate of primary interest is gender. Next, consider other possible explanatory variables for fev1. Variables such as age or height come to mind. We arrange these covariates in a diagram with arrows indicating influences from one variable to another, such as depicted in Figure 6.1.1.

We see from the diagram that there are arrows from all covariates to the outcome because we argue that all covariates have a potential influence on fev1. Moreover, there are arrows between some of the covariates, namely from gender to height and from age to height because we believe both gender and

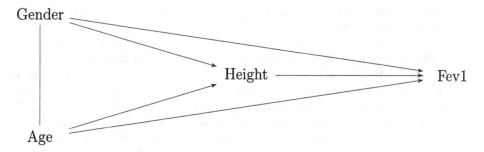

Fig. 6.1.1. Path diagram for imaginary investigation of lung function.

age to have an effect on height. These arrows have a direction because the effects obviously cannot be turned around, because height obviously has no effect on either gender or age. On the other hand, the line between gender and age has no arrow, indicating an association that may happen to show in the data but has no causal interpretation.

If we performed a simple comparison of lung function for men and women (typically a t-test) we imagine that we will get a result indicating that men have a somewhat higher value of fev1 than women. This corresponds to looking at the simple model illustrated by the diagram:

$$\text{Gender} \longrightarrow \text{Fev1}$$

This sex difference may well be caused by the inherent difference in height between men and women so that the model

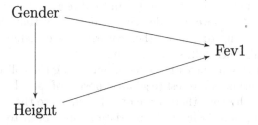

may in fact be simplified to

$$\text{Gender} \longrightarrow \text{Height} \longrightarrow \text{Fev1}$$

indicating that gender may have no independent effect on fev1, that is, no effect that does not "pass through" the variable height. In such a situation, we say that height is an *intermediate* variable (or *a mediator*) for the effect of gender on fev1.

If we include age in the analysis, the diagram becomes that of Figure 6.1.1 and the difference between men and women as expressed by the direct effect of gender on fev1 may change somewhat unless the age distribution for the two sexes are similar.

Diagrams as the one in Figure 6.1.1 are known as directed acyclic graphs (DAGs), although the connections between variables in DAGs are always directed. Such diagrams have been introduced to depict conditional independence properties of models for high-dimensional outcomes (e.g., Lauritzen, 1996) and have later found their way into epidemiology (Pearl, 1995; Jewell, 2004, Ch. 8). Construction of such a diagram, of course demands a theoretical knowledge of the problem under investigation and of the various explanatory variables under consideration. Some general guidelines can be given by considering a time-aspect of the covariates. This can give rise to hierarchical categories of covariates such as

1. Very basic-type data: gender, age, number of siblings, hair color etc.
2. Acquired demographic-type data: social group, working status, marital status, number of children
3. Height, weight, health measurements, treatment, exposure
4. Outcome

This hierarchy is constructed so that we may expect arrows from lower levels to higher levels, whereas between variables on the same level, we may or may not see chance relations. Following the definition of an intermediate variable above, we see that covariates on a higher level may be intermediate variables for those at a lower level.

If there is an arrow from a particular covariate pointing directly towards the outcome, we say that the covariate has a *direct* effect on the outcome. It may also have *indirect* effects going through intermediate variables on its way to the outcome. The sum of the direct and indirect effects is called the *total* effect. Based on the above considerations we can say that the direct effects may change according to which other covariates are included in the model whereas the total effect will be more stable.

When conducting an investigation and analyzing the collected data, some covariates are of primary interest (e.g., an exposure of some kind), as explained in Section 6.1.1, whereas others are more of a nuisance that have to be dealt with in an appropriate fashion. A covariate related both to the exposure of interest as well as to the outcome is called a *confounder*, provided that it is not a mediator for the exposure. For instance, in Figure 6.1.1, age is a confounder for the effect of gender, whereas height is not. Confounders should be corrected for when evaluating the effect of an exposure, in fact, Clayton and Hills (1993, Ch. 14) discuss a confounder as a variable one would have controlled for, had one been able to design the proper experiment. Failure to do so will result in biased estimates because the effects from uncontrolled confounders will contaminate the estimate of the exposure. Unfortunately, we never know if we have managed to identify all possible confounders and, therefore, the research process may continue to refine the models and create more precise results.

6.1.3 Initial model building

Having identified covariates of interest and examined a diagram of interdependencies, we are now ready to form an initial model, relating the outcome to those covariates that can answer our specific question and fulfill the purpose of the investigation. A warning is in order here: if you use models with too many covariates (or covariates with very flexible effects using many parameters) the results may become very imprecise. On the other hand, leaving out potential confounders may result in bias. The dilemma is to find a reasonable trade-off between bias and precision, a task that is impossible with few observations. A rule of thumb says that for quantitative outcomes you have to have as least ten times as many observations as parameters in your model. For a binary outcome the factor 10 should refer to the size of the smallest category (either 0 or 1) whereas in survival analysis, it refers to the number of failures (e.g., Harrell, 2001, Ch. 4). The factor is therefore often denoted "events per variable," abbrieviated EPV. We believe such a strict lower limit to be unwise because it may prevent proper adjustment for important confounders. If the choice is between abstaining from the inclusion of important explanatory variables and violating this rule, we believe the latter choice to be the more sensible, although the results should be accompanied by a cautious remark on the possible instability of results. According to simulation studies (Vittinghoff and MacCulloch, 2006), the rule may be relaxed without any drastic consequences in the form of bias or misleading confidence intervals. In particular, identification of important predictors seems to be trustworthy even if the EPV factor is halved.

The next question is *how* to enter each covariate in the linear predictor and how to relate the linear predictor to the outcome. The last question is the most straightforward to answer inasmuch as the possibilities are limited to specific link functions, that is, known functions including no parameters (the identity function, the logarithm, the logit etc.). Important issues to keep in mind are that the link function corresponds well with the type of outcome and that it leads to useful and simple interpretations. Chapters 3 – 5 have discussed the most common choices of link function for quantitative, binary, and survival time responses whereas in Chapter 7 we introduce a number of alternatives.

The combination of covariates into a linear predictor is a more difficult task and it is impossible to lay out quite general principles for this process. Some examples have been given throughout the previous chapters and we here summarize some of the issues. First, we must differentiate between the different types of covariates, that is, binary, categorical with more than two categories, or quantitative.

For binary covariates, there is only one possibility, namely to introduce a parameter to describe the difference in the linear predictor between its two levels. For categorical covariates with more than two levels (say $k + 1$, e.g., $0, 1, \cdots , k$), we likewise generally introduce k parameters, each describing the difference in the linear predictor between level j ($j = 1, \cdots, k$) and level 0 (the chosen reference level). Recall from Section 3.2 that the choice of reference category does not affect the model as such but only its appearance (i.e., which estimates appear in the output). For covariates with sparse categories, however, we should consider the possibility of collapsing some of the categories in order to avoid very unreliable results. Which categories to consider collapsing should be determined according to a combination of two aspects: the distribution of subjects in the categories (i.e., the number in each category) and theoretical knowledge of the meaning of these categories so as to make sure that categories will only be collapsed if it makes sense in connection with the problem under investigation. For instance, for the categorized version of body mass index considered in Section 3.2.1, it obviously does not make sense to collapse categories "normal weight" and "obese" while keeping "overweight" as a separate category.

Including quantitative covariates as part of the linear predictor is more tricky and may involve many considerations of theoretical as well as practical issues. It is advisable to treat covariates somewhat differently according to their status, that is, whether they are covariates with a known effect from previous studies, covariates of primary interest in the present investigation, or possible confounders of no particular interest in their own right.

A covariate known previously to have an effect on the outcome under consideration should (at least as a starting point) be included in the way that it has been used previously. Alternative descriptions of the effect of such a covariate should only be considered if the previously used approach can be demonstrated to be erroneous or suboptimal (either due to previous inconsistencies or due to changes in the interpretation because of inclusion of new covariates related to it).

For the covariates of main interest in the present investigation, we may have some theoretically justified anticipation of the sign or even the size of a possible effect, but usually we have very little knowledge about the specific form of the relationship (notable exceptions being problems from physiology or pharmacokinetics). We advise the first step to be construction of informative plots to give a first impression of the relationship, if any, for the whole dataset or in each of the treatment groups separately. Such pictures, typically in the form of scatterplots or plots of averages for one or more groupings of the covariate, have been discussed in Chapter 4 in connection with the various types of outcomes. It should be borne in mind, though, that such pictures represent only *marginal* relationships between covariate and outcome and may be changed (a little or quite considerably) by the various other covariates to be included in the model. In order to judge the proper form of the *conditional* relationship between the two, given other relevant covariates, we instead use residual plots to see whether we need to modify the model; see Section 6.1.5.

When modeling the effect of a quantitative covariate of main interest, it is generally recommended to keep it as simple as possible, at least initially. For quantitative covariates, the simplest possible effect is a linear effect. Slight deviations from linearity in marginal plots do not necessarily indicate true deviations from linearity but may simply be due to a disturbing effect from other covariates associated with the one under consideration. Residual plots will have to be examined to see if the deviation persists.

If deviations from linearity are strong and of a systematic nature (a clear bending downwards or upwards), a transformation of the covariate may be considered necessary. Theoretical knowledge of the problem may give a reasonable suggestion as to which kind of transformation to use, but in the absence of such knowledge, the covariate may be categorized in a number of categories and its effect visualized by a step function. The number of categories may depend upon the number of subjects in the sample as well as on theoretical arguments concerning the covariate itself (e.g., traditional thresholds for body mass index in the definitions of overweight and obesity as used in Sections 3.1.1 and 3.2.1, or thresholds for the normal range of bilirubin as used in Section 4.2.3). The form of the step function may now indicate which kind of transformation is reasonable. The advice is to stick to simple transformations, typically logarithms (of any base, Appendix B) or the square root, but in special situations functions such as the reciprocal (the function $f(x) = 1/x$) or functions of exponential type (such as $f(x) = 10^x$) may be used. If we have many observations, we may even use the categorized version of the covariate in an initial model or a spline function or fractional polynomials as discussed in Section 4.2. For the covariates of primary interest, we do not recommend to present the estimates using automatic smoothing such as a Lowess curve, because this will prevent a simple communication of the effect.

Finally we have to deal with a number of possible confounders (as defined in Section 6.1.2) or simply other covariates with a possible effect on the outcome. We have to adjust effectively for confounders because any residual influence may be mistaken as an effect of one of the main covariates of interest, because of the correlation to the confounder (by definition). Therefore, flexible smooth curves may be considered here (e.g., linear splines or fractional polynomials). Whereas this may provide a fairly accurate adjustment, we should at the same time take care to avoid overfitting inasmuch as this may cause effects to be "stolen" from the covariates of interest (e.g., Harrell, 2001, Ch. 5).

As discussed in Section 6.1.2, confounders are defined to be predictors of the outcome as well as associated with the covariate of interest (e.g., an exposure). This, formally, means a predictor of the outcome that is not simultaneously correlated to the exposure is not a confounder. However, as demonstrated by, for example, Gail, Wieand, and Piantadosi(1984), failure to include a predictor for the outcome in a model with a nonlinear link function may still lead to bias in the exposure effect. It may, further lead to a decreased precision: a larger standard deviation for the estimated effect of the exposure. We, therefore, expand the general advice on which variables to include in an initial model to all possible predictors of the outcome, unless they are intermediate variables from the exposure to the outcome.

6.1.4 Strategy of analysis

Having decided upon a reasonable functional form for the effect of the relevant explanatory variables (e.g., simple linear, linear spline, step function according to the choice of some thresholds, etc.) the next step will be to build a model with some or all of these variables as covariates.

Many statistical software packages offer automatic covariate selection, based on different philosophies: forward selection, backward elimination, or the "best subset" model. We do not recommend these methods and only describe them in a digression at the end of this section. Instead, an initial model may be built by performing steps fully controlled by the investigator and supplemented by model checks and diagnostics along the way (see Section 6.1.5). For convenience, the variable of main interest in the following is denoted "a treatment" or "an exposure" even though it may as well be some characteristic of the subjects.

One preliminary step in the model-building process is to enter each covariate in turn in a model together with the treatment and perhaps also including important covariates known from previous studies to have an effect. In this initial step we may identify variables with a possible effect on the outcome. By comparing the effects of treatment in each of these models (as well as in the model including only treatment) we also get an idea of possible confounding. We recommend all of the variables found of importance in such a screening to be entered in an initial model, along with the variables known previously to have an effect. Also, variables of primary interest in the investigation may be entered even if found nonsignificant in such an initial screening.

The model derived in this fashion should then be subjected to model checking and diagnostics along the lines of Section 6.1.5 before proceeding. This is important in order to identify possible misspecifications of the covariate effects, remembering that the functional form of these effects was determined from simpler investigations not including other covariates.

If the model is found to be a reasonable description of the data, the next step may be to make certain model simplifications, typically deletion of covariates from the model. From Section 2.3.3 we know the general ideas and traditional methods regarding the technical aspects of testing hypotheses. We have seen that testing involves choosing a level of significance and that this level of significance may be interpreted as the risk of rejecting a true hypothesis (error of type I), that is, the risk of finding an effect that in fact is not present. On the other hand, an often much greater risk is that of accepting a false hypothesis (error of type II), failing to detect an effect that is actually present but may be too small to be identified with the given amount of data.

A common strategy in statistical analyses of multiple regressions models, (i.e., models including many covariates) is to exclude any covariate with no significant effect on the outcome, at least if they are not predefined to be variables of special interest. However, because a nonsignificant covariate is not necessarily without effect on the outcome (seen in the light of a type II error as explained above), this may be a dangerous route to follow. Each time we eliminate a covariate on the basis of a test, we run the risk of leaving out a potentially important predictor, and more so if we have a limited amount of data. Part of the effect otherwise explained by this covariate is now explained by the remaining covariates in the model and another part of the effect will not be explained at all. If the covariate eliminated is closely correlated with one or more covariates remaining in the model, almost all of its predictive ability will be "taken over" by these, leading to a bias in the resulting estimates. Simulation studies show this effect to be substantial especially in situations with many covariates (e.g., Harrell, 2001, Ch. 4). A sound principle is to keep the covariates of interest in the model, at least until it feels safe to conclude that their effect, if any, is too small to be of any substantial interest.

This risk of bias has led to a general recommendation of not reducing the model at all, but to stick to the initial model (of course provided that model checks do not contradict this). Whereas this will, indeed, reduce the risk of bias, it may on the other hand give rise to larger standard deviations of the estimates leading to the traditional dilemma with a trade-off between bias and precision.

We recommend a compromise between the two extremes in which we reduce the model by omitting insignificant variables provided that this does not induce substantial changes in the effects of the covariates of interest. It then remains to be determined what is meant by a substantial change and this may to some extent depend on the circumstances. A threshold of 10% seems to be reasonable in most situations (e.g., Jewell, 2004, Ch. 9).

Moreover, in the model selection process, model checks should be routinely performed to ensure that omission of covariates does not induce violations of assumptions. We collect principles for model checks in Section 6.1.5.

Digression. Automatic variable selection

In the forward selection procedure, the process starts out with an empty initial model. All covariates are now screened one at a time for effect on the outcome and the one found to be the most significant is entered into the model. In this process it is assumed that all covariates are transformed in a way so that they can be entered directly in the linear predictor. Also note that including interactions in this process requires that they are constructed as new covariates and that inclusion of such interaction covariates is extremely dangerous and may lead to all kinds of ridiculous results.

Having identified the most significant covariate, the next step is to look through all models with two covariates, namely the one found in the previous step plus one of the remaining. Again the choice is to include the covariate that has the most significant effect on the outcome, only now adjusted for the first covariate. This iterative process of selecting the most significant covariate from the remaining variables is continued until none of the remaining covariates is found significant.

The level of significance in this iterative process is often somewhat higher than the usual, meaning that variables enter the model even if they are nonsignificant at the traditional level.

In the backward elimination procedure, the process is the opposite. The process starts with an initial model including all possible covariates considered to be relevant for the specific question (a "full model", although we should take proper precautions not to include more than the amount of data can support). The variables are now removed sequentially from the model, in each step eliminating the one with the largest P-value. This process stops when all covariates left in the model are significant at some prechosen level. A hybrid process is to allow either an exclusion or an inclusion in each step.

A competing procedure for model selection is simply fit all possible models constructed from the available covariates ("all subsets regression") . If there are n_c possible covariates to choose from, this gives a total of 2^{n_c} different models to consider (if only models without interactions are considered). Each model can then be evaluated according to some criterion (of which several exist) and the most successful candidate chosen for interpretation and future use. The most widely used criterion is the Akaike's information criterion (abbreviated AIC; see, e.g., Harrell, 2001, Ch. 9), a measure of the goodness-of-fit of the model, that is, a trade-off between complexity of the model and precision of the estimates. The determination coefficient that describes the amount of explained variation (the quantity R^2, as discussed in Chapter 4), should under no circumstances be used for this purpose inasmuch as model complexity does not influence this quantity and hence it will always point to the most complicated model (i.e., the one including all covariates) as the best one.

If applying an automatic procedure it is strongly recommended to use only part of the available data, say two thirds, and leave the last third for evaluation of the selected model. This cross-validation principle will most often show that the covariates in the model are not quite as strong predictors as they were first seen to be, a phenomenon called *shrinkage*. If the predictive ability of the model on the remaining third of the data is very different from expected (based on the findings from the dataset used for identification of the model), it is a hint that we should not trust our model.

Automatic model-finding processes suffer from high instability, in the sense that a particular transformation of a single covariate or a slight change in a few observations may lead to a completely different model. Furthermore, such automatic procedures run a high risk of identifying covariates to be important predictors even though they are in fact of little or even no importance at all.

However, the worst "feature" of the automatic selection procedures is that they treat all covariates in the same manner, no matter whether they are variables of main interest, basic-type variables, or covariates that are tried out for the sake of completeness. This means that in the process of comparing P-values for entering or eliminating covariates from the model, a truly important variable of main interest (e.g., the exposure itself) may disappear from a model with too many interrelated covariates. ⬦

6.1.5 Model checks and diagnostics

In Chapters 3 to 5, we have shown a number of examples of various types of models and analyses of these. In this connection it was emphasized that it ought to be an integral part of any statistical analysis to examine the appropriateness of the model because gross deviations from the model assumptions may lead to unreasonable and erroneous conclusions.

We here briefly sum up the various ways that such model checks can be carried out. They are to a certain extent dependent upon the type of outcome, thus not all methods described below are equally informative or even applicable in all situations. In Sections 6.2.1–6.2.3 some of the most important of these methods are used in examples covering the three main types of outcome: quantitative, binary, and survival time.

Our opinion is that the most important tool for assessment of the model is diagnostic plots and, in particular, plots of residuals against covariate values. Such plots are used to check whether the covariate effect is correctly specified. Whereas these may be readily constructed for quantitative data, they demand a little extra for binary data and for survival times, as explained in Section 4.1.2, respectively, 4.1.3. These residual plots should ideally look chaotic, that is, with no obvious systematic structure such as trends (linear or curved), trumpets and the like. For binary data and survival times, this assessment requires that the plots are supplemented with a smoothing curve, but a smoother is also useful (though not mandatory) for quantitative outcomes.

Other types of residual plots are also called for in particular situations. For instance, for quantitative data, we may investigate an assumption of constant standard deviation by plotting residuals against predicted values. For more information, the reader is referred to the relevant sections such as Sections 4.1.1, 5.1.1 and 5.1.2.

Residual plots may be supplemented by numerical tests for model fit. The specific nature of such tests depends on the particular type of model, but the general idea is to look at a more general model (relaxing one or more of the assumptions of your original model) and then perform a test for the reduction from the general model to the more restrictive model. Such tests, as well as tests based on "$(O - E)^2 / E$", are referred to as a *goodness-of-fit test*.

If clear systematic structures are present in any of the residual plots, or if a goodness-of-fit test shows inadequacy of the proposed model, it must be revised. The residual plots will show which aspects should be modified and the process of modification can then follow the general rules as laid out in Section 6.1.3.

Whereas residual plots may detect an inadequacy of the proposed model to describe the collected data, we may also reverse the concepts and ask if there are observations that do not fit well with the model. This is done by making *diagnostic plots*, the nature of which will depend on the particular kind of model. The general idea is to look for observations with large residuals. Such observations may be called *outliers* and they ought to be investigated more closely, partly because they may provide new information (we may discover that they were taken under special circumstances, the effect of which we had not thought about previously) and partly because they may distort the conclusion by having an unduly large influence.

What to do about such outliers is another matter. Some general rules apply, however. Do not exclude outliers simply because they are "misbehaved" but exclude them only:

- If they are erroneous
- If the circumstances are so special that it might have been used as an exclusion criterion (and then remember to leave out also all other observations with the same circumstances) and limit the conclusions accordingly
- If they have an unduly large influence on the results due to an extreme value of a covariate (or perhaps an extreme combination of covariate values), in which case all other observations showing this type of covariate pattern should be excluded (this is actually just another form of an inclusion criterion).

Observations may be influential without showing up as outliers. In small to moderate-sized samples, it is therefore wise to investigate the influence of each single observation and take action as mentioned above if very influential observations are detected. For detection of outliers and influential observations, it is generally advisable to use the leave-one-out residuals as described in Section 2.3.2. These exist for quantitative and binary outcomes and are better suited for detection of atypical/unusual observations although the similarity to traditional residual plots will often be close, especially for large datasets.

If outliers are retained in the data, the model may have to be modified, for example, by including an extra covariate describing the special circumstances found in the outlying observations. However, because this may be a chance finding, it should be investigated further in a subsequent study before we can really trust such an effect.

6.1.6 Collinearity

During the analyses of data, including changes made in the model as a consequence of model checks and testing of preplanned hypotheses, one may encounter problems of various kinds such as large changes in parameter estimates when removing (or changing the scoring of) another covariate, ridiculously large standard deviations for estimated parameters, or signs of a few extremely influential observations. Such problems make it very hard to draw precise conclusions regarding the effects of any particular covariate and, in extreme situations, computer programs may even issue a warning saying that some numerical instability has occurred, for example, division by a near-zero value.

A model exhibiting such problems may still be perfectly valid for prediction purposes, at least when the covariate values for the new subject are comparable to those that appear in the dataset used for estimation. It may, however, at the same time be totally useless for the scientific purpose of determining whether it is covariate x_1 or x_2 that carries the effect. This problem occurs in situations where x_1 and x_2 are highly correlated and in that case it is easily detectable. However, it may also occur in situations where no single correlation between any two covariates is exceptionally large, for example, if one variable is approximately the sum of two of the others. We say that we have an approximate linear constraint between the covariates in this case, $x_1 + x_2 - x_3 \approx 0$, and we use the term *ill-conditioned* or *collinearity* for the data at hand. Such a situation may easily go undetected and only present itself as increased standard deviations for the estimated parameters. If a few observations deviate from the near-constraint, these will have an overwhelming effect on the result of the estimation, because these observations will carry the only available information on how to separate the influence of the variables in question.

A quite common situation is a multiple regression analysis with too many covariates in the model, showing all covariates to be insignificant when evaluated by separate tests but, at the same time, clearly demonstrating the ability to predict the observed outcome. This tells us that at least some of the covariates carry information, perhaps in unison, but that at the same time, every single one of them may be dispensed with as long as we keep all the others in the model.

For scientific purposes, such ill-conditioned data are annoying. Various methods have been implemented in the main statistical software packages to allow for detection of problems. Typically, they pinpoint certain near-to-linear constraints on the covariates and the next step must be either to eliminate some of those covariates involved in such a linear constraint or perhaps combine closely related covariates into a common scale (e.g., frequency of intake of a number of food items). An example may be a study on children where it may be extremely difficult to single out the effects of age, height, and weight inasmuch as they more or less increase at the same rate during childhood. Shifting focus to age and body mass index (combining the two correlated covariates height and weight into one single new covariate, body mass index) may help somewhat, although not entirely, because body mass index is known to be increasing with age in childhood as well. A possible solution could be to use weight or body mass index in the form of a Z-score, indicating the normalized deviation from an age-dependent average body mass index. However, such an approach requires that the dependence between body mass index and age is considered known (or can be estimated sufficiently precisely from the data).

6.1.7 Interactions

In all of the above subsections, we have discussed only models in which each covariate enters additively. That is, even if the effect of a single covariate may be described by a complicated spline function, this spline function is subsequently added to the effects of all the other covariates to form the linear predictor. In other words, the effect of one covariate is assumed to stay the same no matter how the values of all the remaining covariates change. This assumption is the assumption of no interaction as explained in detail in Section 5.2.

Models with no interactions are relatively simple because the effect of each covariate can be interpreted independently of the value of every other. The effect of a covariate may depend upon other variables being *present* in the model (confounding) but it does not change according to the *value* of these other covariates. For instance, the effect of the mother's weight on the weight of a newborn may diminish if we also include parity in the model, but this does not mean that the effect of mother's weight changes with parity.

Models with interactions are more complicated to understand and communicate because they involve specification of effects that vary according to the value of one or more other covariates. Also, the diagrams (DAGs) introduced in Section 6.1.2 do not immediately accomodate interactions. For these reasons, interactions should not be entered uncritically in the model. They make the models much more complicated and put a higher demand on the sample size because they include more parameters. Only prespecified interactions should be considered: interactions that have an intuitive scientific interpretation (experience shows a formidable ability to explain chance interactions found to be significant). Often, interactions with basic variables such as exposure, treatment, gender and age may be worthwhile considering. When entering interactions in the model, take care to be parsimonious in order to obtain a test with reasonable power. This may, for instance, imply collapsing some categories of a categorical covariate in the specification of an interaction between this and other covariates (see Section 5.2.4 for more details and examples).

6.2 Examples

In this section, the principles for model building, outlined in Section 6.1, are illustrated by discussing three examples in detail. These three examples have all been used for illustration and motivation in previous chapters and represent the three main types of outcome variables covered. Thus, in Section 6.2.1 we study Example 1.1 including the quantitative outcome, vitamin D, Section 6.2.2 discusses Example 1.4 with the binary outcome postsurgery complications, and in Section 6.2.3 we go through Example 1.3 dealing with the survival time outcome, time to treatment failure, among patients with PBC.

6.2.1 The vitamin D example

In the previous chapters we have repeatedly returned to Example 1.1 from Section 1.1 concerned with body mass index and vitamin D concentration for women.

The objectives of this study were to determine the vitamin D status among women from different countries in Europe, and in particular to identify determinants that could explain the discrepancy among the four countries. Such determinants could be age, body mass index, sun exposure habits, and intake of vitamin D (from the food and from possible supplements).

Table 6.2.1. Median values for vitamin D concentration and potential explanatory variables for the women in four European countries

Country	Number	Vitamin D	Age	Body Mass Index	Vitamin D Intake
Denmark	53	47.80	71.51	25.39	8.29
Finland	54	46.60	71.92	27.98	12.41
Ireland	41	44.80	72.05	26.39	5.46
Poland	65	32.50	71.69	29.37	5.16

Table 6.2.1 shows medians (nmol/L) for vitamin D concentration, as well as for age, body mass index (BMI) (kg/m^2), and vitamin D intake (nmol/L). We saw in Sections 3.1.1, 3.2.1, and 4.1.1 that body mass index was negatively associated with vitamin D status. This fact is also reflected in Table 6.2.1 from which we see that the Polish women have the highest level of BMI and by far the lowest level of vitamin D. We may therefore conjecture that the difference between countries is caused by this difference in body mass index.

Following the arguments from Section 3.1.1 (regarding symmetric distributions and constant standard deviation) we use a logarithmic transform of vitamin D in the analyses to follow. The model for comparing the four countries (C) with respect to logarithmic vitamin D concentration (Y) is described by the very simple diagram

$$\text{Country} \rightarrow \text{Vitamin D}$$

and applying methods from Section 3.2.1 yields a highly significant result $(P < 0.0001)$, stating that Poland has indeed a lower mean than the other three countries.

If we assume that all of the difference among countries is mediated by BMI, the model would be

$$\text{Country} \rightarrow \text{BMI} \rightarrow \text{Vitamin D}$$

but it is probably more realistic to assume that body mass index can only account for some of the discrepancy between countries, so that we are rather dealing with the model

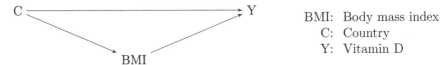

BMI: Body mass index
   C: Country
   Y: Vitamin D

In fact, the results from this latter model show that only a small part of the difference between vitamin D concentrations in the four countries may be accounted for by the differences in body mass index even though the body mass index is a strong predictor $(\widehat{b} = -0.0115(0.0035), P = 0.0012)$. Table 6.2.2 shows that the estimated differences among countries, adjusted for body mass index (i.e., differences among women in different countries conditioned to have the same body mass index) are only moderately different from the estimated marginal differences. Likewise, there is still a highly significant difference among countries $(P = 0.0002)$, so there is plenty of room for looking for other explanatory variables.

Table 6.2.2. Marginal estimated differences among countries and estimated differences adjusted for the effect of body mass index.

Comparison	Marginal Differences	Adjusted Differences
Denmark vs. Poland	0.142 (0.063, 0.221)	0.114 (0.035, 0.193)
Finland vs. Poland	0.168 (0.090, 0.246)	0.161 (0.084, 0.238)
Ireland vs. Poland	0.171 (0.086, 0.256)	0.141 (0.056, 0.226)

As mentioned previously, such explanatory variables could be age (A), sun exposure habits (S), and intake (I) of vitamin D (from food and possible supplements). These may all be influenced by the country of residence, so they are to be regarded as intermediate variables between country (C) and outcome (Y, i.e., vitamin D concentration). The diagram for the situation would be as illustrated in Figure 6.2.1.

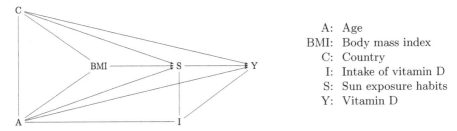

A: Age
BMI: Body mass index
   C: Country
   I: Intake of vitamin D
   S: Sun exposure habits
   Y: Vitamin D

Fig. 6.2.1. Diagram of model for explanation of country differences in vitamin D concentration.

In order to pursue the search for variables that can explain the differences among countries, we try to include all of the variables from Figure 6.2.1. Three of the variables are quantitative: body mass index (BMI), age (A), and vitamin D intake (I) and we have to decide how to model the effects of these. Figure 6.2.2 shows initial (marginal) graphical investigations where the logarithmic vitamin D concentration (the outcome) is plotted against each quantitative covariate, without adjustment for other potential covariates. For body mass index, it seems reasonable to start with a linear effect (as we have previously done in Section 5.3.1) and likewise for age (which hardly has an effect at all in this narrow age range). For vitamin D intake, the effect seems to level off for large values and a logarithmic transformation of this explanatory variable seems to be more reasonable if the effect is to be modeled linearly. This is in some sense also more "logical" inasmuch as the units for this variable are the same as for the outcome.

Sun exposure habits is a categorical variable with three levels (prefer staying in the sun, stay sometimes in the sun, avoid staying in the sun). Table 6.2.3 shows median values of body mass index and vitamin D concentration, subdivided according to sun habits. We note a tendency for higher vitamin D levels for women preferring to stay in the sun and likewise, the lowest vitamin D level is found for women avoiding the sun. There does not seem to be any clear association between body mass index and sun habits.

Table 6.2.3. Median values for vitamin D and body mass index, according to sun exposure habits.

Sun Habits	Number	Vitamin D	Body Mass Index
Prefer sun	39	43.70	28.78
Sometimes in sun	104	41.30	26.90
Avoid sun	70	38.30	27.28

We may also investigate the association between country and sun habits. If Polish women tended to avoid the sun, this could be the explanation for their lower level. In Table 6.2.4 this is actually seen to be the case although Irish women show the same pattern. The conjecture could be that the combination of avoiding sun and having a high body mass index could account for the low level among Polish women.

Table 6.2.5 shows the estimates in the model including all of the above mentioned covariates (Model 1). Age has next to no effect at all, thus we choose to exclude this from the analysis. The resulting estimates appear in Table 6.2.5 in the column "Model 2" and we note that this hardly changes the estimates. In Model 2, the variable "sun" has a P-value of 0.25 and in Model 3, it is excluded. Note that this exclusion leads to a rather large change in the estimated difference between Finland and Poland ($(0.0860 - 0.0747)/0.0747 =$

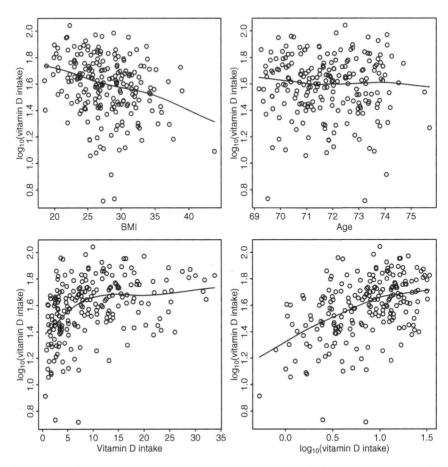

Fig. 6.2.2. Scatterplot, with superimposed smoother, of vitamin D concentration ($\log_{10}$-transformed) versus each of the quantitative variables (in addition plotted against logarithmic (base 10) values of vitamin D intake).

Table 6.2.4. Number of women according to country and sun exposure habits

Sun habits	Denmark		Finland		Ireland		Poland	
Prefer sun	15	(28.3%)	15	(27.8%)	4	(9.8%)	5	(7.7%)
Sometimes in sun	24	(45.3%)	25	(46.3%)	21	(51.2%)	34	(52.3%)
Avoid sun	14	(26.4%)	14	(25.9%)	16	(39.0%)	26	(40.0%)
Total	53		41		65		54	

15%), and we may, therefore, want to retain it in the model, if this parameter is of main interest.

Table 6.2.5. Estimates from the model indicated by the diagram in Figure 6.2.1 (Model 1), and simplifications of this (Model 2 and Model 3).

Variable	Model 1 $\widehat{b}$	Model 1 SD	Model 2 $\widehat{b}$	Model 2 SD	Model 3 $\widehat{b}$	Model 3 SD
Body mass index	−0.00978	0.00317	−0.00983	0.00316	−0.00927	0.00313
Age	−0.00394	0.00948				
Vitamin D intake $(\log_{10})$	0.255	0.036	0.255	0.036	0.258	0.035
Sun						
Prefer sun	0.0430	0.0368	0.0435	0.0367		
Sometimes	0	—	0	—		
Avoid sun	−0.0195	0.0301	−0.0215	0.0297		
Country						
Denmark	0.0964	0.0367	0.0959	0.0366	0.1090	0.0357
Finland	0.0764	0.0373	0.0747	0.0370	0.0860	0.0362
Ireland	0.1408	0.0389	0.1382	0.0384	0.1407	0.0385
Poland	0	—	0	—	0	—

All models from Table 6.2.5 show — not very surprisingly — that the intake of vitamin D has a very significant positive effect on the outcome. However, inclusion of this important covariate still cannot account for the differences between the countries ($P = 0.0013$ for the effect of country in the adjusted model).

Before we proceed we have to make sure that Model 3 from Table 6.2.5 is reasonable. Figure 6.2.3 shows residual plots for all the explanatory variables considered, as well as residuals plotted against predicted values. For the quantitative covariates, a smoother has been added to aid the search for patterns of deviations from the model. We find all plots to show no structure at all, indicating that the model has no obvious flaws. A few outliers are present, though. In particular one woman from Finland and one from Poland have rather large negative residuals. Both women tend to avoid the sun but otherwise there are no common characteristics for the two. Note that the residuals used in these plots are the ordinary residuals $y_i - \widehat{m}_i$ with units identical to the units of the outcome. We have also made plots using other kinds of residuals, and their appearance is similar (not shown).

We now turn to consider possible interactions. With a total of six covariates there may be many of these but we remember from Section 6.1.7 only to consider those that may be anticipated from a theoretical point of view. Two of these come into mind, involving country on the one hand and sun

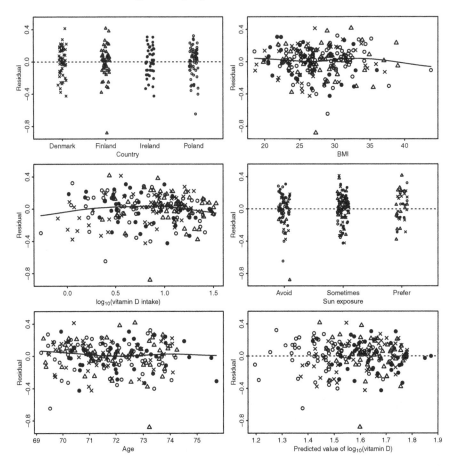

Fig. 6.2.3. Residual plots for model 3 from Table 6.2.5. Symbols used: Denmark (×), Finland (△), Ireland (•) and Poland (◦).

exposure habits (S) or vitamin D intake (I) on the other hand. Inasmuch as the aim is to explain the differences among countries, it may at first seem somewhat strange to include interactions involving country. However, such an interaction (or two) may actually (provided that it is big enough) be the very explanation of the differences among countries. This is most easily seen in the case of interaction between country and sun exposure habits: the effect of sun exposure habits is expected to vary among countries because the sun is not equally strong in all countries. If the differences among countries were only present among women who preferred to stay in the sun, and if the difference were compatible with weather conditions in the countries, this might explain the differences.

The same arguments may hold for vitamin D intake (I). Due to possible differences in the vitamin content of otherwise identical food items we could expect this variable to have different impacts in different countries. In order to see whether this can explain the differences in different countries, we need very precise measurements of food consumption, presumably also concerning other vitamins or tracers.

In order to investigate graphically whether such interactions may be present and how they are to be modeled, we may use two approaches. The first one inspects the marginal relationship between vitamin D concentration and the covariate whereas the other looks at residuals from Model 3 above. The former approach is more directly interpretable in terms of relation between covariate and outcome. For vitamin D intake, this is seen in the left panel of Figure 6.2.4 which indicates slightly different effects of vitamin D intake among the four countries. However, this approach suffers from the fact that we have not adjusted for any other covariates (in this case body mass index). Therefore, the residual approach shown in the right panel of Figure 6.2.4 is to be preferred. Here, the residuals are plotted against logarithmic vitamin D intake for each country and the figure seems to show no clear systematic patterns.

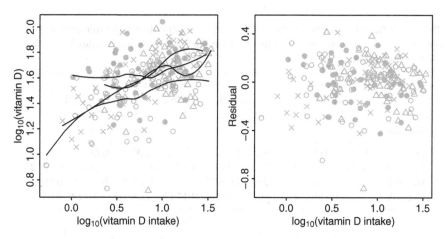

Fig. 6.2.4. Scatterplot investigating a possible interaction between country and logarithmic vitamin D intake, with smoothers according to country. Left panel: Marginal effect. Right panel: Residual effect, adjusted according to Model 3 from Table 6.2.5. Symbols used: Denmark ($\times$), Finland ($\triangle$), Ireland ($\bullet$) and Poland ($\circ$).

Likewise, we could investigate a possible interaction between country and sun exposure habits but inasmuch as these are both categorical we do not have to investigate the functional form. We may, however, argue that an interaction between four countries and three levels of sun exposure habits involves several degrees of freedom and, following the lines of Section 5.2.4, we may therefore want to collapse categories (for sun habits) when looking at interactions. In the light of the numbers in Table 6.2.3 there is, however, no obvious choice for this collapsing so we stick to the full representation of the interaction.

Table 6.2.6 shows the estimates from the model with both of the above mentioned interactions. The results show that the effect of vitamin D intake is stronger in Denmark than for the rest of the countries. In particular, Finland and Ireland show small and insignificant effects. The overall interaction between country and vitamin D intake is strongly significant ($P = 0.0031$). The interaction between sun habits and country is also significant, although only borderline ($P = 0.026$). Figure 6.2.5 shows a graphical illustration of the estimates, and the effect is seen to be quite difficult to interpret. A cautious interpretation might be that the effect of sun habits is only seen for Finland and Poland, and in somewhat different ways (Finnish women having large values for both "sometimes" and "prefer" whereas Polish women only have large values for "prefer"; there are only five women in this group). For Denmark we see hardly any effect but for Ireland the relationship between sun exposure and vitamin D seems to be reversed. We can offer no explanation for this except for the fact that the group "prefer sun" contains only four Irish women.

Table 6.2.6. Estimates from the model (Model 4) including two interactions: Country with sun habits and intake. The common effect of body mass index is estimated to −0.0090 (0.0031).

| Variable | Vitamin D Intake ($\log_{10}$) | | Sun Habits | | | | | |
| | | | Sometimes in Sun | | Prefer vs. Sometimes | | Avoid vs. Sometimes | |
	$\hat{b}$	SD	$\hat{b}$	SD	$\hat{b}$	SD	$\hat{b}$	SD
Denmark	0.4365	0.0617	1.6318	0.0369	0.0699	0.0594	0.0042	0.0616
Finland	0.1321	0.0869	1.6724	0.0400	−0.0191	0.0588	−0.1425	0.0612
Ireland	0.1149	0.0810	1.6207	0.0395	−0.093	0.0998	0.0960	0.0613
Poland	0.2453	0.0574	1.5266	0.0312	0.1737	0.0886	−0.0424	0.0475

The conclusion to our analysis of the vitamin D study is somewhat unsatisfactory because we have not been able to explain the differences in vitamin D concentration between the four countries. We have found body mass index and vitamin D intake to be important predictors, the latter with an effect depending on country. Even though sun habits were not marginally important, it showed significance in an interaction with country. However, there is still a large difference between countries even for women who avoid staying in the sun, therefore this does not help in explaining the differences among countries. On the contrary, it seems to suggest even bigger differences among countries if we try to explain the very different patterns according to sun habits.

Finally, we investigate whether there are influential observations in the dataset. Figure 6.2.6 shows a plot of Cook's distance (the combined measure

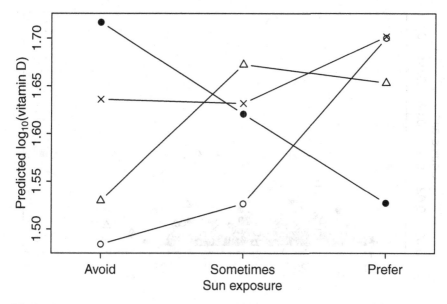

Fig. 6.2.5. Illustration of the interaction between sun habits and country, from Model 4 in Table 6.2.6. Predicted values for median body mass index and vitamin D intake. Symbols used: Denmark ($\times$), Finland ($\triangle$), Ireland ($\bullet$) and Poland ($\circ$).

for changes in the estimated effects due to deletion of individual observations; see, e.g., Section 4.1.1). We note a single somewhat influential subject (the largest Cook distance, approximately 0.1). This is a woman from Finland avoiding the sun and we have discussed her previously in connection with the residual plots in Figure 6.2.3. She has a much lower observed vitamin D concentration (5.2) than predicted (33.3). Her influence is particularly large for the interaction parameters involving Finland, that is, the parameters describing the differences among Finland and the other countries regarding the effect of vitamin D intake (left panel of Figure 6.2.7) and "avoiding sun" (right panel of Figure 6.2.7).

Conclusion

The overall conclusion from this example is that we have not been able to explain the differences among countries. We have detected an interaction between country and sun habits, with no clear interpretable pattern. Because of this unconvincing pattern, we here report the results from a model excluding this interaction. Apart from a difference among countries, the final model therefore includes an effect of body mass index with $\widehat{b} = -0.0096(0.0031)$ and an effect of vitamin D intake that varies from one country to another. The estimates of this latter effect are seen in Table 6.2.7. Because all of the analyses were carried out on a logarithmic scale for level of vitamin D, it remains

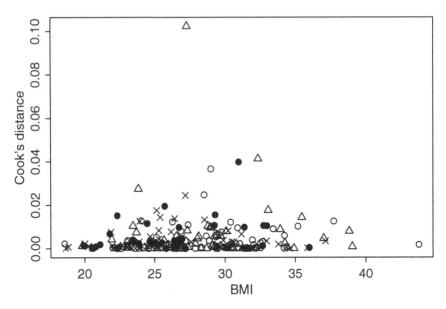

Fig. 6.2.6. The influence measure Cook's distance versus body mass index. Symbols used: Denmark ($\times$), Finland ($\triangle$), Ireland ($\bullet$) and Poland ($\circ$).

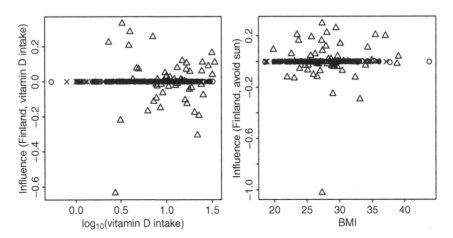

Fig. 6.2.7. Influence measures for selected estimated effects: interactions among Finland and the other countries regarding effect of vitamin D intake and "avoiding sun". Symbols used: Denmark ($\times$), Finland ($\triangle$), Ireland ($\bullet$) and Poland ($\circ$).

to transform back to the original scale (see Appendix B). The effect of a one-unit increase in body mass index corresponds to multiplying the vitamin D level by $10^{-0.0096} = 0.978$, with a corresponding 95% confidence interval of $(10^{-0.0157}, 10^{-0.0036}) = (0.965, 0.992)$. This means that, for women from all countries, an increase in body mass index of one unit (e.g., approximately 3 kg for a women measuring 1.65 m) gives an estimated decrease in vitamin D level of 2.2%, with confidence interval from 0.8% to 3.5%.

For the effects of vitamin D intake, the estimates are recalculated in Table 6.2.7 to give the effect of doubling vitamin D intake. An example of this calculation, for Danish women, is $2^{\hat{b}} = 2^{0.4349} = 1.352$.

Table 6.2.7. Estimated effects on the original scale, ignoring the interaction between country and sun habits.

Country	$\hat{b}$	Estimate for Vitamin D Intake 95% CI	Ratio	Effect of Doubling the Vitamin D Intake 95% CI
Denmark	0.4349	(0.3126, 0.5571)	1.352	(1.245, 1.468)
Finland	0.1744	(0.0028, 0.3461)	1.129	(1.005, 1.267)
Ireland	0.0918	(-0.0671, 0.2507)	1.066	(0.957, 1.186)
Poland	0.2263	(0.1140, 0.3386)	1.170	(1.085, 1.262)

Table 6.2.7 shows that a doubling of the vitamin D intake would on average increase the vitamin D level in the blood by only 6.7% for an Irish woman but with 35.2% for a Danish woman.

6.2.2 The surgery example

Recall Example 1.4 from Section 1.1 involving 691 patients, undergoing either orthopedic, gynecological or abdominal surgery. The purpose of the study was to determine whether some types of neuromuscular blocking agents (NBA) were more prone to postsurgery pulmonary complications than others. Furthermore, it was of interest to know whether residual neuromuscular block (RNB, measured by some clinical tests following operation, but here indicated by a measure of neuromuscular function called TOF-ratio) was a risk factor for complications, and in particular so for Pancuronium (which, by the way, is the only long-acting drug among the three).

The outcome of interest is the binary variable

$$y_i = \begin{cases} 1, & \text{if subject } i \text{ experiences a postsurgery complication,} \\ 0, & \text{otherwise.} \end{cases}$$

The number of complications (the actual counts as well as the percentage of the corresponding group) for each of the three neuromuscular agent groups appear in Table 6.2.8. Based on this table, the three agents appear to have quite similar risks of postoperative complications, perhaps with a slightly increased risk for Pancuronium.

Table 6.2.8. Complications in relation to type of neuromuscular blocking agent (NBA).

NBA	Number	Complications (%)
Pancuronium	230	19 (8.3)
Vecuronium	230	14 (6.1)
Atracurium	231	13 (5.6)
Total	691	46 (6.7)

The study was conducted as a block randomized study with surgery groups as blocks. This means that patients from each surgery group were randomized to receive one of the three neuromuscular blocking agents (Pa, At, or Ve). In principle, therefore, there should be no relation between type of surgery and blocking agent and a valid inference for assessing the effect of NBA is to follow the discussion of Section 3.2.2 and do a simple comparison of the three estimated probabilities of Table 6.2.8. This results in a chi-squared test statistic of 1.466, which under the hypothesis of no difference between the three neuromuscular blocking agents is distributed as $\chi^2(2)$, giving $P = 0.48$, that is, no detectable difference.

Due to drop-outs there is, however, a tiny difference in the distribution of NBA in the three surgery groups as seen in Table 6.2.9. We may therefore see a slight confounding from type of surgery on the effect of NBA because we know from Sections 3.1.2 and 3.2.2 that type of surgery (S) has a clear impact on the risk of complications (Y) in the sense that abdominal surgery has a larger risk of complications than the two other surgery groups.

Table 6.2.9. Number of patients according to surgery type and neuromuscular agent.

Surgery Group	Neuromuscular Blocking Agent Pancuronium	Atracurium	Vecuronium	Total
Orthopedic	72 (35.0%)	66 (32.0%)	68 (33.0%)	206 (100%)
Gynecological	75 (31.3%)	84 (35.0%)	81 (33.8%)	240 (100%)
Abdominal	83 (33.9%)	80 (32.7%)	82 (33.5%)	245 (100%)
Total	230	230	231	691

It is also suspected that age (A) and the duration of the anesthesia (D) could also affect the probability of a complication. Further variables that might come into consideration (but are not considered here) include gender, general health status of the patient, weight, smoking habits, and body temperature.

Our main interest lies in the effect of the neuromuscular blocking agent (NBA) and residual neuromuscular block (RNB) on the risk of complications (Y), and because it is likely that NBA may influence RNB, the diagram will initially look like:

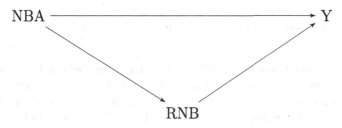

RNB is an intermediate variable for the effect of NBA on the risk of complication, therefore it should not be entered in the model when the aim is to evaluate the effect of NBA. On the other hand, including RNB in the model can answer our second question, namely whether a difference between NBA groups (had there been any) could be explained by an induced risk of RNB. Expanding the model with all of the covariates mentioned so far, we get the diagram:

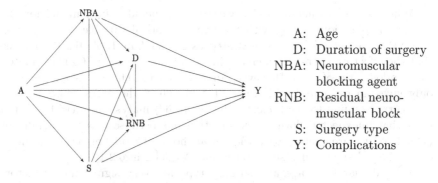

A: Age
D: Duration of surgery
NBA: Neuromuscular blocking agent
RNB: Residual neuromuscular block
S: Surgery type
Y: Complications

For assessment of the effect of NBA, we should omit the intermediate variables D and RNB, so that the model becomes that of Figure 6.2.8.

Because the outcome is a binary variable (complication 0: no, 1: yes), we model the expectation $E(y_i) = \text{pr}(y_i = 1)$ using the traditional logit link, as explained in detail in Sections 3.1.2 and 4.1.2. The linear predictor on this logit scale has to be a function of the three variables in Figure 6.2.8 (i.e., A, S, and NBA). The categorical variables S and NBA each have three levels and their effects are modeled by choosing a reference category and estimating the difference between this reference level and the other two levels. The variable

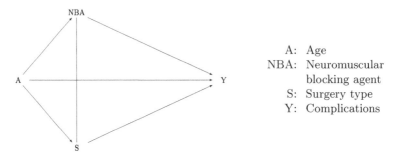

Fig. 6.2.8. Model diagram for initial model without intermediate covariates.

age (A) is a quantitative variable, and we must decide how to enter it into the linear predictor. It is a common belief that older patients have a higher risk of complications, but whether this effect is gradual (so that age could be modeled as having a linear effect) or whether it is only an effect seen above some threshold (such as, e.g., 60 years, a commonly chosen threshold) remains to be investigated.

We therefore initially choose the effect of age as a linear spline (i.e., a broken line; see Section 4.2.1), with a break at the age of 60. This means that age gives rise to two covariates, namely age x_i itself as well as the variable defined from age as

$$x_i^+ = (\text{age} - 60)I(\text{age} > 60).$$

When these two age-related covariates are included in a model for the risk of complications, along with the two categorical variables surgery type and NBA, we get the results presented as Model 1 in Table 6.2.10. We see that the effect of a ten-year increase in age before the age of 60 is estimated as an odds ratio of 1.78. However, for ages beyond 60, a ten-year increase only gives an estimated odds ratio of 1.45. Thus, the extra component in age (corresponding to the break at the age of 60) makes the curve bend in a somewhat unexpected downwards direction but because it is not significant ($P = 0.58$) we are content with the initial choice of modeling age by a linear effect. This changes our results to those of Model 2 in 6.2.10.

We see that both age and surgery type are very significant predictors for the probability of a complication. For abdominal patients the odds of a complication are estimated to be six to eight times as high as for the other two surgery groups, and ten years of age increase the odds by more than 50%. These effects are conditional upon the other two covariates being held fixed, but irrespective of the value of these fixed values. For instance, the effect of age is interpreted as the odds ratio for complication between two individuals with an age difference of ten years having had the same type of surgery (S) and the same type of neuromuscular blocking agent (NBA). We have included no interactions in the model, therefore this odds ratio is assumed to be the

Table 6.2.10. Estimates from Model 1 with linear spline (break at 60 years) in age, and from Model 2 with linear effect of age.

Variable	Model 1 OR (CI)	P	Model 2 OR (CI)	P
Surgery type		<0.0001		<0.0001
Abdominal vs. Orthopedic	8.11 (3.22, 20.45)	<0.0001	8.32 (3.31, 20.95)	<0.0001
Gynecological vs. Orthopedic	1.25 (0.36, 4.29)	0.73	1.27 (0.37, 4.37)	0.81
NBA type		0.48		0.45
Atracurium vs. Vecuronium	1.02 (0.45, 2.33)	0.96	1.03 (0.45, 2.34)	0.95
Pancuronium vs. Vecuronium	1.51 (0.71, 3.24)	0.29	1.52 (0.71, 3.26)	0.28
Age, *10 years increase*			1.61 (1.30, 1.98)	<0.0001
before age 60	1.78 (1.16, 2.74)	<0.0088		
beyond age 60	1.45 (0.95, 2.21)			

same no matter at which surgery type and which blocking agent (NBA) we are looking.

We may well question such an assumption of no interaction, in particular between the two important covariates, age and type of surgery. Figure 6.2.9 shows residuals from Model 2 of Table 6.2.10, plotted against age and with a superimposed smoother for each of the three types of surgery. We are concerned about a possible pattern in these residuals and whether such a pattern might be different in the three groups.

Figure 6.2.9 does not suggest any clear patterns in age and neither does it suggest that the age effects differ from one surgery group to another. Including an interaction between age and surgery type in our model yields the separate estimates of the age effect in the three surgery groups as shown in Table 6.2.11, and even if these seem to be quite different, this difference does not reach significance ($P = 0.45$), possibly because we have too few observed complications. Note that, in this situation, it would be considered a fishing expedition to perform a subgroup analysis and interpret the formal significances in two of the surgery groups and the nonsignificance in the third. Actually, from Table 6.2.11 we see that even if the insignificant age effect in the gynecological group corresponds to the lowest estimated effect among the three, the highly significant age effect in the abdominal group is only estimated a little larger whereas the boundary significant effect in the orthopedic group is by far the largest of the three. This has to do with the age distribution among the patients experiencing complications in the three groups.

Even though the interaction between surgery and age is not significant, this is not the same as saying that the age effects are necessarily identical in the three groups. The reason is of course that we may well have overlooked something due to too small a sample size (a type II error). In order to decide whether anything important may have been overlooked we instead have to

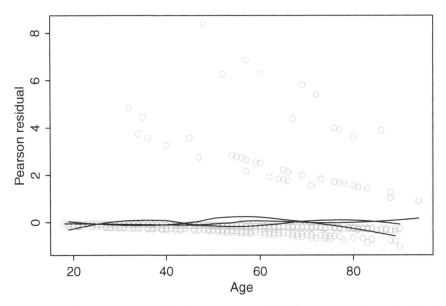

Fig. 6.2.9. Scatterplot of residuals from the model of the right-hand panel of Table 6.2.10 versus age, with superimposed smoothers according to surgery type.

look at estimated differences between age effects. For instance, the difference between the age effect in the orthopedic group and the gynecological group is estimated to be 0.591 with an estimated SD of 0.539 (i.e., with the confidence interval (−0.466, 1.647)). This means that the age effect could have an odds ratio up to a factor $\exp(1.647) = 5.19$ higher in the orthopedic group compared to the gynecological group. We are not in a position to decide whether this may be important but it looks like a large possible discrepancy that cannot be ruled out.

Table 6.2.11. Estimated age effects for each surgery group separately, adjusted for NBA.

Surgery Group	$\widehat{b}$ (SD)	OR (CI) for 10 Years of Age	P
Orthopedic	0.947 (0.459)	2.58 (1.05, 6.34)	0.039
Gynecological	0.356 (0.283)	1.43 (0.82, 2.48)	0.21
Abdominal	0.446 (0.122)	1.56 (1.23, 1.98)	0.0003

Inasmuch as the principal aim of this study was to evaluate the performances of the three different NBA, it is of primary interest to see to which extent this is affected by the modeling of the age effect, especially because we have seen that we cannot feel certain about the modeling of the age effect due to an insufficient amount of data. Table 6.2.12 summarizes the odds ratio estimates between the three neuromuscular blocking agents for different models, and fortunately, we notice a very stable estimation of the differences between the three blocking agents.

Table 6.2.12. Estimated odds ratios between NBA groups from models with different age adjustments.

Model	Atracurium vs. Vecuronium	Pancuronium vs. Vecuronium	Pancuronium vs. Atracurium
Linear age effect	1.03 (0.45, 2.34)	1.52 (0.71, 3.26)	1.48 (0.68, 3.20)
Linear spline for age	1.02 (0.45, 2.33)	1.51 (0.71, 3.24)	1.48 (0.68, 3.20)
Age–surgery interaction	1.03 (0.45, 2.35)	1.52 (0.71, 3.25)	1.47 (0.68, 3.18)

The tempting conclusion seems to be that there is no difference among the three neuromuscular blocking agents. However, as always this conclusion should not be taken on the basis of a significance test alone but always supplemented with a careful consideration of the confidence intervals from Table 6.2.12. If these include values of interest (i.e., values that would have been interesting if they were actually the true differences) our conclusion must be that the study is inconclusive. For example, the comparison between Pancuronium and Atracurium includes an odds ratio of more than three which can hardly be called a small effect. In this situation, therefore, the conclusion is not just that there are no significant differences among the neuromuscular blocking agents but rather that, based on these data, there is insufficient information to conclude whether there might be a difference among the neuromuscular blocking agents.

Among the three NBA, it is known that Pancuronium behaves differently from the other two by being of a so-called long-acting type whereas the other two are short-acting. This makes it interesting to look specifically at two of the three differences and maybe even collapse the two short-acting into one group (seen from Table 6.2.12 that this is at least not spoken against). This does not change the results much, though. We find an estimated OR for complications for long-acting drug versus short-acting drugs to be 1.50 with confidence intervals (0.78, 2.87) and $P = 0.22$.

This seems to conclude our assessment of differences among NBA and at this stage, it would be sensible to perform a model check and search for influential observations. In order not to overload this section with information, we have chosen to present this only for the model that follows after including additional covariates.

Intermediate explanatory variables

In this example, we have two explanatory variables that are intermediate for the neuromuscular blocking agent (which is the covariate of primary interest), namely RNB (residual neuromuscular blockade) and duration of anesthesia. Even if the general recommendation is to avoid the inclusion of such intermediate covariates, the idea pops up that the different NBA may modify the effect of one of these variables. It might, for example, be the case that the long-acting drug Pancuronium could be especially hazardous in terms of complication risk in the presence of RNB, even if Pancuronium as such did not imply an increased risk of getting a RNB. Such a result would be of clinical relevance because it would mean that one should be especially observant with patients receiving this particular neuromuscular blocking agent. Therefore, even if RNB is an intermediate variable for NBA, it may be relevant for the evaluation of the NBA to include it in an interaction with RNB.

Because of the similarity between the two short-acting blockers Atracurium and Vecuronium, we simplify the analyses that follow by collapsing these into one, so that instead of NBA, we now have the categorical covariate long-act on two levels (Pancuronium or one of the other two).

Residual neuromuscular blockade may be modeled in different ways. It originates from a quantitative variable (called TOF-ratio) measuring the depression of nerve stimulation on a scale between 0 and (ideally) 1. However, from clinical experience, it is often dichotomized with a threshold of 0.7, values below this threshold being considered dangerous for subsequent development of complications. We therefore start out by modeling this covariate as a linear spline with a break at 0.7.

Unfortunately, 15 patients have missing values for this covariate and because it is an intermediate variable, this could have potentially harmful consequences for the analyses. As mentioned in Section 6.1.1, the important consideration here is to make sure that the cause is not related to the outcome. Unfortunately, we do have a problem here, because 4 of the 15 missing values (26.7%) occur among the patients with a complication. In the total sample, we see complications for only 46 patients out of 691 (only 6.7%).

We might, therefore, consider imputation of these values. This would require modeling of the TOF-ratio, with covariates such as age, duration of anesthesia, and so on, and subsequently sampling from the resulting conditional distribution. However, we choose not to do so. This is partly in the light of the small proportion of missing values (approximately 2%) and partly because such an imputation would be beyond the scope of this book. We do, however, emphasize that the analyses including this intermediate variable should be interpreted cautiously.

It turns out that the break at 0.7 in the linear model for the effect of RNB (TOF-ratio) does not show an interaction with long-act, $P > 0.2$. Nor is it significant, so we proceed with a model including both TOF-ratio and duration as linear effects, the former with an interaction with long-act. The estimates from this model appear in Table 6.2.13. The interaction between long-acting and TOF-ratio gives $P = 0.007$ and it is seen to be the long-acting drug Pancuronium, which shows a somewhat stronger effect of TOF-ratio than the other two drugs.

Table 6.2.13. Estimates in a model including duration of anesthesia and TOF-ratio, the latter with an interaction with long-act.

Variable	$\widehat{b}$ (SD)	OR (CI)	P
Surgery type			<0.0001
Abdominal vs. Orthopedic	2.274 (0.506)	9.71 (3.60, 26.18)	<0.0001
Gynecological vs. Orthopedic	0.789 (0.671)	2.20 (0.59, 8.20)	0.24
Age, 10 years	0.459 (0.116)	1.58 (1.26, 1.98)	<0.0001
Duration of anesthesia, 1 hour	0.470 (0.160)	1.60 (1.17, 2.19)	0.0033
Long-act vs. short-act at TOF-ratio 0.7	1.055 (0.571)	2.87 (0.94, 8.80)	0.065
TOF-ratio, 0.1 increase			
Pancuronium	−0.501 (0.163)	0.61 (0.44, 0.83)	0.002
Other two	0.344 (0.257)	1.41 (0.85, 2.33)	0.18

Residual plots for this model are shown in Figure 6.2.10. We note a downwards slope for the residuals in the Pancuronium group when TOF-ratio becomes small and when duration of anesthesia becomes large. This suggests that we have overfitted these effects because we observe fewer complications than expected under these circumstances otherwise considered to be dangerous. However, as apparent from Figure 6.2.10, the effect is due to very few observations. As was the case for the example in the previous Section 6.2.1, we also here made plots based on leave-one-out residuals with almost identical results (not shown).

An overall goodness-of-fit test may be performed by subdividing the expected probabilities from the final model into 10 groups and comparing observed and expected number of complications in these groups by a chi-squared test. The observed and expected numbers are given in Table 6.2.14. The resulting test statistic is 3.877 which evaluated in a Chi-squared distribution with 8 degrees-of-freedom gives $P = 0.87$. This test is known as the *Hosmer and Lemeshow goodness-of-fit test* (Hosmer and Lemeshow, 2000, Ch. 5). Note that it may depend somewhat on the precise categorization into ten groups and may be implemented a little differently in different statistical software.

Because of the relatively large size of the dataset we do not expect any single observation to have a large influence on the results. However, we briefly investigate this by looking at a plot of Cook's distance (upper-left corner of Figure 6.2.11) and changes in selected estimated parameters, namely for the

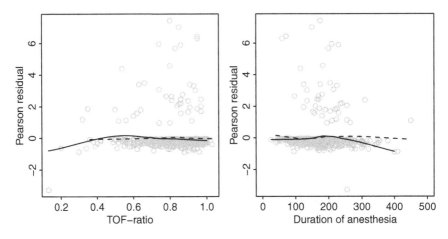

Fig. 6.2.10. Residual plots for model from Table 6.2.13.

Table 6.2.14. Observed and expected number of complications in ten subgroups according to predicted values.

Deciles of Predicted Probabilities of Complication	Number of Subjects	Number of Complications Observed (O)	Expected (E)	$\frac{O-E}{\sqrt{E}}$
1	67	0	0.208	-0.456
2	68	0	0.458	-0.676
3	68	0	0.779	-0.883
4	67	1	1.093	-0.089
5	68	3	1.571	1.140
6	68	3	2.189	0.548
7	67	2	3.118	-0.633
8	68	4	4.895	-0.405
9	68	10	8.518	0.508
10	67	19	19.171	-0.0390

effect of age, duration of anesthesia, and the interaction between TOF-ratio and long-acting NBA. We note a single quite influential observation with a Cook value above 0.1. This corresponds to an abdominal patient aged 67, with a duration of anesthesia of 255 minutes. In spite of a TOF-ratio of only 0.13 and the fact that Pancuronium (the long-acting neuromuscular blocking agent) was used, this patient experienced no complication. We therefore see the large influence on the interaction term (≈ 1) in the lower-right corner. We also note that practically all the subjects with any noteworthy influence on the estimated effect of age (and most of those with an influence on the effect of duration) are subjects experiencing a complication. This is because complications occur rather rarely so that conclusions rely more on these than on the noncomplications. We may want to take the consequence of the single very influential observation and limit the analysis to the subjects with TOF-ratio above, say 0.2. However, because the TOF-ratio is an intermediate variable, that would be questionable and such a selection may lead to biased results. Intuitively, if the long-acting drug leads to many low TOF-ratios (with complications) and these were all removed from the dataset, the long-acting drug would no longer seem dangerous. Instead, the consequence of such an influential observation should be to carry out a larger investigation and thereby, it is hoped, be able to model the effect of TOF-ratio in a more satisfactory way.

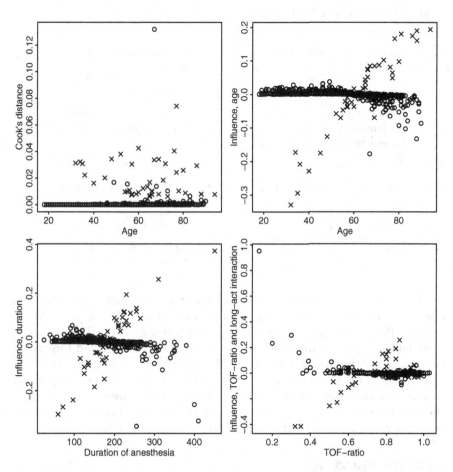

Fig. 6.2.11. Influence diagnostics. Cook's distance and influence on selected parameter estimates: the effect of age, duration of anesthesia, and the interaction between long-act and TOF-ratio; ×: patients with complications, ○: patients without complications.

Conclusion

Because the model checks and the search for influential observations revealed no drastic problems with our model, we conclude that the results stated in Table 6.2.13 could be the final results from these analyses. The differences among the three neuromuscular blocking agents was the focus of the analysis, thus the main finding is that Pancuronium increases the risk of a complication for patients having a low TOF-ratio. If we remove the insignificant effect of the TOF-ratio for the short-acting drugs, we get slightly modified odds ratio estimates as seen in Table 6.2.15.

Table 6.2.15. Odds ratios for the final model including only effect of TOF-ratio for Pancuronium.

Variable	OR (CI)	P
Surgery type		<0.0001
Abdominal vs. Orthopedic	9.15 (3.42, 24.48)	<0.0001
Gynecological vs. Orthopedic	2.02 (0.55, 7.46)	0.29
Age, 10 years	1.55 (1.24, 1.94)	<0.0001
Duration of anesthesia, 1 hour	1.52 (1.12, 2.06)	0.0072
Long-act vs. short-act at TOF-ratio 0.7	1.62 (0.82, 3.23)	0.17
TOF-ratio, 0.1 increase, Pancuronium	0.61 (0.45, 0.84)	0.0024

The six curves in Figure 6.2.12 illustrate the estimated probability of a complication for the three surgery groups, two curves for each according to whether Pancuronium (the long-acting drug) had been used. The estimated probabilities are calculated for a patient aged 60 years having had surgery for two hours, and they are plotted against the value for the TOF-ratio. Note that corresponding to the results from Table 6.2.15, only the curves corresponding to Pancuronium show an effect of the TOF-ratio. We investigated whether the structure of those curves was much affected by the single influential observation and, fortunately, that turned out not to be the case.

6.2.3 The PBC-3 trial

Recall from Section 1.1.1 that PBC-3 was a multicenter randomized clinical trial conducted in six European hospitals with patient accrual between January 1983 and January 1987. In this period, 349 patients with the liver disease primary biliary cirrhosis (PBC) were randomized to either treatment with Cyclosporin A (CyA, 176 patients) or placebo (173 patients). PBC is a slowly progressing liver disease with patients diagnosed at varying disease stages,

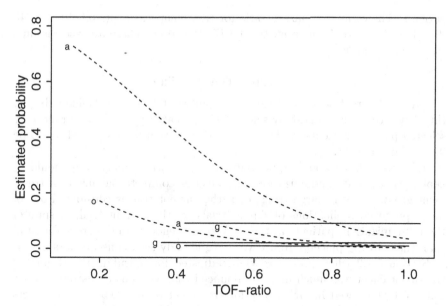

Fig. 6.2.12. Illustration of estimated probabilities of a complication, for the three surgery groups, according to whether Pancuronium has been used. Estimated probabilities are plotted against values of the TOF-ratio. Solid line: Pancuronium, from top to bottom: abdominal, gynecological, orthopedic.

thereby making populations of patients with PBC rather heterogeneous. The purpose of the trial, as explained in Section 1.1.1, was to study the effect of treatment on "time to failure of medical treatment" defined as either death or liver transplantation. Patients were followed from randomization until treatment failure, drop-out, or 1 January 1989; 90 patients (CyA: 44, placebo: 46) had an observed treatment failure and 4 patients were lost to follow-up before 1 January 1989. For the sake of simplicity, we will "no treatment failure" by "survival" in what follows.

At time of entry, a number of clinical and biochemical variables were scheduled to be recorded in all patients, however, some laboratory tests are missing in a few patients as further described below. At the same time, a liver biopsy was also scheduled but this was for various reasons only taken in 82% of the patients in the placebo group and 85% of the CyA-treated patients. Missing data was therefore more severe for histological variables (i.e., those obtained from the liver biopsy).

Inasmuch as this is a randomized study, a simple and "correct" analysis of the data would be that of a simple comparison between the survival times in the two treatment groups (taking proper account of censoring as explained in earlier chapters). Thus, the two-sample logrank test and the Cox regression model including treatment as the only covariate were discussed in Section 3.1.3 and showed no difference in survival between CyA- and placebo-treated patients. The estimated hazard ratio for treatment was $\exp(-0.059) = 0.943$ (0.624, 1.426) and the logrank test 0.077, $P = 0.78$. These analyses assume the simple diagram:

Treatment $\rightarrow$ Time to failure.

The resulting treatment effect can be considered the *marginal* effect, that is, (literally) comparing randomly selected CyA-treated patients with randomly selected placebo patients. In fact, the randomization allows this effect to be interpreted causally.

Even though one could argue that this is *the* correct analysis, it should be kept in mind that randomization only ensures complete balancing of treatment groups for very large trials, or if the current trial is considered one of many potential replications of similar trials. In the current trial, in spite of the randomization, patients in the CyA group tended to be more severely ill than those in the placebo group. We have already seen consequences of this in Section 5.1.2 where we noted that, adjusted for bilirubin, the estimated treatment effect was much more pronounced than without adjustment. Thus Table 5.1.11 showed hazard ratios for treatment around 0.67. These effects are now to be interpreted conditionally on bilirubin, that is, comparing randomly selected CyA and placebo patients with the same level of bilirubin, and assuming that this effect is the same no matter the bilirubin value (the assumption of no interaction as discussed in Section 5.2.2). This leads us to consider the "natural history of PBC," that is, what we would expect to see in the placebo group. Survival will be affected by liver function, L:

Liver function $\rightarrow$ Time to failure

and possibly also by the basic variables gender, G, age, A, and hospital, H. However, although gender and age may affect the outcome, time to treatment failure (Y) both directly and via liver function, it is likely that the only effect of hospital on the outcome will be through liver function, gender, and age. This is because hospitals may recruit from different patient populations, but given liver function, gender and age there should be no effect of hospital on the outcome. This leads us to the diagram:

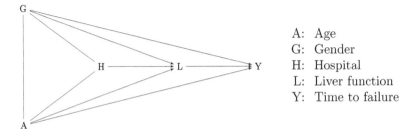

A: Age
G: Gender
H: Hospital
L: Liver function
Y: Time to failure

Next, we wish to add treatment (T) to the diagram. Treatment will affect the survival time (the effect of interest) and if randomization were completely succesful then treatment should have no association with other explanatory variables, leading to the diagram:

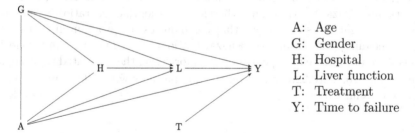

A: Age
G: Gender
H: Hospital
L: Liver function
T: Treatment
Y: Time to failure

According to this diagram, the effect of treatment on survival time can be studied without consideration of other explanatory variables. However, in the current study, treatment may be associated with both age and liver function due to incomplete randomization. Randomization was blocked on both gender and hospital therefore there is by definition no association between treatment and these two variables. This leads to the diagram in Figure 6.2.13.

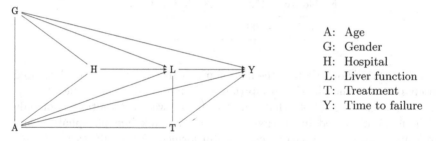

A: Age
G: Gender
H: Hospital
L: Liver function
T: Treatment
Y: Time to failure

Fig. 6.2.13. Model diagram for the PBC-3 study.

According to the diagram in Figure 6.2.13, an initial analysis of the effect of treatment on the outcome should take liver function and age into account but not gender and hospital. However, because gender may have a direct effect on the survival time, we would recommend (see Section 6.1.4) evaluating how sensitive the estimated treatment effect is to deletion of gender from the model. Liver function is not measured directly but only via biochemical markers such as bilirubin, albumin, alkaline phosphatase (alkph), aspartate transaminase (ast), and via histological stage. Therefore, we consider how the distribution of these variables may differ between the two treatment groups and, on the other hand, how these variables affect survival.

Table 6.2.16 shows the results for histological stage and 6.2.17 for the other variables. It can be deduced from Table 6.2.16 that out of those with a biopsy, 58.4% of CyA-treated patients are in the more severe stages 3 or 4 whereas that is only the case for 50% in the placebo group. Also, that table shows that patients in stages 2 or 3 have significantly better survival than the reference group, stage 4. Note also the ridiculously small $\hat{b}$ and large SD for stage 1. This is because no treatment failures were seen in that stage, making the estimated hazard ratio 0 and, therefore, the log(hazard ratio) is "minus infinity." The numbers for stage 1 that come out of the program in that case have no meaning (but the other log(hazard ratios), stage 2 versus 4 and stage 3 versus 4 are not affected by this). Adjusted for stage, the estimated treatment effect is $\hat{b} = -0.092(0.229)$ based on the 291 patients with a liver biopsy (77 treatment failures).

Table 6.2.16. PBC-3 study: distribution (%) of histological stage in treatment groups and its (unadjusted) effect on survival.

Stage	Placebo (%)	CyA (%)	Cox Model $\hat{b}$	SD
1	14.5	13.6	−16.48	609.6
2	26.6	21.6	−1.67	0.32
3	17.9	21.0	−0.98	0.28
4	23.1	28.4	Reference	
No biopsy	17.9	15.3	Not included	
Total	100	100		

Table 6.2.17 shows that all the liver markers are worse among CyA-treated patients than in the placebo group (lower albumin and higher values for the other three markers). Note that, due to very skewed distributions, not only bilirubin, as discussed in Section 4.1.3, but also alkaline phosphatase and aspartate transaminase have been log-transformed. Although, as mentioned earlier, there are no requirements on the distribution of a covariate, in the initial modeling of the effects of those markers we use log-transformed versions. Subsequently, during the model checking, we study whether this provides a reasonable description of the hazard rate. As expected, the fraction of females is about the same in both groups. The table also shows the estimated treatment effect after adjustment for each of the other variables. Albumin, bilirubin (as we know), ast and gender are significantly associated with survival whereas alkph and age are not. The treatment effect after adjustment is everywhere increased compared to the unadjusted estimate of $\hat{b} = -0.059 (0.211)$, most pronounced after adjustment for bilirubin. The numbers of missing values are small: albumin (6), bilirubin (0), alkph (0), and ast (1).

Returning to the diagram in Figure 6.2.13, and interpreting "liver function", L as joint effects of the markers bilirubin, albumin, alkph, and ast (and, perhaps, histological stage), we estimate the treatment effect adjusted for these covariates and for age (although the age distributions seem rather similar in the two treatment groups). Note that, even though gender according

Table 6.2.17. PBC-3 study: distribution of covariates in treatment groups, their (unadjusted) effect on survival, and the treatment effect after adjustment for each covariate.

Variable	Placebo Mean	SD	CyA Mean	SD	Covariate Effect $\hat{b}$	SD	Treatment Effect $\hat{b}$	SD
Albumin(g/L)	39.3	5.3	37.5	5.8	−0.129	0.020	−0.294	0.218
log(bilirubin)(μmol/L)	3.14	0.99	3.26	1.05	1.01	0.099	−0.399	0.215
log(alkph)(IU/L)	6.64	0.76	6.66	0.71	0.246	0.145	−0.073	0.211
log(ast)(IU/L)	4.39	0.57	4.43	0.56	0.968	0.205	−0.104	0.212
Age (years)	54.0	10.0	54.2	10.0	0.0124	0.0109	−0.056	0.211
Gender (% females)	85.6		85.2		−0.674	0.249	−0.065	0.211

to Table 6.2.17 is significant, this need not have consequences for evaluation of the treatment effect, inasmuch as gender is, formally, not a confounder (because of the lack of association between gender and treatment). As a safeguard, however, as recommended, we evaluate how sensitive the estimated treatment effect is to inclusion of gender in the model. Table 6.2.18 shows the results. A number of models were fitted. In Model 1 both age and the four biochemical markers were included. This model, based on 341 patients with 87 treatment failures, gave a treatment effect of −0.568 whereas, in Model 2, eliminating age which has similar distributions in the two treatment groups changed this to −0.604. In Model 3, age is included and the two insignificant markers, alkph and ast, are eliminated. Here, the estimated treatment effect is −0.544 (based on 343 patients with 88 events). Keeping only bilirubin and albumin as adjustment variables (Model 4) the treatment effect is −0.574. Model 5 includes all markers, age, and histological stage (dichotomized as 3 or 4 versus 1 or 2) and is based on only 285 patients with 74 events. Here, the estimated treatment effect is −0.543 with a SD somewhat larger than in Models 1–4, namely 0.243. Adding gender to Model 1, the treatment effect changes from a hazard ratio of $\exp(-0.568) = 0.57$ to $\exp(-0.531) = 0.59$, a change of only 3.7% on the hazard ratio scale. Therefore, gender is, indeed, not needed as an adjustment variable when assessing the effect of treatment.

Because no interactions were considered of special interest in this study, we do not pursue a study of interactions between treatment and other variables. Note that, even though bilirubin has a profound influence on survival this does not call for a special investigation of a potential treatment interaction.

Model checking

To evaluate the results, the assumptions of the models must be checked. We focus on Model 1 and examine the assumptions of proportional hazards and linear effects on the log(hazard rate) of the quantitative covariates. Because treatment is the covariate of primary interest we first study the proportional

Table 6.2.18. PBC-3 study: effects on survival of covariates and treatment.

Variable	Model 1 $\widehat{b}$ (SD)	Model 2 $\widehat{b}$ (SD)	Model 3 $\widehat{b}$ (SD)	Model 4 $\widehat{b}$ (SD)	Model 5 $\widehat{b}$ (SD)
Treatment	−0.568	−0.604	−0.544	−0.574	−0.544
	(0.224)	(0.227)	(0.223)	(0.224)	(0.243)
Albumin	−0.070	−0.086	−0.073	−0.091	−0.060
	(0.024)	(0.023)	(0.023)	(0.022)	(0.026)
log(bilirubin)	1.036	0.974	1.071	0.959	0.962
	(0.128)	(0.127)	(0.112)	(0.107)	(0.157)
log(alkph)	−0.111	−0.146			−0.053
	(0.160)	(0.161)			(0.180)
log(ast)	0.290	0.122			0.335
	(0.243)	(0.132)			(0.270)
Age (years)	0.039		0.038		0.039
	(0.013)		(0.012)		(0.015)
Stage (3–4 vs. 1–2)					0.809
					(0.348)

hazards assumption for treatment. The assumption is that the hazard ratio for treatment is constant over time or, in other words, that there is "no interaction between treatment and time." Therefore, one way of checking this assumption is to introduce such an interaction and study whether the added flexibility provides a model with better fit. A simple way of doing this is to add a covariate of the form

$$I(i \text{ is treated with CyA})f(t) \tag{6.2.1}$$

to Model 1. The results from this approach will to some extent depend on the choice of the function $f(t)$ in (6.2.1), however, the sensitivity tends not to be great; see Table 6.2.19. According to this table, the proportional hazards assumption is not questionable for any of the covariates. The table also shows the treatment effects estimated allowing the effect of each covariate (except treatment), in turn, to have a time-varying effect. It is seen that these treatment effects are quite insensitive to this extra flexibility of the model.

For treatment we further evaluate the assumption graphically without having to specify a parametric alternative to proportionality via a function $f(t)$. This builds on another way of relaxing the proportional hazards assumption for treatment, which is to study the *stratified Cox model* (5.1.4) where the log(hazard rate) for patient i is

$$l_i(t) = \log(h_{0j}(t)) + b_{\text{alb}}\text{Albumin}_i + \cdots + b_{\text{age}}\text{Age}_i, j = 0, 1, \tag{6.2.2}$$

where $j = 1$ if i was treated with CyA and $j = 0$ if i belonged to the placebo group. In (6.2.2), $h_{00}(t)$ is an unspecified baseline hazard for placebo-treated

Table 6.2.19. PBC-3 study: tests for proportional hazards for treatment and other covariates.

Covariate, x	$f(t)$	Effect of $xf(t)$				Treatment Effect	
		$\widehat{b}$	SD	$(\widehat{b}/\text{SD})^2$	P	$\widehat{b}$	SD
Treatment	$\log(t)$	0.093	0.257	0.13	0.72		
Treatment	t	0.031	0.180	0.03	0.86		
Albumin	$\log(t)$	0.034	0.027	1.54	0.22	−0.573	0.224
$\log$(bilirubin)	$\log(t)$	−0.092	0.130	0.51	0.48	−0.553	0.225
$\log$(bilirubin)	t	−0.073	0.092	0.62	0.43	−0.548	0.225
$\log$(alkph)	$\log(t)$	−0.023	0.172	0.02	0.89	−0.568	0.224
$\log$(ast)	$\log(t)$	−0.402	0.268	2.25	0.13	−0.550	0.224
Age	$\log(t)$	0.024	0.013	3.62	0.06	−0.570	0.225
Model 1						−0.568	0.224

patients (with all other covariates being 0), just like the baseline hazard in Model 1. However, in (6.2.2) the baseline hazard for CyA-treated patients is no longer bound to $h_{00}(t)$ as $\exp(b_{\text{CyA}})h_{00}(t)$ but instead it is allowed to vary freely; that is, no restrictions are imposed on $h_{01}(t)$. The stratified Cox model was fitted to the data which provided effects for the five quantitative covariates close to those shown in Table 6.2.18. Figure 6.2.14 shows a plot of the estimated cumulative baseline hazard $\widehat{H}_{01}(t)$ for CyA against that for placebo $\widehat{H}_{00}(t)$ just as the corresponding Figure 3.1.7 which showed unadjusted cumulative hazards. When proportional hazards is a reasonable assumption, the plot will approximate a straight line through the point (0,0) with slope $\approx \exp(b_{\text{CyA}})$. This is more or less what we see in Figure 6.2.14. Similar plots could be made for each of the five quantitative covariates from Model 1. To do so would require stratification into suitable intervals (as we did for bilirubin in Figure 3.2.7) and fitting a stratified model allowing an unspecified baseline hazard in each stratum. We have chosen not to present these graphs in the text but leave this investigation as an exercise.

Digression. Time-dependent covariates

The added covariate in (6.2.1) is an example of a time-dependent covariate and one important feature of the Cox regression model (and other hazard regression models; see Section 7.5) is its ability to cope with such covariates. The variable "treatment $\times f(t)$" is a very simple example of a time-dependent covariate because, for a given treatment group, its value at any time t is *known in advance*; that is, it is nonrandom. Another example of a time-dependent covariate that develops deterministically over time would be "current age" which is simply "age at entry $+t$."

In the PBC-3 study, patients were scheduled to be seen at follow-up visits to the treating hospital during the course of the trial. At such visits, blood samples were taken and updated measurements of the biochemical variables, such as bilirubin and albumin, are therefore available. However, when evaluating the effect of treatment,

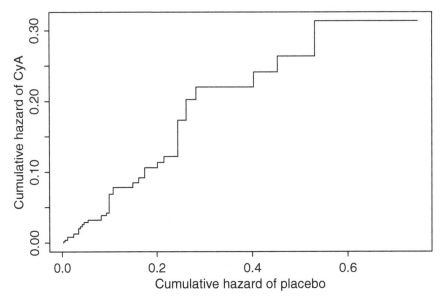

Fig. 6.2.14. PBC-3 stratified Cox model: cumulative baseline hazard for CyA patients plotted against that for placebo-treated patients.

which is the main purpose of the trial, such time-dependent covariates should not be considered because they may be intermediate variables between treatment and survival (Section 6.1.2). Analysis of the effect of such variables may, on the other hand, be very useful in understanding both the natural course of the disease and how treatment may affect survival. A further difficulty in connection with this kind of truly random time-dependent covariate is that the survival probability can no longer be computed from the hazard function: equations such as (3.1.21) no longer hold. This is because the probability of still being alive at some later point in time will depend not only on current values of covariates but also on their future development, so, a joint model for the time-dependent covariate and its effect on the hazard function is needed. Such joint models are beyond the scope of the present book and the reader is referred to Wulfsohn and Tsiatis (1997) or Henderson, Diggle, and Dobson (2000).

Notice the difference between a time-dependent covariate and a covariate with a time-dependent effect. The basic assumption in the Cox regression model is proportional hazards, that is, a time-constant hazard ratio for each covariate. Such an assumption may still be valid even though a covariate may depend on time. In Section 7.5.2, we study a hazard model where the effects of covariates are allowed to be time-varying (on an additive scale). ⋄

We next turn to an examination of linearity of the effects of the quantitative covariates. We examine this assumption by adding a linear spline function (Section 4.2.1) to Model 1 for each covariate, in turn, and study how this affects both the fit of the model and the estimated treatment effect. The covariate intervals in which the effect is assumed linear were chosen to have endpoints (r_1, r_2) close to the tertiles of the covariate distribution. That is, for a covariate x we include the term

$$b_0 x_i + b_1(x_i - r_1)I(x_i > r_1) + b_2(x_i - r_2)I(x_i > r_2)$$

in the linear predictor. Table 6.2.20 shows the results. Although the linearity assumption is, formally, rejected at the 5% level for log(ast), it is seen that nowhere does the inclusion of the linear splines change the treatment effect much.

Table 6.2.20. PBC-3 study: tests for linearity for quantitative covariates.

Covariate (Cutpoints)	$\hat{b}_0$ (SD)	$\hat{b}_1$ (SD)	$\hat{b}_2$ (SD)	P for Linearity	$\hat{b}_{CyA}$ (SD)
Albumin (30,40)	−0.054 (0.122)	−0.034 (0.145)	0.067 (0.092)	0.77	−0.572 (0.225)
log(bilirubin) (10,40)	−1.226 (1.055)	2.821 (1.288)	−0.696 (0.480)	0.09	−0.568 (0.225)
log(alkph) (500,1200)	0.456 (0.654)	−0.647 (0.924)	−0.079 (0.749)	0.61	−0.577 (0.225)
log(ast) (60,120)	3.273 (1.318)	−3.986 (1.685)	0.695 (0.963)	0.047	−0.533 (0.226)
Age (50,60)	0.024 (0.035)	0.039 (0.065)	−0.043 (0.065)	0.79	−0.572 (0.226)

As an overall evaluation of the model, Figures 6.2.15 – 6.2.19 show plots of standardized pseudo-residuals against covariates for the timepoints 0.71, 1.18, 2.16, and 3.19 years. It is seen that the smooth curves through the residuals are close to 0 with few exceptions for the largest timepoint (3.19 years) and for the most extreme values of albumin, log(bilirubin), and log(ast).

We, finally, looked at deletion diagnostics for Model 1 and a single influential point for the effect of albumin was detected, Figure 6.2.20. This is a patient failing at 2.5 years with a high albumin level of 56.7 g/L. Eliminating this observation would reduce the effect of albumin by $0.46 \times SD(\hat{b}_{alb}) = 0.011$; see Figure 6.2.20. No other estimates would be affected by more than about 0.3 SD, if deleted.

Conclusion

In the models analyzed in Table 6.2.18, the insignificant marginal hazard ratio for treatment, 0.943, changed into significant values ranging from $\exp(-0.604) = 0.55$ to $\exp(-0.544) = 0.58$. Even though the marginal estimate is a valid one due to the randomized design we would argue that the

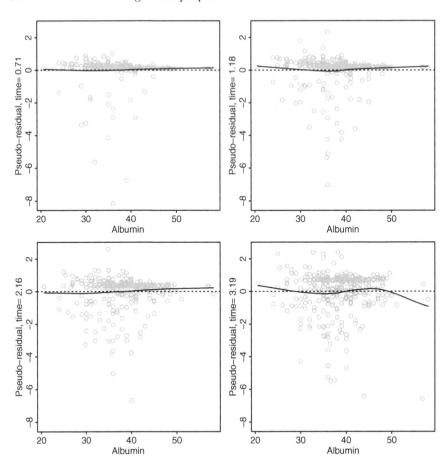

Fig. 6.2.15. PBC-3: pseudo-residuals from Model 1 plotted against albumin for the timepoints 0.71, 1.18, 2.16, and 3.19 years.

adjusted estimates are more correct because they address the influence of the not quite successful randomization. Based on the model diagram and on the fact that removing age (which has little association with treatment) from the model, the treatment effect changes somewhat, we prefer the fully adjusted Model 1. Alternatively, one could quote Model 5 also adjusting for histological stage. However, in that case one would have to address the large number of missing values, for example, via some sort of multiple imputation. Table 6.2.21 shows hazard ratios with confidence limits for the covariates in Model 1. For the three covariates that have been log-transformed, hazard ratios and confidence limits corresponding to a doubling of the covariate have been calculated from Table 6.2.18 as explained in Appendix B.

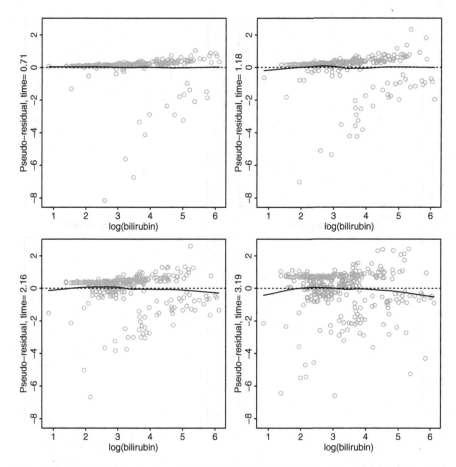

Fig. 6.2.16. PBC-3: pseudo-residuals from Model 1 plotted against log(bilirubin) for the timepoints 0.71, 1.18, 2.16, and 3.19 years.

Table 6.2.21. PBC-3 study: estimated hazard ratios (with 95% confidence limits) for covariates in Model 1.

Covariate		Hazard Ratio	(95% Confidence Limits)
Treatment	(CyA vs. placebo)	0.567	(0.365,0.879)
Albumin	(per 10 g/L)	0.494	(0.310,0.789)
Bilirubin	(per doubling)	2.05	(1.72,2.44)
Alkaline phosphatase	(per doubling)	0.924	(0.745,1.150)
Aspartate transaminase	(per doubling)	1.22	(0.872,1.72)
Age	(per 10 years)	1.48	(1.16,1.89)

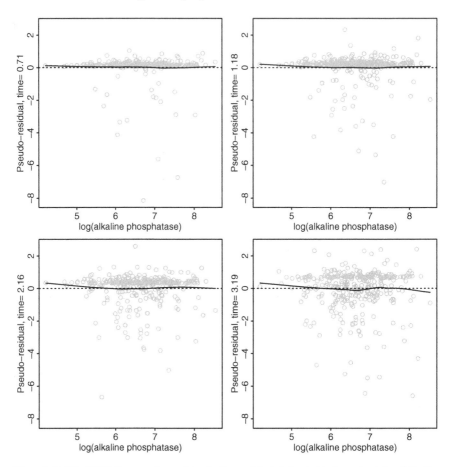

Fig. 6.2.17. PBC-3: pseudo-residuals from Model 1 plotted against log(alkaline phosphatase) for the timepoints 0.71, 1.18, 2.16, and 3.19 years.

6.3 Sample size determination

So far, n has just denoted the number of individuals in our dataset and not much attention has been devoted to the way in which this sample size was determined. However, when planning investigations, it is important to assess the "necessary" size of the study. If new data collection is involved, costs will increase with sample size. If treatments are being compared in a clinical trial then it would be unethical to let the trial continue for such a long period that too many patients are treated with an inferior drug. Even if an existing database is going to be used to study a new question, then it is important to evaluate whether the question may, at all, be satisfactorily addressed.

By "necessary" size we mean that the sample should be sufficiently large to address the scientific question of interest. Technically, this means that the

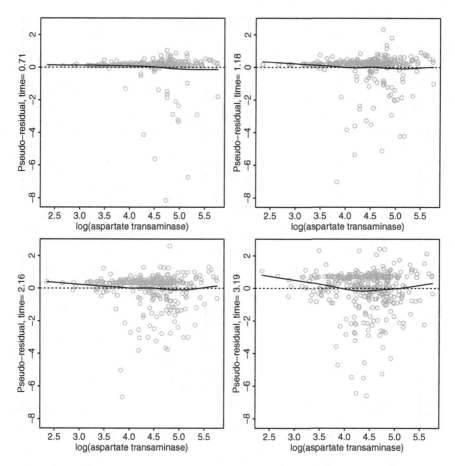

Fig. 6.2.18. PBC-3: pseudo-residuals from Model 1 plotted against log(aspartate transaminase) for the timepoints 0.71, 1.18, 2.16, and 3.19 years.

power for a relevant alternative of interest, that is, an important difference not to be overlooked, should be sufficiently large. We focus on the simple two-sample situation (Section 3.1) and only add a few remarks on a single quantitative covariate with a linear effect (Section 4.1). In both of these situations, only one parameter is involved. It may seem rather modest and unrealistic to focus on such simple situations but we do, in fact, recommend to base sample size determination on the identification of one (or a few) core two-sample problem(s) to make sure that the sample size suffices to address those satisfactorily. This is also in line with our recommendation not to design too complicated studies attempting to answer many questions at a time (Section 6.1).

The sample size may, alternatively, be determined to obtain a desired precision (SD) of a parameter estimate. In our opinion, this situation occurs quite

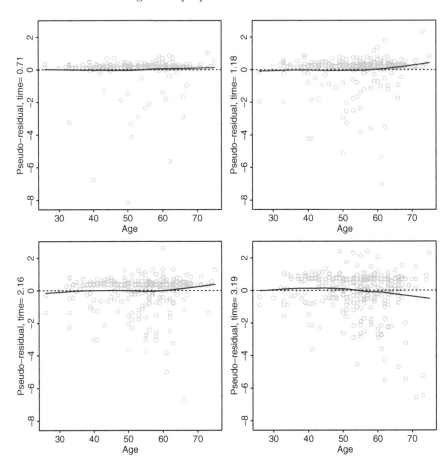

Fig. 6.2.19. PBC-3: pseudo-residuals from Model 1 plotted against age for the timepoints 0.71, 1.18, 2.16, and 3.19 years.

infrequently in practice and is not further discussed. We only briefly comment on situations where the effect of interest is adjusted for other covariates, situations that will typically require larger samples. It is a consequence of the fact that adjustments require larger samples that a randomized study is to be preferred to an observational study. This is because a randomized study will reduce or even eliminate the need for adjustment for other covariates, and thereby also reduce the demand on the sample size. Even more important, it will increase the validity of the conclusions from the study. However, randomized designs are of course not always feasible, for example, in investigations aimed at studying a harmful effect of a substance such as tobacco.

For the one-parameter situation, a simple formula is available for the necessary sample size n as a function of the desired power $1 - \beta$, and the relevant effect size b_0 (and a few more quantities; see below). For more complicated

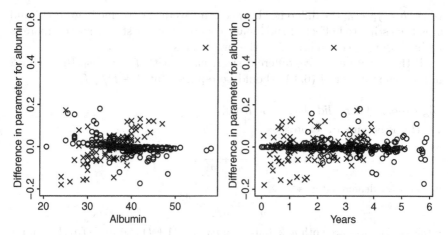

Fig. 6.2.20. PBC-3: deletion diagnostics from Model 1 for the effect of albumin plotted against albumin or against time.

situations, no general formulas exist and the necessary sample size will depend on many more aspects of the data, including the joint distribution of all covariates and their postulated effects on the outcome. In such situations, a general way of approaching the problem is to use simulations, that is, to randomly generate many datasets with the required specifications, to compute the relevant test statistic on each generated dataset, and simply evaluate the fraction of repetitions for which the test statistic is significant. This fraction will estimate the power for the chosen sample size. Even though this sounds easy in principle, it may be difficult in practice to specify all aspects of the situation. Of course, simulations may also be used in the simple one-parameter situation as an alternative to using the formulas presented in the following. In addition, many computer programs are available (both commercial and freely available) for doing sample size calculations.

As in earlier chapters, we highlight similarities among the techniques for quantitative, binary, and survival time outcome variables and present test statistics for these three types of data with exactly the same structure. This means that the way in which the necessary sample size is determined based on the formulas follows precisely the same pattern in all cases. We therefore first present the formulas and subsequently explain how they are used.

Quantitative outcome

The two-sample problem is here the comparison of two mean values. For *equal group sizes* the relevant t-test statistic (3.1.6) from Section 3.1.1 is

$$t = \frac{\bar{y}_1 - \bar{y}_0}{s\sqrt{\frac{1}{n/2} + \frac{1}{n/2}}} = \sqrt{n}\frac{\widehat{b}}{2s}, \qquad (6.3.1)$$

where $\widehat{b} = \bar{y}_1 - \bar{y}_0$, the difference between the average outcome in groups 1 and 0, is the estimated effect of the binary covariate under study. Furthermore, s is the (assumed common) SD in the two groups.

If the two groups have different sizes, n_0, n_1 with $f = n_1/n_0$, the factor 2 in the denominator of (6.3.1) should be replaced by $(1 + f)/\sqrt{f}$.

Digression. Where did that come from?

This is because the expression

$$\frac{1}{n_0} + \frac{1}{n_1}$$

in the t-test denominator is

$$\frac{1}{n/2} + \frac{1}{n/2} = \frac{4}{n}$$

if the sample sizes are both $n/2$, but when $n_0 = n/(1+f)$ and $n_1 = fn/(1+f)$, the expression becomes

$$\frac{1+f}{n} + \frac{1+f}{fn} = \frac{(1+f)^2/f}{n}.$$

◇

Binary outcome

For binary data, the most obvious way to compare the outcome in two groups is directly to use the two proportions of 1-outcomes, $\widehat{p}_0$ and $\widehat{p}_1$. The resulting test statistic follows from the construction of a confidence interval for the risk difference (Section 3.1.2). In the case of equal group sizes, the test statistic is

$$\frac{\widehat{p}_1 - \widehat{p}_0}{\sqrt{\frac{\widehat{p}_0(1-\widehat{p}_0)}{n/2} + \frac{\widehat{p}_1(1-\widehat{p}_1)}{n/2}}} = \sqrt{n}\frac{\widehat{b}}{\sqrt{2}\sqrt{\widehat{p}_0(1 - \widehat{p}_0) + \widehat{p}_1(1 - \widehat{p}_1)}} \approx \sqrt{n}\frac{\widehat{b}}{2s}. \quad (6.3.2)$$

In (6.3.2), $\widehat{b} = \widehat{p}_1 - \widehat{p}_0$ is the estimated risk difference, and $s = \sqrt{\bar{p}(1 - \bar{p})}$ (with $\bar{p} = (p_0 + p_1)/2$, the average probability of a 1-outcome). In previous chapters, focus has been on log(odds ratios) when analyzing binary outcomes. The corresponding test statistic follows directly from the confidence interval (3.1.19) for the log(odds ratio)

$$\frac{\log\left(\frac{\widehat{p}_1}{1-\widehat{p}_1}\right) - \log\left(\frac{\widehat{p}_0}{1-\widehat{p}_0}\right)}{\sqrt{\frac{2/n}{\widehat{p}_1(1-\widehat{p}_1)} + \frac{2/n}{\widehat{p}_0(1-\widehat{p}_0)}}} \approx \sqrt{n}\frac{\widehat{b}}{2s}, \quad (6.3.3)$$

where now $\widehat{b}$ is the estimated log(odds ratio) and $s = 1/\sqrt{\bar{p}(1 - \bar{p})}$.

In the case of different group sizes, $n_1 = fn_0$, the factor 2 in the denominators of (6.3.2) and (6.3.3) should be replaced by $(1 + f)/\sqrt{f}$, similarly to the case of quantitative data.

Survival data

For survival data, the two-sample logrank test (3.1.32) cannot directly be written in the same form as (6.3.1)–(6.3.3). However, a simple approximation (Schoenfeld, 1983) based on a model with a *constant* hazard (see Section 7.5.1) is available. As above, we study two groups where (possibly censored) survival times are observed, and we wish to compare the survival time distributions in the groups via the log(hazard ratio). Let $\widehat{b}$ be the estimated log(hazard ratio) and q the *average failure probability*. This will depend on a number of aspects of the study. First, it depends on the survival functions in the two groups to be compared, for example, expressed as the median survival times. Typically, patients are recruited to a survival study over a certain *accrual period* and subsequently followed through a *follow-up period* and q also depends on the lengths of these accrual and follow-up periods as explained in more detail below; see Equation (6.3.7). In the case of equal sample sizes, the test statistic that approximates the logrank test is simply:

$$\sqrt{n}\frac{\widehat{b}}{2s} \tag{6.3.4}$$

with $s = 1/\sqrt{q}$. For different group sizes, $n_1 = fn_0$, we again replace the factor 2 in the denominator of (6.3.4) by $(1 + f)/\sqrt{f}$.

General approach

We have seen that the relevant test statistic for the two-group comparison in all cases takes the same simple form (6.3.1)–(6.3.4). This test statistic follows approximately a standard Normal distribution under the hypothesis H_0 of no difference between the two groups ($b = 0$), and it is approximately Normal with mean $\sqrt{n}b_0/(2s)$ and SD$= 1$ under the alternative hypothesis $b = b_0$. It follows that the same approach for sample size calculations can be used, at least approximately, for all three types of outcome. This approximation turns out to be sufficiently good for practical purposes, partly because the n that comes out of a sample size determination should always be considered "an order of magnitude" and not a precise number. Thus, sample size calculations leading to, for example, $n = 120$ or $n = 150$ should not be considered entirely different. This has to do with the uncertainty attached to some of the quantities that enter into the considerations introduced in what follows.

   This is the general approach common to the three types of outcome considered: for a given level of significance, α (in practice almost always $\alpha = 0.05$) we wish to address one of the following problems.

1. For given effect size b_0 and given power $1 - \beta$, find the sample size n for which the power is $1 - \beta$.
2. For given sample size n and effect size b_0 find the power of the test for this alternative.

3. For given sample size n and power $1 - \beta$ find the effect size b_0 for which the power is $1 - \beta$.

The three quantities n, b_0, and β are related through the formula

$$n = \frac{(z_{1-\alpha/2} + z_{1-\beta})^2 \frac{(1+f)^2}{f} s^2}{b_0^2}. \tag{6.3.5}$$

Digression. From where does that formula come?

We want, for all types of outcome, the sample size n (for equal-sized groups, $f = 1$) to be so large that the test statistic

$$t_n = \sqrt{n} \frac{\widehat{b}}{2s}$$

is (numerically) larger than $z_{1-\alpha/2}$ with probability $1 - \beta$ when the true effect size is b_0. We look at the case where $b_0 > 0$ (the case $b_0 < 0$ is completely analogous). In this case

$$\mathrm{pr}(|t_n| > z_{1-\alpha/2}) \approx \mathrm{pr}(t_n > z_{1-\alpha/2}) = \mathrm{pr}(t_n - \sqrt{n}\frac{b_0}{2s} > z_{1-\alpha/2} - \sqrt{n}\frac{b_0}{2s}). \tag{6.3.6}$$

When $b = b_0$, the distribution of $t_n - \sqrt{n}b_0/(2s)$ is standard Normal, so the probability in (6.3.6) is $1 - \beta$ when

$$z_{1-\alpha/2} - \sqrt{n}\frac{b_0}{2s} = z_\beta = -z_{1-\beta},$$

and (6.3.5) follows (for $f = 1$). $\diamond$

In (6.3.5), z_p is the pth percentile in the standard Normal distribution (i.e., $z_{0.975} = 1.96$ when $\alpha = 0.05$) and the factor depending on f (ratio between the two sample sizes) is equal to 4 when $f = 1$ (equal group sizes). This means that it is easy to find n from b_0 and β, and b_0 from n and β whereas finding β from n and b_0 involves solving an equation based on $z_{1-\beta}$. We see that using (6.3.5) requires specification of f, α, and s plus two of the three quantities n, b_0, and β. In randomized studies, f will usually be set to $f = 1$ because this will minimize the total number of subjects to be recruited. In observational studies, f will reflect the exposure distribution which, obviously, need not be a 50–50 distribution. The significance level α is, as mentioned, almost always set to $\alpha = 0.05$ (see also Section 2.3.3).

The value of s has quite different meanings for the three types of outcome. For quantitative data, s is the standard deviation in each group, so, in order to determine the necessary sample size, a value of s must be set. Some times, s may be known from previous research in the area. Alternatively, a *pilot study*, that is, a small study such as the one planned with, say 5–20 individuals, may be performed from which s may be estimated. It is seen that, not surprisingly, a larger s leads to a higher necessary sample size n, as it is more difficult to see a difference between two groups when the outcome is highly variable within groups.

For binary data, s depends on $\bar{p}$, the average outcome probability. This means that an estimate of $\bar{p}$ is needed to do the sample size calculation (we need to know approximately how frequent is the outcome under study). Again, previous knowledge or pilot studies may provide an estimate for this. Finally, for survival data, the situation is more complicated and the quantity, $s = 1/\sqrt{q}$ is a bit harder to assess. As for binary data, one needs to evaluate the absolute failure risk, for example, expressed as the *median survival time* M_0 in the control group . The median survival time in group 1 is then approximately (if the hazard rates are constant) $M_1 = M_0/\exp(b_0)$ and the average median survival time is $\bar{M} = (M_0 + M_1)/2$. If patients are accrued for a period of length A and subsequently followed up for a period of (at least) length F (so that the total study time is $F + A$), then the average failure probability is

$$q = 1 - \exp\left(-\log(2)\frac{F}{\bar{M}}\right)\frac{1 - \exp(-\log(2)\frac{A}{\bar{M}})}{\log(2)\frac{A}{\bar{M}}}. \tag{6.3.7}$$

It follows from (6.3.7) that small $\bar{M}$ (short time to failure, i.e., many observed failures) and large A, F (longer study duration) will increase the average failure probability; see Figure 6.3.1 which shows q as a function of $\bar{M}$ for selected values of A, F.

If the sample size n is to be determined based on relevant values for b_0 and for the power $1 - \beta$, then it is usually required that the power should be no smaller than 0.8. If $1 - \beta = 0.8$ then, after all, the study has a "1 in 5 risk" of being inconclusive, that is, to yield an insignificant result even if the alternative hypothesis $b = b_0$ is true, because the type II error probability β is 0.2 in this case. It will, therefore, rarely be relevant to conduct a study if the power is below 0.8.

The parameter for which it is most difficult to assign a value is probably the effect size b_0 which should be a "relevant" difference, "not to be overlooked" and is often referred to as the minimum relevant difference, MIREDIF. As seen in (6.3.5), only the ratio between b_0 and s is needed. Therefore, for quantitative data one sometimes specifies b_0 as a multiple of the standard deviation, for example, one argues that a relevant difference could be one or 1.5 times the SD.

Digression. Other designs

Closely connected to the determination of sample size is the possibility of choosing a design in which the subjects act as their own control (e.g., a cross-over study with two treatments given in two consecutive periods of time, a before-and-after treatment study, or a comparison of measuring techniques applied simultaneously, e.g., on each arm or leg). Such a paired design will decrease the demand on sample size because the relevant measure of variation s for quantitative outcomes changes from the between-subject variation to the within-subject variation (multiplied by

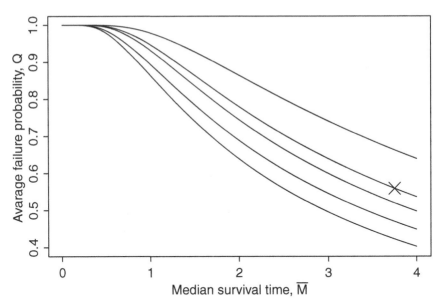

Fig. 6.3.1. Average failure probability, q (6.3.7) as a function of (average) median survival time $\bar{M}$ for different values of accrual period A and follow-up time F (from top to bottom): $A = F = 4$, $A = F = 3$, $A = 3, F = 2$, $A = 2, F = 3$, and $A = F = 2$. The cross marks a point referred to in the example below.

$\sqrt{2}$), which is typically smaller. However, a paired design may not always be feasible. This is not the kind of study of primary interest in this book where we focus on situations with only one response variable observed in each individual (see, however, Sections 5.4 and 8.1). $\diamond$

Examples

We now go through a few worked examples of sample size or power calculations based on Equation (6.3.5).

1. Suppose that some quantitative outcome variable has a standard deviation of 40 in the relevant patient population and that a clinically relevant difference between a treated group and an untreated control group is $b_0 = 15$. If half the patients are treated $f = 1$, then the necessary total sample size to detect this difference with a power of 0.80 (i.e., $z_{1-0.8} = z_{0.2} = 0.84$) is

$$n = \frac{(1.96 + 0.84)^2 4(40)^2}{15^2} \approx 223.$$

If, instead the relevant difference had been expressed (more modestly) as one half SD the required sample size would have been

$$n = \frac{(1.96 + 0.84)^2 4}{0.5^2} \approx 125.$$

2. Suppose that 75% of a given population are nonsmokers and have a 5-year risk of developing a given disease of about 0.1. We wish to design a cohort study to assess whether the risk among smokers could be 0.05 higher than for nonsmokers. We want the power to detect this difference to be as high as 0.9 (i.e., $z_{1-0.9} = z_{0.1} = 1.28$). In this case, only $f = 1/3$ of the subjects will be exposed, $\bar{p} = (0.10 + 0.15)/2 = 0.125$, and s^2 becomes 0.125 times 0.875. The required sample size is

$$n = \frac{(1.96 + 1.28)^2 \frac{4^2}{3}(0.125 \cdot 0.875)}{(0.15 - 0.10)^2} \approx 2449.$$

Had the same effect size instead been formulated as an odds ratio of 1.59 $(=(0.15/0.85)/(0.1/0.9))$ then we would have found the similar result

$$n = \frac{(1.96 + 1.28)^2 \frac{4^2}{3}}{(0.125 \cdot 0.875)(\log(1.59))^2} \approx 2380.$$

This means that ≈ 600 smokers and 1800 nonsmokers should be recruited and followed for 5 years.

Had we only been able to recruit, say 80% of the required individuals (i.e., 480 smokers and 1440 nonsmokers) then the power β (based on the risk difference) would have been the solution to the equation

$$480 + 1440 = \frac{(1.96 + z_{1-\beta})^2 \frac{4^2}{3}(0.125 \cdot 0.875)}{(0.15 - 0.10)^2},$$

that is, $z_{1-\beta} = 0.91$ or $1 - \beta = 0.82$. Similarly, we can compute the effect size for which we would still have 90% power based on the smaller sample size as the value of the risk difference b_0, solving

$$480 + 1440 = \frac{(1.96 + 1.28)^2 \frac{4^2}{3}(0.125 \cdot 0.875)}{b_0^2},$$

that is, $b_0 = 0.056$, so that we would only be able to detect a somewhat larger difference.

3. Suppose that the median lifetime with traditional treatment is $M_0 = 3$ years and that a relevant treatment effect to detect is a hazard ratio of $\exp(b_0) = 1/1.5$ leading to $M_1 = 4.5$ years and $\bar{M} = 3.75$ years. If the study is planned with $A = 3$ years of accrual and a further $F = 3$ years of follow-up then the average failure probability (6.3.7) is 0.559 (see the cross in Figure 6.3.1), and the required sample size for a power of 80% becomes

$$n = \frac{(1.96 + 0.84)^2 4}{(0.559 \cdot \log(1.5))^2} \approx 341$$

or $341/36 = 9.5$ new patients per month during the accrual period.

A single quantitative covariate with a linear effect

In our view, the two-sample problem discussed above is the most important situation for sample size calculations. As mentioned in the introduction to this section, a relevant two-sample problem may often be identified even in studies focusing on more complicated situations. However, if a study deals with a linear effect of a quantitative covariate then the relevant sample size formula can be rewritten into an expression like (6.3.5) (Vaeth and Skovlund, 2004). This amounts to setting $f = 1$ and b_0 equal to $2s_x b_x$ where s_x is the SD of the quantitative covariate x, and b_x is the effect size for the slope parameter. In addition to the parameters that must be identified before sample size determination in the 2-sample problem, the variation of the covariate s_x must be assessed (or the x-values may be determined by design). A pilot study may be one way of setting a value for s_x. Finally, instead of evaluating a relevant difference b_0 between two groups, a relevant slope b_x must be evaluated.

Adjustment for confounders

For a situation where the effect of interest is to be adjusted for $n_c - 1$ other explanatory variables the sample size calculations presented above tend to give too small a value. If that calculation results in a certain value n then according to Hsieh, Bloch, and Larsen (1998) the necessary sample size should approximately be $n/(1 - r_{n_c}^2)$ where r_{n_c} is the "multiple correlation coefficient" between the covariate of interest and the remaining $n_c - 1$ covariates. This parameter will often not be easy to specify in advance. However, when a study is to be conducted in a population where the confounder distribution is known then it may be possible to approximate r_{n_c}.

Digression. "Post hoc" power calculations

Sometimes, it is advocated that power calculations are useful when reporting results from a study. We believe this to be fundamentally wrong. In our view, power and sample size calculations are important when planning studies as discussed in the beginning of this section whereas, for reporting results, confidence intervals should be used to quantify the uncertainty associated with the conclusions from the study. By definition, a confidence interval gives the range of parameter values compatible with the data observed and with this knowledge it is unimportant to assess what the power would have been, had the true parameter value been this or that. In fact, Hoenig and Heisey (2001) showed that giving the power corresponding to the *estimated* parameter value provides no extra information than presenting the *P*-value. ◇

6.4 Exercises

Exercise 6.1. Draw a model diagram for the fetal death Example 1.2 from Section 1.1.1, using the variables age, number of fever episodes and parity, and fetal death as outcome.

Exercise 6.2. Draw a model diagram for the tryptase dataset 3 from Example 1.12, using the variables age, gender, and ASA as covariates and using the baseline tryptase as outcome.

Exercise 6.3. Draw a model diagram for the tryptase dataset 2 from Example 1.12, using the variables age, gender, control, ASA, and reaction tryptase as covariates and using "positive" as outcome variable.

1. If we aim at investigating the effect of ASA group and age on the probability of a positive allegy test, should we then include gender in the model?
2. Same question for reaction tryptase.

Exercise 6.4. Recall the surgery Example 1.4. Assume that we want to set up a new investigation to study the difference in complication probabilities for Pancuronium and Atracurium. Find the number needed in each group if the specifications are:

1. Power 80% to detect an odds ratio of 2 between the two blocking agents, assuming the complication risk for Atracurium to be 2%.
2. Power 90% to detect if the risk for the Pancuronium group is 50% increased in relation to the risk for Atracurium (which is again assumed to have a complication risk of 2%).

Exercise 6.5. Recall the tryptase Example 1.12 and suppose that we are going to design a new study for studying the age effect on the baseline tryptase value.

1. Find the power for detection of a difference in baseline tryptase of a size equal to 25% of its SD, when comparing two age groups of size 50.
2. Find the power for detecting a slope of 0.05 for the relation between age and baseline tryptase in a linear regression analysis, using a total of 100 patients, with an age distribution corresponding to the one observed in the tryptase dataset 3.

Exercise 6.6. Recall the study of malignant melanoma Example 1.10 and consider designing a new study aimed at determining a possible effect of radical surgery (as in the example) versus conservative surgery.

1. How many patients must be recruited per year to two groups of equal size for detecting a difference corresponding to a hazard ratio of 1.5 with a power of 80%, assuming an accrual period of 3 years, a subsequent follow-up period of 3 years, and assuming that the median survival time for the radical surgery group is as in the example.

2. If randomization is planned to be unequal by recruiting twice as many patients to the conservative group as to the radical group how much would we then have to increase the total number of patients recruited per year in order to achieve the same goals as in the above question?

Exercise 6.7. Use data from the PBC-3 Example 1.3 to perform a model check in Model 1 from Table 6.2.18.

1. Stratify into suitably chosen intervals for albumin and study the cumulative baseline hazards.
2. Do the same for age and bilirubin.

7

Alternative outcome types and link functions

In previous chapters we have focused on quantitative data with a linear mean, binary data with a logistic link, and proportional hazards models for survival data. In this chapter we first study two "new" datatypes. The first is *multinomial* data (Section 7.1) where the outcome is a categorical variable with more than two levels. This includes both the case where the categories are ordered (*ordinal* data, Section 7.1.1) and where they are unordered (*nominal* data, Section 7.1.2). The second type is *counts* (Section 7.2) and we study models based on both the Poisson and the Binomial distribution.

Next, we briefly discuss alternative models for both quantitative (Section 7.3) and binary data (Section 7.4), as well as for survival data (Section 7.5). Sections 7.3–7.5 may be a bit more difficult to read than most previous sections because our focus is now on more technical aspects of the models to be presented.

Common to all of the models studied in this chapter is the presence of a linear predictor. This means that much of the discussion can build on previous chapters.

7.1 Multinomial outcome

One of the main examples of outcome types we have discussed in previous chapters is *binary data*, that is, a categorical variable with two categories, and *logistic regression* has been a major topic. (In Section 7.4 we study models for a binary outcome with link functions other than the logit function.) The present section introduces a new type of outcome: a categorical variable with three or more categories. We refer to such data as *multinomial*.

For multinomial data one distinguishes between the two situations where either the categories are ordered, or they are not. These two situations are referred to as *ordinal* and *nominal* data, respectively. An example of an ordinal variable is a disease stage that can be seen as a categorization of a quantitative variable which is impossible — or at least very hard or expensive — to quantify numerically, such as progression of cancer. Another example could be a variable with levels fatal stroke, nonfatal stroke, or no stroke. In both examples, categories are ordered but it is not obvious how to assign a meaningful numerical value to each subject. Examples of nominal variables include blood type according to the AB0 system (types A, B, AB, or 0), job category, and choice of health insurance plan. In practical applications, ordinal outcome variables seem to be much more frequent, and in Section 7.1.1 that situation is covered in detail. Nominal outcome data are then discussed more briefly in the subsequent Section 7.1.2. We show that, in both sections, the simple logistic regression model from previous chapters constitutes an important starting point and, in fact, both *ordinal logistic regression* (Section 7.1.1) and *polychotomous logistic regression* (Section 7.1.2) can be approximated by a number of ordinary logistic regressions. In fact, in practical applications reported in the literature, multinomial outcome data have often been transformed to binary data by combining categories. The current section discusses potential models where this simplification need not be done .

7.1.1 Ordinal outcome

Examples of ordinal data were given in the introduction to Section 7.1. We saw that, even though we cannot assign a meaningful number to each category, we can at least rank them (i.e., arrange them, e.g., in an increasing order according to degree of severity). In general, however, we cannot say anything about the distance between successive levels. When the levels originate from categorization of a measured quantitative variable, we may of course allocate meaningful numbers to each category, for example, the midpoint of the interval for that category, or the average of the observations belonging in the interval.

In Example 1.9 in Section 1.5, we described an investigation of 127 subjects with liver disease. For each of these subjects, the degree of fibrosis y_i was determined on a four-point scale (0,1,2,3). Because these four categories are only verbally described (i.e., with no quantitative assessment), we regard the scale as ordinal.

An assessment of liver fibrosis involves a liver biopsy which is an invasive procedure with potentially serious side effects, thus we are very motivated to replace this with markers that may be quantified from blood samples. Three such markers are available in this study: ha, p3np, and ykl40. In Figure 7.1.1 the distribution of these markers is seen to be fairly skewed, so that averages and standard deviations will not be reasonable summary statistics. Instead, Table 7.1.1 presents medians and quartiles for these markers. Figure 7.1.1 and Table 7.1.1 both indicate a trend in the distributions of the markers, such that high values seem to be associated with higher degrees of fibrosis. We seek a model to describe this relation, so that we may use the values of the three markers for prediction of the degree of liver fibrosis.

The blood markers are of a quantitative nature, so an obvious first choice for a linear predictor would be

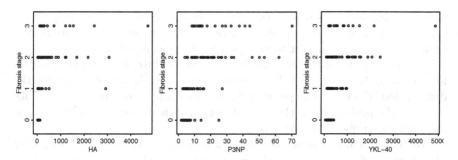

Fig. 7.1.1. Distribution of blood markers according to degree of fibrosis.

Table 7.1.1. Medians and interquartile ranges of three blood markers according to degree of fibrosis.

Degree of Fibrosis	Count	Median (Interquartile Range)		
		ha	p3np	ykl40
0	27	27.5 (25.0–37.0)	5.00 (3.2–6.2)	174.0 (135.0–270.0)
1	40	42.0 (27.0–94.5)	5.90 (4.6–8.4)	270.0 (150.0–498.0)
2	42	211.5 (109.0–460.0)	15.85 (9.7–24.6)	466.0 (330.0–1067.0)
3	20	242.5 (148.5–954.5)	14.55 (11.3–30.7)	676.0 (327.5–1137.5)

$$\mathrm{LP}_i = a + b_1 x_{i,1} + b_2 x_{i,2} + b_3 x_{i,3}, \qquad (7.1.1)$$

where the explanatory variables x_1, x_2 and x_3 denote the value of the markers ha, p3np, and ykl40, respectively. These markers appear only as covariates, therefore there is no formal requirement regarding their distributions. Concerns regarding influential observations and/or the linearity assumption implied in (7.1.1) may, however, require transformation of the explanatory variables as we show below.

In order to build a model for the degree of liver fibrosis, we have to establish a link between this linear predictor and the ordinal outcome y_i. Because the categories 0 through 3 do not contain quantitative information, it makes little sense to consider the mean value of y. On the other hand, the information contained in y is more refined than that of a binary variable, so we are faced with a dilemma. If we stick to the models considered so far in this book, we may either reduce y to a binary variable by collapsing categories (but note this may be done in three distinctly different ways) or we may pretend that we are dealing with quantitative information (which may be reasonable in some situations with many response categories that may more or less be considered equidistant).

None of these possibilities is optimal in this example. The former implies a loss of information and a choice of threshold, whereas the latter assumes that it makes sense to speak about a mean value of the degree of fibrosis, based on the categories 0 to 3 (or some other arbitrarily chosen scoring, e.g., 0,1,4,9, leading to different models). Later in this section, we compare results obtained using two different ways of scoring these categories.

The main focus of this section, however, is to illustrate some possibilities for analyzing the data directly as ordinal outcomes. In order to specify the distribution of y on a four-point scale, we need a total of three probabilities (because the probability of the last category will then be determined from the fact that the probabilities have to sum to one).

We let $p_{i,j}$ denote the probability that patient i is observed as having liver fibrosis on level j (i.e., $p_{i,j} = \text{pr}(y_i = j)$) and define the cumulative probabilities "from the top" as

$$q_{i,3} = p_{i,3} \qquad \text{probability of category 3,}$$
$$q_{i,2} = p_{i,2} + p_{i,3} \qquad \text{probability of category 2 or above,}$$
$$q_{i,1} = p_{i,1} + p_{i,2} + p_{i,3} \qquad \text{probability of category 1 or above.}$$

Each of these three cumulative probabilities corresponds to a chosen threshold for y: $q_{i,3}$ corresponds to cutting between categories 2 and 3, $q_{i,2}$ corresponds to cutting between categories 1 and 2, and $q_{i,1}$ corresponds to cutting between categories 0 and 1. Therefore, we have a choice of three different logistic regressions, linking one of the above probabilities to the linear predictor using a logit link, as outlined in Section 4.1.2. This corresponds to a dichotomization of y according to the chosen threshold. Any of these logistic regressions may be worthwhile considering, but the amount of results and conclusions may be a bit overwhelming. However, if the three analyses differ only slightly, we can condense and strengthen the information and at the same time retain important results.

Let us review the results that we get from a single logistic regression, for example, the one based on cutting between categories 1 and 2. The observations are then binary and the model can be formulated as a single linear predictor for the logit-transformed probability of a 1 (here chosen to be the highest categories, i.e., categories 2 and 3)

$$\text{LP}_i = \text{logit}(q_{i,2}) = \log\left(\frac{q_{i,2}}{1 - q_{i,2}}\right)$$
$$= a + b_1 x_{i,1} + b_2 x_{i,2} + b_3 x_{i,3} \qquad (7.1.2)$$

and the results are stated in Table 7.1.2.

We note that for two of the covariates, we get estimates extremely close to zero and correspondingly, the odds ratios associated with these covariates are very close to 1. This does not necessarily mean that these covariates do not contribute to the prediction of the outcome but may simply be due to an inappropriate scaling of the covariates. If we look at the distribution of the covariates as illustrated in Figure 7.1.1, we note two important features. One of these is the skewness in the covariate distributions that was already

Table 7.1.2. Estimates in a logistic regression, using threshold between 1 and 2.

	ha	p3np	ykl40
Estimate, $\widehat{b}_j$	−0.0002 (0.0007)	0.2298 (0.0525)	0.0028 (0.0009)
Odds ratio, $\exp(\widehat{b}_j)$	0.9998	1.2583	1.0028
CI for Odds ratio	(0.9985, 1.0011)	(1.1353, 1.3947)	(1.0011, 1.0045)

mentioned above. The second feature is that the covariates have very different ranges, two of them (ha and ykl40) having maximum values around 5000 and the third (p3np) having a maximum of approximately 70. The estimates from Table 7.1.2 refer to the change in outcome for a one unit change in the covariate, thus we certainly would expect the coefficients of ha and ykl40 to be very close to zero inasmuch as a one-unit change on a scale up to 5000 hardly matters at all, even though the covariate might be closely related to the outcome.

A simple remedy would be to scale the covariates, for example, dividing each covariate value by 100 or even 1000. This would correspond to simply multiplying the estimates and the SD by the same factor and change the interpretation accordingly. Thus, for a change of 100 units in ykl40, we would have an estimate of 0.28(0.09), corresponding to an odds ratio of 1.32, that is, a 32% increased odds of having fibrosis above the chosen threshold.

An alternative to a simple rescaling of the covariates would be to use percentage scales, that is, to perform a logarithmic transformation of the covariates so that a one unit change will correspond to multiplication of the covariate by some constant (which is the base of the chosen logarithm, Appendix B). Making a logarithmic transformation of the covariates also has the effect of making the distributions more symmetric as seen from Figure 7.1.2. This limits the influence of single observations, as discussed in Section 4.1.3.

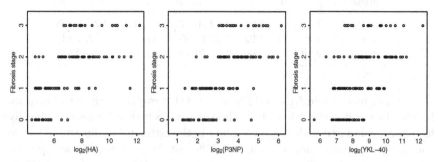

Fig. 7.1.2. Distribution of the logarithm of the blood markers according to degree of fibrosis.

Based on these arguments, we prefer to use all three covariates on a logarithmic scale. However, because this choice has implications for the model fit (it is a new model assuming linearity on a new scale), we should, as always, perform model checks. We return to this below. In order to ease the later interpretation, we choose logarithms with base 2, so that a "one-unit increase in the logarithm" corresponds to multiplication by a factor 2 on the original scale.

Using these $\log_2$ transformed covariates, we get the estimates as presented in Table 7.1.3. We see that a doubling of a single covariate yields odds ratios of 1.79, 3.57, and 1.69 respectively, so that a doubling of all three covariates simultaneously gives an odds ratio of $1.79 \times 3.57 \times 1.69 = 10.80$.

Table 7.1.3. Estimates in a logistic regression, using threshold between 1 and 2, with logarithmic covariates ($\log_2$).

	ha	p3np	ykl40
Estimate $\widehat{b}_j$	0.584 (0.064, 1.104)	1.272 (0.437, 2.106)	0.526 (0.018, 1.035)
Odds ratio $\exp(\widehat{b}_j)$	1.79 (1.07, 3.02)	3.57 (1.55, 8.21)	1.69 (1.02, 2.81)

In the above analysis we chose a specific threshold in order to make a simple logistic regression. However, this choice was arbitrary and could have been made in two other ways, producing three sets of such estimates as shown in Table 7.1.4 and illustrated graphically in Figure 7.1.3.

Table 7.1.4. Estimates in separate logistic regressions for different thresholds, using logarithmic covariates ($\log_2$).

Threshold	Odds Ratios ha	p3np	ykl40
3 vs. 0–2	1.30 (0.88, 1.91)	1.62 (0.82, 3.21)	1.52 (0.95, 2.42)
2–3 vs. 0–1	1.79 (1.07, 3.02)	3.57 (1.55, 8.21)	1.69 (1.02, 2.81)
1–3 vs. 0	2.09 (0.89, 4.90)	1.75 (0.69, 4.40)	1.98 (1.01, 3.89)

We note from Table 7.1.4 and Figure 7.1.3 that even though the odds ratios for the three different choices of the threshold seem rather different (especially for p3np), compared with the uncertainty in the estimates as illustrated by the confidence intervals, they are not that different. We can obtain more precise estimates if we are willing to assume that the odds ratios for each covariate do not depend on the chosen threshold. This corresponds to looking at a single model, in which the linear predictor in (7.1.2) is extended to all thresholds, by changing only the intercept term and letting the influence of the covariates (the coefficients b_1, b_2, and b_3) be identical for all thresholds.

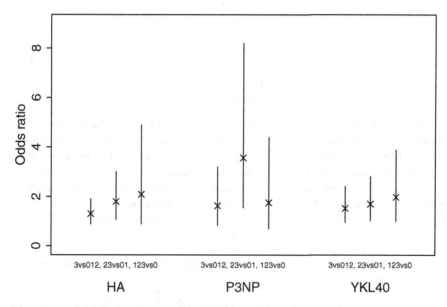

Fig. 7.1.3. Odds ratio estimates (with 95% confidence intervals) for separate logistic regressions.

The resulting model is the *proportional odds model for cumulative logits*, specified for $j = 1, 2, 3$ by

$$\text{LP}_{i,j} = \text{logit}(q_{i,j}) = \log\left(\frac{q_{i,j}}{1 - q_{i,j}}\right) = \log\left(\frac{\text{pr}(y_i \geq j)}{\text{pr}(y_i < j)}\right)$$
$$= a_j + b_1 x_{i,1} + b_2 x_{i,2} + b_3 x_{i,3}, \qquad (7.1.3)$$

or, on the original probability scale:

$$q_{i,j} = q_j(x_i) = \frac{\exp(a_j + b_1 x_{i,1} + b_2 x_{i,2} + b_3 x_{i,3})}{1 + \exp(a_j + b_1 x_{i,1} + b_2 x_{i,2} + b_3 x_{i,3})}. \qquad (7.1.4)$$

Note that in this model, the bs are independent of j (the threshold), whereas the intercept a is not! This means that on the logit scale, the linear predictors corresponding to the three possible thresholds are parallel (with a suitable high-dimensional definition of parallel), with levels defined by the a-parameters, which simply reflect the distribution between low and high categories in relation to the chosen threshold. These will therefore be monotonically decreasing with j, because the probability of being above the threshold decreases with increasing threshold. This ensures that the probabilities of the individual categories, given as successive differences between the qs as shown in (7.1.5) are all positive, so that the model is well defined:

$$p_{i,3} = q_{i,3},$$
$$p_{i,2} = q_{i,2} - q_{i,3},$$
$$(7.1.5)$$
$$p_{i,1} = q_{i,1} - q_{i,2},$$
$$p_{i,0} = 1 - q_{i,1}.$$

The results from model (7.1.3) are presented in Table 7.1.5. The intercepts bear no relation to the effect of the covariates, but merely reflect the distribution of subjects over categories. They are needed for predicting probabilities and in order for them to make sense, we have centered the covariates so that a zero value of all covariates corresponds to an individual with ha= 100, p3np= 10 and ykl40= 500. The estimated intercepts are then $\hat{a}_1 = 2.592(0.343)$, $\hat{a}_2 = 0.173(0.253)$, and $\hat{a}_3 = -2.592(0.347)$.

Table 7.1.5. Estimates from the proportional odds model (7.1.3), using logarithmic covariates ($\log_2$).

Marker	Effect of Doubling	Effect of 1 SD on log-scale	P-Value
ha	1.48 (1.07, 2.04)	1.52	0.019
p3np	2.28 (1.37, 3.79)	1.69	0.0016
ykl40	1.72 (1.24, 2.39)	1.46	0.0011

The results in Table 7.1.5 indicate that all three blood markers make an independent contribution to the prediction of degree of liver fibrosis. We may formulate the effect of a single blood marker (e.g., ykl40) to say that a patient with a value of ykl40 twice as high as another patient has a 72% increased odds for having fibrosis of a high degree, provided that the two subjects are identical with respect to the two other blood markers.

Comparison of the odds ratios for the three markers suggests that p3np is the most important one for predicting liver fibrosis. This cannot be inferred from these crude estimates, however, because a factor two may not be regarded as the same amount for all blood markers. Actually, from Figure 7.1.2, we note that on the logarithmic scale, the range of ha and ykl40 is approximately twice as large as for p3np and doubling of p3np is therefore a priori expected to produce a larger effect. If a comparison has to be made, it is therefore customarily done by considering *standardized coefficients* produced by converting the covariates into Z-scores by scaling them with their own standard deviation. The corresponding odds ratios are shown in the middle column of Table 7.1.5. These should be used for comparison only, and only if the data have been chosen randomly from a well-defined population, inasmuch as they have a correlationlike interpretation and therefore depend on the distribution of the covariates (see Section 4.1.1). If we believe the subjects to

be sampled randomly from the population of liver patients, we may compare
the three estimates, and based on these, we still find p3np to be the most
important predictor, although the difference is now very small.

Note, however, that based on the P-values, ykl40 seems to be the most
important predictor. It should be borne in mind, though, that the P-value is
merely an indication of the strength of the evidence of a relationship, not of
its size.

Now we turn to model checking. We have several features that we should
investigate: the linearity of the effect of the covariates (on the logarithmic
scale), the proportional odds assumption (the assumption that odds ratios
are identical for all thresholds), and the ability of the model to predict the
degree of fibrosis (a goodness-of-fit check).

Scale of the covariates

We have already discussed the choice of scale for the covariates and chosen
the logarithmic scale due to ease of interpretation and as a way to avoid
problems with undue influence from single observations. We have no knowledge, however, of whether the model with untransformed covariates (or some
other covariate transformation than the logarithm) performs better in this
particular situation.

In order to investigate the adequacy of the chosen scale, we could either
construct residual plots, model the covariate effects using splines as discussed
in Section 4.2.1, or calculate numerical tests for goodness-of-fit in competing
models.

Residuals for ordinal regression models generalize those from logistic regressions that have been presented in Section 4.1.2. We are now dealing with a
set of $k+1$ indicators, one for each attainable category $I(y_i = 0), \dots, I(y_i = k)$,
therefore we define $k+1$ standardized residuals (i.e., divided by their estimated
standard deviation) for each subject by

$$r_{i,j} = \frac{I(y_i = j) - \widehat{\mathrm{pr}}(y_i = j)}{\sqrt{\widehat{\mathrm{pr}}(y_i = j)(1 - \widehat{\mathrm{pr}}(y_i = j))}}.$$

Here, $\widehat{\mathrm{pr}}(y_i = j)$ is obtained by substituting estimated values for the $a-$ and
$b-$ parameters into Equations (7.1.4) and (7.1.5). These residuals may be examined graphically using methods illustrated previously for binary outcomes.

Because of these several categories, residual plots become numerous. Thus
in our situation we have 4 residuals for each individual and each of these has
to be plotted against 3 covariates, giving a total of 12 plots, which are shown
in Figures 7.1.4–7.1.6. These figures do not suggest any major violations of the
model assumptions, possibly with an exception for p3np (Figure 7.1.5) which
shows a slight increasing tendency for large values, indicating that the probability of having fibrosis of degree 2 is estimated a little too low for high values
of p3np. In the upper-left panels of each of these three figures, we see (the

same) three large residuals. These correspond to three patients with fibrosis
degree 0, having rather large values for all three blood markers and therefore
predicted to have a higher degree of fibrosis. A similar explanation holds for
the one or two large values for fibrosis degree 1 (upper-right panels) whereas
for the lower-left panels, the two largest residuals correspond to patients with
fibrosis degree 2, having rather low values of all three markers and therefore
expected to have also a lower degree of fibrosis. For the lower-right panels,
the many large residuals correspond to patients with fibrosis of degree 3, and
their large size reflects the fact that the estimated probability for this stage
does not become very large even for high values of the markers.

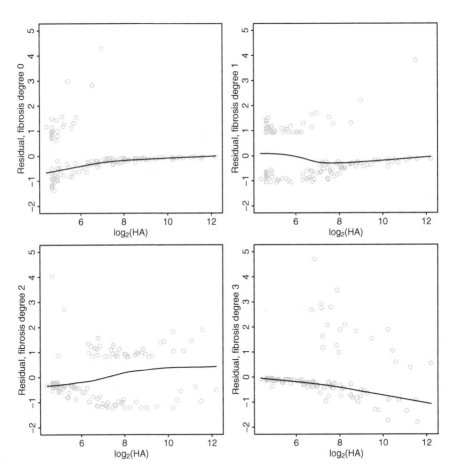

Fig. 7.1.4. Residuals plotted against the blood marker $\log_2(\text{ha})$.

Also, based on $-2\log L$, the model with logarithmic covariates performs
much better than the one with untransformed covariates (246.466 versus

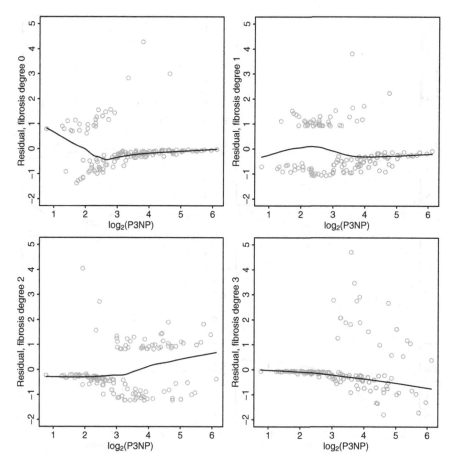

Fig. 7.1.5. Residuals plotted against the blood marker $\log_2(\text{p3np})$.

271.42). Goodness-of-fit tests may be performed for each fibrosis category j separately, by dividing the predicted probabilities $\widehat{\text{pr}}(y_i = j)$ into, for example, decile intervals (i.e., containing approximately one tenth of the total number of observations, here 13) and comparing the observed and expected number of cases with this particular fibrosis degree as described in Section 6.2.2. It may also be performed for the three cumulated probabilities $\widehat{q}_{i,j} = \widehat{\text{pr}}(y_i \geq j)$ giving a more direct connection to the estimated parameters. For the sake of brevity, we refrain from performing these tests.

The proportional odds assumption

The proportional odds assumption claims that no matter which of the three thresholds we choose as a cutpoint for a logistic regression model, the effect of the covariates will be the same. This assumption can be checked by testing

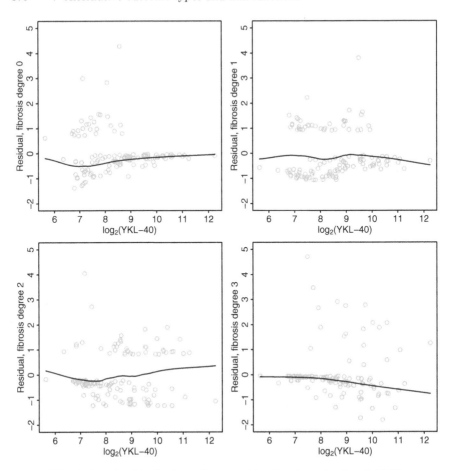

Fig. 7.1.6. Residuals plotted against the blood marker $\log_2(\text{ykl40})$.

the model against a more liberal alternative. The obvious choice of model extension would be to relax the assumption of identical covariate effects for all thresholds, to give the more general linear predictor

$$\text{LP}_{i,j} = \text{logit}(q_{i,j}) = \log\left(\frac{q_{i,j}}{1 - q_{i,j}}\right)$$
$$= a_j + b_{1,j}x_{i,1} + b_{2,j}x_{i,2} + b_{3,j}x_{i,3}, \qquad (7.1.6)$$

in which the three regression coefficients are allowed to depend on the threshold. In Table 7.1.4, we presented estimates obtained from the separate logistic regressions, carried out successively for each choice of threshold. Because this involves the fitting of three different models to the same data by defining three different versions of the same outcome variable, it will not be the same as fit-

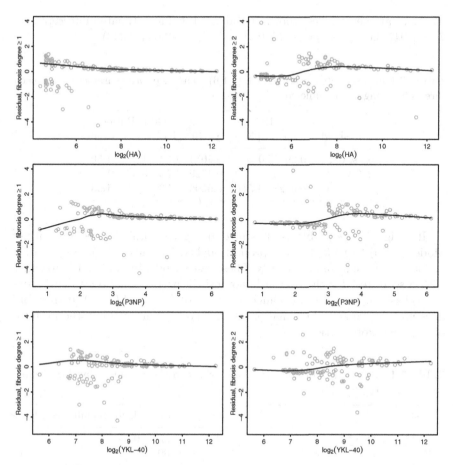

Fig. 7.1.7. Residuals for cumulative probabilities, plotted against the blood markers.

ting the single model (7.1.6) to all data, because this provides a model for all four probabilities simultaneously without combining any of the categories.

Unfortunately, model (7.1.6) has some built-in problems, inasmuch as the estimated probabilities obtained by successive differencing as shown in (7.1.5) are now not guaranteed to produce positive values.

This is due to the fact that the linear predictors on the logit scale, corresponding to the three possible thresholds are no longer parallel and, therefore, intersect at some point. If an intersection occurs in the observed range of the covariates, negative estimated probabilities will occur. In the fibrosis example, we get one such negative probability corresponding to the individual with the lowest value of p3np. Even if we can perform the estimation under restrictions to ensure positivity of all probabilities, it clearly shows the inadequacy of model (7.1.6). The estimates (without imposing this restriction) are nevertheless shown in Table 7.1.6. The estimated intercepts are $\hat{a}_1 = 2.947(0.611), \hat{a}_2 = 0.284(0.285)$, and $\hat{a}_3 = -2.054(0.246)$.

Table 7.1.6. Estimates from model (7.1.6), with separate parameters for each threshold, using logarithmic covariates ($\log_2$).

Threshold	Estimates			Odds Ratios		
	ha	p3np	ykl40	ha	p3np	ykl40
3 vs. 0–2	0.2931	0.4573	0.4057	1.34	1.58	1.50
2–3 vs. 0–1	0.4373	1.2712	0.4529	1.55	3.57	1.57
1–3 vs. 0	0.5828	0.7471	0.6596	1.79	2.11	1.93

If we ignore the problems of estimated negative probabilities, we can use Model (7.1.6) to make tests of proportionality, for each covariate separately and for all of them simultaneously. These tests appear in Table 7.1.7, together with a score test for the overall hypothesis of proportional odds. This score test is based upon the local change in likelihood in Model (7.1.6). It therefore does not involve actual estimation in this model, thus avoiding the problem of negative probabilities.

Table 7.1.7. P-values for the hypothesis of proportional odds using logarithmic covariates ($\log_2$).

Test	ha	p3np	ykl40	Simultaneously
Wald, one at a time	0.085	0.024	0.55	—
Wald, one at a time, with restriction	—	<0.0001	—	—
Wald, all	0.79	0.22	0.69	0.12
Wald, all, with restriction	0.82	0.21	0.66	<0.0001
Likelihood ratio	0.57	0.31	0.97	0.185
Likelihood ratio, with restriction	—	0.31	—	0.197
Score	—	—	—	0.138

The conclusion seems to be that proportional odds are reasonable, although some deviation is seen for the predictor p3np. Table 7.1.4 tells us that p3np gives by far the best discrimination when the threshold is between 1 and 2, although the confidence intervals are rather wide. This difference in performance for the different thresholds is the cause of the (slight) problems with proportional odds for this covariate.

Using the proportional odds model, we can calculate predicted probabilities for each subject and category, that is, estimates of $p_{i,j}$. If the model is adequate for the data, $\hat{p}_{i,j}$ should be large whenever the subject has fibrosis of category j. In Figure 7.1.8, we have, for each category j, taken averages over $\widehat{p}_{i,j}$ for each group of patients according to their actual degree of fibrosis. This gives four averages for each category, one corresponding to the correct category and the three remaining corresponding to misclassification probabilities. In the figure, the averages corresponding to the same actual degree of fibrosis are connected and the values corresponding to the correct degree are marked with a dot. For instance, we see that patients having fibrosis of degree 0 have the highest average estimated probability for this stage (immediately followed by patients with actual degree 1) and that they are lowest in estimated probability for degree 3. This is what we would hope for for all of the estimated probabilities but, unfortunately, it is not quite the case because the average of the estimated probabilities for degree 3 is largest for patients with actual degree 2.

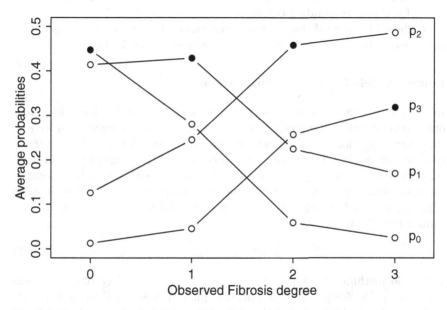

Fig. 7.1.8. Average probabilities of the different degrees of fibrosis, contrasted to the actual observed degrees. Correctly classified groups are marked with a dot.

The continuation ratio

Thus far, we have only discussed the proportional odds model (and extensions of this to nonproportional odds) where the link function is the cumulative logit (i.e., the logit of the successively cumulated probabilities). Another approach to ordinal data is to look at the *continuation ratio* approach in which we are modeling the conditional probabilities of each category, given that we are not in a category below; that is,

$$h_{i,j} = \text{pr}(y_i = j | y_i \geq j)$$
$$= \frac{\text{pr}(y_i = j)}{\text{pr}(y_i \geq j)}, \quad j = 1, 2, 3.$$

In this case the most obvious link function to use is the logarithm leading to

$$\log(h_{i,j}) = \text{LP}_{i,j} = a_j + b_1 x_{i,1} + b_2 x_{i,2} + b_3 x_{i,3}.$$

The resulting model may be thought of as a discrete time survival analysis where the conditioning is translated to a discrete hazard; that is, given that you are alive up to now, what is the risk of dying in the next time interval. This gives an interpretation of a regression coefficients b as a log(discrete hazard ratio) for the corresponding covariate x.

It should be noticed that, in the continuation ratio model, the direction of the ordering is now used explicitly (conditioning is on "the past").

Linear models for mean fibrosis grade

Let us finally study a linear model for the "mean fibrosis" value. This, obviously, requires that a numerical score is attached to each category, a procedure that cannot be done in a unique way due to the semiquantitative nature of the four categories. To illustrate the method and its simplicity and shortcomings, two such scorings are considered: a linear score where the categories are equidistant ($y_i = 0$, 1, 2, or 3) and an exponential score where they are equidistant on a log-scale ($y_i = 1$, 2, 4, or 8). Table 7.1.8 shows the results from fitting the model

$$\text{E}(y_i) = a + b_1 x_{i,1} + b_2 x_{i,2} + b_3 x_{i,3} \tag{7.1.7}$$

for the logarithmic covariates $x_1 = \log_2(\text{ha}/100)$, $x_2 = \log_2(\text{p3np}/10)$, and $x_3 = \log_2(\text{ykl40}/500)$. It is seen that, in a qualitative sense, the results resemble those obtained from fitting the ordinal logistic regression model (7.1.3), in that all three markers significantly raise the mean fibrosis grade. The P-values in this table tend to be smaller than those obtained from ordinal logistic regression.

Figure 7.1.9 shows the estimated probabilities of exceeding each of the three thresholds based on the model (7.1.7) plotted against the estimated probabilities based on the ordinal logistic regression model (7.1.3). For those based on the model for $\text{E}(y_i)$, the probabilities $\text{pr}(y \geq j \mid x_1, x_2, x_3)$ were calculated assuming a Normal distribution for the fibrosis grade with a mean equal to the linear predictor and using the residual SD given in the table. It is seen that, for the score 0, 1, 2, 3, the predicted probabilities are close to those obtained using the more satisfactory model (7.1.3) and those based on

Table 7.1.8. Results from fitting linear regression models for the mean fibrosis score.

Covariate	Score: 0, 1, 2, 3			Score: 1, 2, 4, 8		
	$\hat{b}$	SD	P	$\hat{b}$	SD	P
Intercept	1.534	0.068		3.583	0.172	
lha	0.141	0.053	0.009	0.337	0.136	0.014
lp3	0.295	0.083	0.0006	0.583	0.212	0.007
lyk	0.201	0.056	0.401	0.0005	0.143	0.006
Residual SD	0.677			1.719		

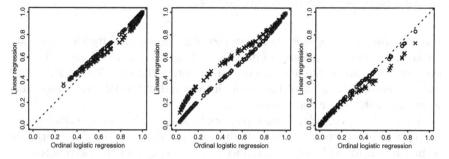

Fig. 7.1.9. Fibrosis data: estimated probability of exceeding each of the three thresholds (from left to right: 1, 2, and 3) based on linear models for the mean fibrosis grade plotted against those based on ordinal logistic regression: o = linear score, x = exponential score. The dashed line is the identity line.

the score 1, 2, 4, 8 seem to differ showing the sensitivity of the results to the chosen way of assigning numerical values to the categories.

To further evaluate the model based on the most obvious choice of scores, 0, 1, 2, 3, Figure 7.1.10 shows residuals from that model plotted against each of the three covariates lyk, lp3, and lha, respectively. Based on these figures, the model seems to provide a satisfactory fit to the data.

In conclusion, the ordinal regression model (7.1.3) is the most natural choice of a model for the fibrosis data and any score attached to the categories is more or less arbitrary. However, the simplicity of a linear model for the mean fibrosis grade remains appealing and even the estimates (at least for the linear score) are easily interpretable, for example, for the p3np marker a doubling increases the mean fibrosis grade by approximately 0.3.

7.1.2 Nominal outcome

As mentioned in the introduction to Section 7.1, ordinal outcome data seem to be more frequent in applications than nominal outcome data (although nominal variables may be common as explanatory variables). For that reason we use the fibrosis example from the previous Section 7.1.1 to introduce

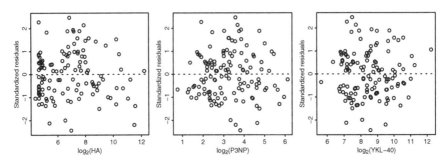

Fig. 7.1.10. Fibrosis data: residuals from Model (7.1.7) (using scores 0, 1, 2, 3) plotted against the covariates lha, lp3, and lyk.

the *polychotomous logistic regression model* for nonordinal multinomial data although the outcome, degree of fibrosis (0, 1, 2 or 3) is, indeed, ordinal. However, in cases where the assumptions of the proportional odds model (7.1.3) are not reasonably fulfilled, the model introduced in the following may serve as an alternative even for ordinal data.

We therefore consider an outcome variable y_i with $(k + 1)$ values g_0, g_1, ..., g_k which need not be ordered. Our aim is to specify the distribution of y_i in relation to explanatory variables $x_{i,1}, \ldots, x_{i,n_c}$ and the polychotomous logistic regression model specifies this using the following log(odds).

$$\log\left(\frac{\mathrm{pr}(y_i = g_j)}{\mathrm{pr}(y_i = g_0)}\right) = a_j + b_{1,j}x_{i,1} + \cdots + b_{n_c,j}x_{i,n_c} = \mathrm{LP}_{i,j}, \quad j = 1, \ldots, k.$$

$$(7.1.8)$$

In (7.1.8) all parameters are interpreted in relation to the same category (g_0) for the outcome y_i. That is, a_j is the log of the odds (when all $x_{i,u} = 0$) that y_i takes the value g_j rather than the reference value g_0, and $b_{u,j}$ is the log of the ratio between odds (associated with a 1-unit increase in $x_{i,u}$) that y_i takes the value g_j, rather than the reference value g_0. Note the difference from (7.1.3) where, for an ordinal y_i (i.e., $g_0 < g_1 < \ldots < g_k$) we studied the model

$$\log\left(\frac{\mathrm{pr}(y_i \geq g_j)}{\mathrm{pr}(y_i < g_j)}\right) = a_j + b_1 x_{i,1} + \cdots + b_{n_c} x_{i,n_c}, \quad j = 1, \ldots, k$$

for the odds that y_i *exceeds* the jth threshold g_j. In (7.1.3), the further assumption that the log(odds ratio) parameters b_u were the same for all thresholds (j) was imposed.

For $k = 1$, (7.1.8) is just the familiar logistic regression model and, in fact, the parameters in the model may be estimated consistently (as defined in Section 2.3) by fitting k simple logistic regression models for binary outcomes (e.g., Begg and Gray, 1984). As an illustration we consider the fibrosis data (Example 1.9), analyzed in Section 7.1.1 and described in Table 7.1.1 and Figures 7.1.1 and 7.1.2. For those data, the intercept a_1 and the three log(odds ratios) $b_{1,1}, b_{1,2}, b_{1,3}$ may be estimated based on a data subset consisting of all patients with fibrosis degree 0 or 1 and, similarly, $a_2, b_{2,1}, b_{2,2}, b_{2,3}$ may be estimated by restricting to patients with fibrosis degree 0 or 2, and so on. Table 7.1.9 shows the results. For the 1 versus 0 and the 2 versus 0 contrasts, estimates are in agreement with what we saw using the ordinal logistic regression model in the sense that higher marker values increase the risks of higher levels of fibrosis. For the contrast between 3 and 0, the simple logistic regression model including all three markers did not converge because of the fact that the distributions of the ha marker in these two fibrosis categories almost do not overlap.

Table 7.1.9. Estimates in a polychotomous logistic regression model for the fibrosis data using logarithmic covariates ($\log_2$). Estimates for 2 versus 0 and 1 versus 0 are obtained via separate simple logistic regressions. The model for 3 versus 0 did not converge; see text.

| | | Odds Ratios (95% ci) | | |
Fibrosis Grade	Intercept (SD)	ha	p3np	ykl40
3 vs. 0				
2 vs. 0	−17.67 (4.85)	5.00 (1.47, 16.95)	1.63 (0.48, 5.49)	2.30 (0.88, 5.97)
1 vs. 0	−7.90 (2.92)	1.37 (0.58, 3.23)	1.57 (0.63, 3.94)	2.03 (0.98, 4.19)

At first glance, it may seem surprising that consistent estimates can be obtained by separate binary logistic regressions because, in general, it is not advisable to select subjects for regression analysis based on their observed outcomes and our recommendation is, indeed, to estimate all parameters simultaneously. It is a consequence of (7.1.8) that the probabilities for the different outcome categories are

$$\mathrm{pr}(y_i = g_j) = \frac{\exp(\mathrm{LP}_{ij})}{1 + \sum_{w=1}^{k} \exp(\mathrm{LP}_{i,w})}, \tag{7.1.9}$$

for $j = 1, \ldots, k$, and

$$\mathrm{pr}(y_i = g_0) = \frac{1}{1 + \sum_{w=1}^{k} \exp(\mathrm{LP}_{i,w})}.$$

When observations of the outcome y_i and explanatory variables $(x_{i,1}, \ldots, x_{i,n_c})$ are available for independent individuals, $i = 1, \ldots, n$, the likelihood function (Section 2.3.4) is easily derived and maximization provides parameter estimates for $(a_j, (b_{1,j}, \ldots, b_{n_c,j}), j = 1, \ldots, k)$. To exemplify, we consider the fibrosis data and, using fibrosis grade 0 as the reference, the estimates in model (7.1.8) including the three markers $\log_2(\mathrm{ha})$, $\log_2(\mathrm{p3np})$, and $\log_2(\mathrm{ykl40})$ are shown in Table 7.1.10. It is seen that, for all three markers, the odds ratio increases with the degree of fibrosis. This is to be expected judged from the results from Section 7.1.1 because a higher degree of fibrosis corresponds to "crossing more thresholds" as a consequence of the ordinal nature of the outcome variable.

Table 7.1.10. Estimates in a polychotomous logistic regression model for the fibrosis data using logarithmic covariates ($\log_2$).

| Fibrosis | | Odds Ratios (95% ci) | | |
Grade	Intercept (SD)	ha	p3np	ykl40
3 vs. 0	−22.10 (4.32)	3.08 (1.14, 8.30)	4.77 (1.31, 17.39)	3.22 (1.34, 7.78)
2 vs. 0	−17.76 (3.71)	2.66 (1.03, 6.89)	4.26 (1.32, 13.80)	2.61 (1.17, 5.83)
1 vs. 0	−7.65 (2.87)	1.67 (0.69, 4.07)	1.34 (0.51, 3.54)	1.80 (0.90, 3.60)
LR test		9.35	15.79	8.09
(*P*-value)		(0.025)	(0.0013)	(0.044)

It should be emphasized that the parameter estimates obtained from separate simple logistic regressions will not be identical to those obtained by estimating all parameters simultaneously. For the 1 versus 0 contrast, estimates are close to those shown in Table 7.1.9 whereas, for the 2 versus 0 contrast, discrepancies are larger. Estimating all parameters simultaneously will generally provide smaller standard deviations and, more important, it enables comparison of estimates for different levels of fibrosis and provides simultaneous (likelihood ratio) tests for all categories for each of the covariates adjusted for the other covariates. Thus, the last line in Table 7.1.10 shows (three-degree-of-freedom) tests for ha, p3np, and ykl40 showing that all markers are significant at the 5% level, most so p3np. It would not be immediate how to conduct such tests if parameter estimates (see Table 7.1.9) were obtained via three separate logistic regression models. Finally, in the fibrosis example, separate estimation had the additional disadvantage that one of the simple logistic regressions could not be fitted.

The fact that parameters in (7.1.8) may be estimated using simple logistic regression models for binary data has the consequence that model checking may, in principle, be performed in those simple models. However, because in general we recommend to fit the model using the likelihood method based on *all* data, the polychotomous regression model (7.1.8) is the one that should be subject to model checking. For that purpose the multinomial outcome y_i may be transformed into $k + 1$ indicators $I(y_i = g_0), \ldots, I(y_i = k)$ and, thereby defining $k + 1$ residuals for each subject by

$$r_{i,j} = I(y_i = g_j) - \widehat{\mathrm{pr}}(y_i = g_j).$$

Here, $\widehat{pr}(y_i = g_j)$ is obtained by substituting estimated values for $a-$ and $b-$ parameters into (7.1.9). These residuals, possibly standardized by dividing by their estimated standard deviation $\sqrt{\widehat{pr}(y_i = g_j)(1 - \widehat{pr}(y_i = g_j))}$ may be examined graphically using methods illustrated previously for binary outcomes.

Let us finally comment on the two different models that we have fitted to the fibrosis data: the proportional odds model (7.1.3) in Section 7.1.1 and the polychotomous logistic regression model (7.1.8) in the current section. Both models specify the probabilities $pr(y_i = g_j)$, however (because of the non-linearity of the logit function), the two models are not nested and, therefore, they cannot be compared via a likelihood ratio test. For an ordinal outcome, we prefer (7.1.3) because it utilizes the ordinal structure in y and always has fewer parameters than (7.1.8). Therefore, it provides a more parsimonious description of the data with parameters that tend to be easier to interpret. On the other hand, the proportional odds assumption may be too restrictive and (7.1.3) may not provide a satisfactory fit to the data, in which case (7.1.8) is an alternative.

7.2 Count outcome

In the fever in pregnancy Example 1.2 in Section 1.1.1, we have thus far studied possible explanatory variables for the risk of fetal death, one of these being the number of fever episodes during pregnancy. In this section we look at the number of fever episodes as the outcome variable and describe analyses relating this to possible explanatory variables.

If a fever episode is regarded as a pregnancy week with occurrence of fever, we can think of the number of fever episodes as a sum of zeros and ones, a one for each week where the woman experienced fever and a zero for each week without fever. For each week, we denote the probability of a fever episode by p (assumed to be identical for all weeks, i.e., independent of gestational age) and if fever episodes occur independently of each other in separate weeks, the resulting sum will follow a Binomial distribution $Bin(c, p)$, as described in Section 2.1.2, where c denotes the number of weeks available for possible fever episodes.

The probability p is small, therefore the Binomial distribution may be approximated by a *Poisson* distribution, as described in Section 2.1.3, so that the probability that y, the number of fever episodes during $c = 14$ weeks of pregnancy, takes the value u may be written as

$$pr(y = u) = \frac{m^u}{u!} \exp(-m), \qquad (7.2.1)$$

where the parameter m is the mean value $m = cp$. We are looking for explanatory variables for this mean value m. One such variable that in particular could be expected to have an effect is the parity (i.e., the number of previous pregnancies for the woman), because children are known to bring home a lot of germs and expose family members to all sorts of common infections. Other possible explanatory variables could be age (which is presumably closely associated with parity) and alcohol and smoking habits.

Table 7.2.1 lists the number of fever episodes according to a simplified description of parity (0: no previous children, 1: one or more previous children). Moreover, the average and squared SD is given, allowing for an immediate assessment of the effect of parity as well as a superficial check of the Poisson assumption (because in a Poisson distribution, the mean equals the squared standard deviation). This table seems to support our suspicion about children attracting infections because the average number of fever episodes is 0.223 for parity ≥ 1 and only 0.172 for parity 0 mothers ($P < 0.0001$). This apparent difference might, however, be due to other reasons, such as older age or higher alcohol consumption.

Table 7.2.1. Number of fever episodes during pregnancy, according to parity. Additional summary statistics.

Parity	Number of Fever Episodes												Average	SD^2	Average Age
	0	1	2	3	4	5	6	7	8	9	10	≥ 12	Average	SD^2	Age
0	4474	731	69	10	2	1	0	0	0	0	0	0	0.172	0.189	27.88
≥ 1	5219	1141	114	10	1	2	1	1	0	0	2	0	0.223	0.264	31.06
Total	9693	1872	183	20	3	3	1	1	0	0	2	0	0.200	0.231	29.63

Let y_i denote the number of fever episodes for the ith woman. We relate $m_i = \mathrm{E}(y_i)$ to a linear predictor, including some of the above-mentioned explanatory variables. The number of fever episodes is obviously nonnegative, thus it is natural to use a logarithmic transformation. However, a large fraction of women will experience no fever episode during pregnancy, that is, $y_i = 0$ (see Table 7.2.1), thus preventing a logarithmic transformation of the observations. The natural choice is therefore to use instead a logarithmic link: define

$$\log(\mathrm{E}(y_i)) = \log(m_i) = \mathrm{LP}_i = a + b_1 x_{i,1} + \cdots + b_{n_c} x_{i,n_c}. \qquad (7.2.2)$$

Due to the logarithmic link, we cannot use the method of least squares to estimate the parameters. Instead we use a full maximum likelihood approach so we have to specify the distribution of y_i, that is, the point probabilities given in Equation (7.2.1) for varying m_i. Subsequently we compare with the results obtained from a Binomial distribution assumption and an approximation with a Normal distribution.

As mentioned above, the mean of a Poisson distributed variable equals the squared standard deviation. Hence we could get a rough idea about the appropriateness of the Poisson distribution from Table 7.2.1. The total average is 0.200 and the squared standard deviation is 0.231 so we have a slightly larger standard deviation than prescribed by a Poisson distribution (the ratio between squared standard deviation and average is $0.231/0.200 = 1.155$). The goodness-of-fit test for the Poisson distribution actually gives a significant result, $P < 0.0001$, stating that the description is not good (a similar result was found for the Binomial distribution in Section 2.3.2). This is to be expected, however, because the mean may depend on covariates (as specified in Equation (7.2.2)) so that the y_is are not identically distributed.

Subdividing according to parity, we get averages and standard deviations as seen in Table 7.2.1 and we note that for parity 0 the correspondence between squared standard deviation and average is now better (the ratio between squared standard deviation and average being $0.189/0.172 = 1.099$), whereas for parity ≥ 1 it is somewhat worse (the ratio being $0.264/0.223 = 1.184$). If it were feasible to subdivide also according to age and alcohol habits, we could imagine that the observed averages and squared standard deviations (variances) would become closer in each stratum. Actually, if the squared standard deviation is much larger than the average in one or more strata, it could well be a sign of an important explanatory variable that was not (yet) taken into account.

Digression. Overdispersion

Inasmuch as the standard deviation is directly linked to the mean in a Poisson distribution, there is no concept such as a residual variation as we have seen it in the case of Normal distributions. Actually this means that we trust the models to include all relevant explanatory variables such that the conditional distributions for given values of all explanatory variables can be taken to be Poisson and show no variation beyond that specified by the mean value. If this is not the case, we talk about overdispersion. Such an overdispersion can be incorporated into the model by assuming the Poisson means m_i (after adjustment for covariates) to have a Gamma distribution. This introduces an additional free parameter to describe the variation, and the resulting marginal distribution is called a *Negative Binomial distribution* . This may also be thought of as adding an error term to the linear predictor from Equation (7.2.2), and assuming that this error is distributed as the logarithm of a Gamma distribution. Gamma distributions resemble logarithmic Normal distributions, thus an assumption of Normality for the error term will result in similar results. ◇

An analysis including alcohol habits (either in five categories or as a quantitative variable with a linear effect), age at conception (as a quantitative variable with a linear effect), and parity (binary variable as described above) showed alcohol habits to be without any effect, probably because very few women drink more than one or two units a week. We therefore only present the results from an analysis with parity and age, as shown in Table 7.2.2.

When fitting the model, we scaled the age variable to be centered at the age of 30 and increasing in units of 10 years. Therefore, the intercept corresponds to the level for a women who got pregnant at the age of 30 and had one or

Table 7.2.2. Estimates in a model with parity and age as explanatory variables for the number of fever episodes during pregnancy.

	Estimate (CI)	Ratio Estimate (CI)	P
Intercept	−1.488 (−1.541, −1.436)	—	—
Parity			
0	−0.300 (−0.390, −0.211)	0.741 (0.677, 0.810)	<0.0001
≥ 1	0	1	—
Age, 10 years	−0.140 (−0.244, −0.035)	0.870 (0.783, 0.965)	0.0088

more previous children. She has an estimated mean number of fever episodes equal to $\exp(-1.4882) = 0.226$.

We note that both parity and age are significant predictors for the number of fever episodes. Thus, women with no previous children have a mean number of fever episodes which is approximately 25% less than women with one or more previous children (the factor being 0.74, i.e., 26% lower), provided that they have the same age. The confidence interval ranges from 19% to 32% lower. Because of the approximate relation between the mean number of fever episodes and the probability of a fever episode in any given week ($m \approx cp$), the same ratio applies to the interpretation of the probability of a fever episode in any given period of pregnancy (e.g., a week).

Similarly, we find that older women have a somewhat lower level of fever episodes. A ten-year increase in age yields an estimated decrease in the mean number of fever episodes of approximately 13% (CI 4–22%), for women with identical parities.

Note that this is in apparent contradiction with the effect of parity because the parity 0 women have an average age of 27.9 whereas the women with parity ≥ 1 have an average age of 31.1 years (see Table 7.2.1). Actually, it is precisely this association between parity and age that results in a significant age effect *when adjusting for parity*. We have an example of two closely related explanatory variables that have opposite effects on the outcome: parity has a positive effect (women with previous children have more fever episodes) whereas age has a negative effect (older women have fewer fever episodes). If we did not adjust for parity and studied the number of fever episodes solely as a function of age, the effect of age would disappear (estimated effect in that model is −0.010 for 10 years of age, $P = 0.84$). The reason is that for this marginal model the mean number of fever episodes for the youngest mothers is lowered because most of them are nulliparous whereas, for the older mothers it is increased because more of these tend to have previous children.

Likewise, in a model including parity as the only explanatory variable, the effect of this would be somewhat less pronounced compared to the model adjusted for age. We can see this from Table 7.2.1 because the effect of parity is here simply estimated as the ratio $0.172/0.223 = 0.7713$, a little closer to 1 than 0.7407 from Table 7.2.2.

Note that the situation described here with effects being present only when adjusting also for other effects is a classical example of confounding and has nothing to do with interaction. There may or may not also be an interaction between parity and age but we have not investigated this yet. Including an interaction term between parity and the linear age effect gives an estimated difference in the age effect of 0.0047 (0.0109), in the sense that the age effect is somewhat more pronounced for the women without previous children. The difference is, however, not significant ($P = 0.66$).

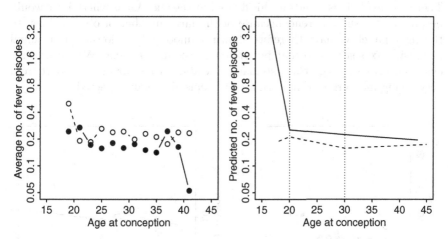

Fig. 7.2.1. Left panel: average number of fever episodes in two-year age groups, with symbols according to parity (parity 1: dots, parity 0: circles). Right panel: predicted values for age effects in the two parity groups as a linear spline with breaks at age 20 and 30 (parity 1: solid curve, parity 0: dashed curve).

We, therefore, conclude that a reasonable model for the number of fever episodes during pregnancy is given by Equation (7.2.3).

$$\log(\mathrm{E}(y)) = \mathrm{LP} = a + b_1 I(\mathrm{parity} = 0) + b_2 \mathrm{Age}. \tag{7.2.3}$$

Model checks

The conclusions presented above rely (as always) on the adequacy of the chosen model. We therefore have to perform model checks to assure ourselves that we have not overlooked important features.

The left panel of Figure 7.2.1 shows the average number of fever episodes in two-year age groups (the outermost age groups cover larger age ranges, 16–20 and 40–45 respectively). We note from this figure that the decline in mean fever episodes with age is not entirely apparent except for the outermost age groups. It is not surprising that the very young mothers may have an infection pattern quite different from more mature mothers thus in order to investigate this effect further, we model age effect as a linear spline with breaks at age 20 and 30. Furthermore, we allow the age effect to be different for the two parity groups, and the resulting predicted mean number of fever episodes is shown in the right panel of Figure 7.2.1. There is found no significant interaction between parity and age in this extended model, either, and the breaks are not significant.

The left panel of Figure 7.2.2 shows a residual plot for the model with a linear effect of age and a parity effect, with no interaction between the two. There are no obvious trends in this figure but the question is whether we would be able to see such a trend because of the large number of observations. In the right panel we have therefore shown a smoothed version of the residual plot, with axes scaled so that possible patterns may appear. We see no such clear patterns to suggest a systematic deviation from our model, apart from very young mothers who have more fever episodes than expected.

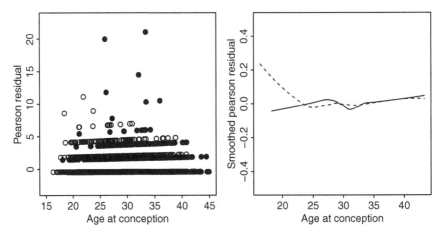

Fig. 7.2.2. Residual plots for the model (7.2.3) Left panel: parity 1: dots, parity 0: circles; right panel: smoothed version according to parity, parity 1: solid curve, parity 0: dashed curve.

We may also perform a goodness-of-fit test for model (7.2.3), along the lines used in Section 6.2.2, by grouping the women according to their predicted mean number of fever episodes. Taking 10 equally sized groups and comparing observed and expected number of fever episodes (totally for women in the group), we get Table 7.2.3 and an overall chi-squared statistic of 7.02. When this is evaluated in a χ^2 distribution with 8 degrees-of-freedom, it yields a

P-value of 0.53 and therefore no indication that the linear predictor is inadequate.

Table 7.2.3. Observed and expected number of fever episodes in ten subgroups according to predicted values.

Predicted Mean Number of Fever Episodes	Number of Women	Number of Fever Episodes Observed (O)	Expected (E)	$\frac{O-E}{\sqrt{E}}$
0.138–0.166	1176	188	187.57	0.031
0.166–0.172	1179	197	199.18	−0.154
0.172–0.177	1179	212	205.56	0.449
0.177–0.183	1177	196	211.40	−1.059
0.183–0.207	1178	239	229.77	0.609
0.207–0.215	1179	273	249.63	1.479
0.215–0.221	1177	229	257.01	−1.747
0.221–0.227	1179	265	264.13	0.054
0.227–0.234	1176	272	270.54	0.088
0.234–0.267	1178	287	283.20	0.226

We may also compare observed and expected values of fever episodes directly in the marginal distribution, as seen in Table 7.2.4. We here get an overall test statistic of 19.97 which is significant in a chi-squared distribution with 2 degrees of freedom ($P < 0.0001$). This means that we do find some signs that the observed number of fever episodes has a distribution which is too wide compared to a Poisson distribution, that is, signs of an overdispersion. This may be explained either by covariates not yet taken into account or by correlation between the occurrence of fever episodes for the same woman in successive weeks.

Table 7.2.4. Observed and expected number of women according to number of fever episodes.

Number of Fever Episodes	Number of Women Observed (O)	Expected (E)	$\frac{O-E}{\sqrt{E}}$
0	9693	9644.63	0.492
1	1872	1923.71	−1.179
2	183	194.44	−0.890
≥ 3	30	14.21	17.545

Comparison to other approaches

As mentioned in the beginning of this section, the Poisson distribution is used here as an approximation to the Binomial distribution. We compare here the above results obtained from the Poisson model (7.2.3) with a similar one assuming the distribution to be $Bin(c = 14, p)$ and choosing the link function to be the logit, with the same linear predictor as given in (7.2.3). Even though the number of fever episodes is restricted to nonnegative integers, we nevertheless also compare to a model assuming Normality, with log-link. The results are shown in Table 7.2.5 which also includes the results from the Poisson model for comparison. We note that there is hardly any difference between the estimates. In fact, the discrepancy between the model fits amounts to less than a quarter of a percent. We could proceed by comparing also with other link functions (e.g., the identity link or a square root link) but by now it has become clear that this will hardly change anything at all.

Table 7.2.5. Comparison of estimates in models assuming Poisson, Normal, and Binomial distributions.

	Parity 0 vs. ≥ 1		Age, 10 Years		Prediction for
Model	Estimate (SD)	P-Value	Estimate (SD)	P-Value	Age 30, Parity 1
Poisson	−0.300 (0.046)	<0.0001	−0.140 (0.053)	0.0088	0.226 (0.214, 0.238)
Binomial	−0.300 (0.045)	<0.0001	−0.139 (0.053)	0.008	0.222 (0.211, 0.234)
Normal, log-link	−0.300 (0.050)	<0.0001	−0.141 (0.058)	0.015	0.226 (0.214, 0.238)

7.3 Quantitative outcome

The models for quantitative outcomes studied thus far have all linked the mean value directly to the linear predictor (i.e., using the "identity link"), perhaps after transformation of the outcome variable. When quantitative covariates are present, this formally has the consequence that negative mean values may be anticipated. In many practical examples the range of the outcome and covariates may prevent this from happening but in some situations, an outcome with positive values can take on values very close to zero (an example might be the concentration of some hormone) and the problem becomes highly relevant.

A possible solution to this problem is to make a transformation of the outcome, typically using a logarithm before linking to the linear predictor and thereby ensuring the positivity of predicted values. This changes the relation between covariate and outcome, because the relation will now be linear on the transformed scale but of exponential type on the original scale. At the same time it will affect the assumption of constant standard deviation of the outcome (we cannot have a constant standard deviation on both scales). It may so happen that these considerations (sensible description of mean and constant standard deviation) are somewhat contradictory. This may be solved by choosing another link function.

The approach using a logarithmic transformation of vitamin D (y_i) when modeling the effect of body mass index x_i has been used previously (e.g., Section 6.2.1). The model can be written as

$$E(\log(y_i)) = LP_i = a + bx_i. \tag{7.3.1}$$

In this section, we compare this with the approach just mentioned, in which we do not transform the outcome, but rather use the logarithm as link function to the linear predictor LP_i, that is, the model

$$\log(E(y_i)) = LP_i = a + bx_i. \tag{7.3.2}$$

In a digression in Section 1.2.2 it was mentioned that the two approaches corresponding to Equations (7.3.1) and (7.3.2) are not identical even though they look rather similar. The difference has to do with the distribution of the outcome y and, as mentioned above, the assumption of constant standard deviation; see also Appendix B. Note that (7.3.2) corresponds to the model (7.2.2) for a Poisson outcome in Section 7.2.

Estimation in regression models with quantitative outcome variables is traditionally carried out using the method of least squares, which is identical to the maximum likelihood method when the outcome is Normally distributed with constant standard deviation. These two assumptions relate to different scales in Equations (7.3.1) and (7.3.2). In Equation (7.3.1) the standard deviation is assumed constant on the logarithmic scale (corresponding to a standard deviation proportional to the mean value on the original scale, i.e., a constant *coefficient of variation*; see the digression below), whereas in Equation (7.3.2) the standard deviation itself is assumed constant on the original scale. Model (7.3.1) may be analyzed using the method of least squares (on the logarithmic scale) whereas in model (7.3.2) the likelihood method will yield another approach (because the mean value is not linearly related to the covariate on the scale of constant standard deviation).

Digression. The coefficient of variation

When measurement error or other types of variation are expressed as percentages, there is an implicit assumption that large levels are associated with large standard deviations, in fact that these are proportional. The coefficient of variation is defined as this constant ratio between standard deviation and mean. Thus, if y_i is a variable measured for subject i with mean value m_i and standard deviation s_i, then expressing s_i as a percentage implies that $s_i = CV m_i$, and the ratio $CV = s_i/m_i$ is denoted the coefficient of variation. It can be shown that if the y_is have a constant coefficient of variation CV (e.g., 8%), then $\log(y_i)$ will have an approximately constant standard deviation equal to 0.08. The approximation is best for small values of CV and becomes unreasonable for values above 25–30%. ◇

We once again use Example 1.1 from Section 1.1 for illustrating the difference between the two approaches corresponding to Equations (7.3.1) and (7.3.2). Furthermore, the simple model relating vitamin D concentration (y_i) to body mass index (x_i), by the formula

$$E(y_i) = LP_i = a + bx_i \qquad (7.3.3)$$

is also included in the comparison. Thus, we use the linear predictor in three different ways, namely as either the simple mean $E(y_i)$, the logarithm of the mean $\log(E(y_i))$, or the mean of the logarithm $E(\log(y_i))$. Note that because we are estimating different models, the parameters a and b in the three linear predictors will not have the same interpretation and their estimates can therefore not be directly compared. However, the parameters in the models (7.3.1) and (7.3.2) involving logarithms will be very close if the standard deviation is small. If we center the covariate at a body mass index of 25, the estimated intercept in the untransformed model with linear predictor (7.3.3) will be the expected vitamin D concentration for a woman with body mass index 25, whereas for the other two models it will be the estimated logarithmic value for such a woman.

The estimate for the untransformed model (7.3.3) with identity link has already been discussed in Section 4.1.1. The estimates were found to be $\widehat{a} = 111.05(18.40)$ and $\widehat{b} = -2.392(0.690)$, using an uncentered version of body mass index. With the body mass index centered at 25, we get instead $\widehat{a} = 51.24(2.95)$. Thus, with the ordinary linear regression on an untransformed scale, the predicted vitamin D concentration for a woman with a body mass index of 25 is 51.24. The estimates from all of the three regressions are collected in Table 7.3.1, along with the estimates from three more models, where body mass index has also been subjected to a logarithmic transformation before entering as a covariate. Moreover, Figure 7.3.1 shows the corresponding estimated relations based on these six models.

We note that all approaches yield very similar descriptions of the relation between vitamin D concentration and body mass index. This is because the outcome as well as the covariate vary in a quite narrow range away from zero, so that the logarithm is reasonably linear in the observed range (Figure B.1).

In Table 7.3.1 we can compare the estimates of the intercept $\widehat{a}$ from rows 1 and 2. For the remaining models, we should compare to $\exp(\widehat{a})$, which are (47.27, 46.58, 50.40, 49.67), respectively. This means that the models using a logarithmic transformation of the vitamin D as outcome predict a lower value for women with a body mass of 25. Actually, they predict lower values in the entire range but because we compare so many similar models in Figure 7.3.1, it is hard to really tell the difference (even more so because of the scaling needed to include the data in the picture as well). We therefore take a closer look at

Table 7.3.1. Parameter estimates in six different models relating concentration of vitamin D (y_i) to body mass index (x_i).

Model	Estimates		
	$\widehat{a}$	$\widehat{b}$	s
1: $E(y_i) = a + b(x_i - 25)$	51.24 (2.95)	−2.392 (0.690)	17.91
2: $E(y_i) = a + b\left(\log(x_i) - \log(25)\right)$	50.61 (2.89)	−63.53 (18.23)	17.88
3: $E\left(\log(y_i)\right) = a + b(x_i - 25)$	3.8558 (0.0629)	−0.0545 (0.01473)	0.3821
4: $E\left(\log(y_i)\right) = a + b\left(\log(x_i) - \log(25)\right)$	3.8411 (0.0618)	−1.4414 (0.3896)	0.3821
5: $\log\left(E((y_i))\right) = a + b(x_i - 25)$	3.9199 (0.0557)	−0.0515 (0.0151)	17.88
6: $\log\left(E((y_i))\right) = a + b\left(\log(x_i) - \log(25)\right)$	3.9054 (0.0562)	−1.3068 (0.3759)	17.91

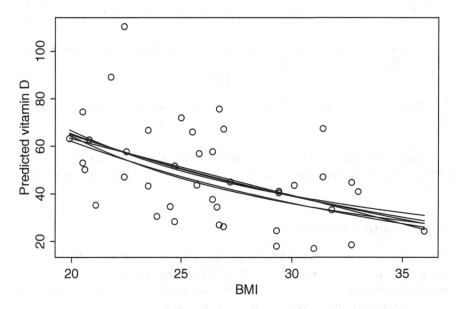

Fig. 7.3.1. Comparison of estimated curves from the six models in Table 7.3.1.

the two graphs corresponding to rows 3 (Equation (7.3.1), dashed line) and 5 (Equation (7.3.2), solid line) of Table 7.3.1. These two curves can be seen in Figure 7.3.2 without the actual data in order for the differences to stand out more clearly. We see that the two curves have almost identical shapes and that the one with a log link on the untransformed outcome is higher for all values of body mass index. This is because the mean is here applied to slightly skewed data, giving higher values.

The estimated standard deviations from Table 7.3.1 can be compared in rows (1,2,5,6) and the standard deviations in rows (3,4) are to be interpreted as coefficients of variation (CV). The average vitamin D concentration is ap-

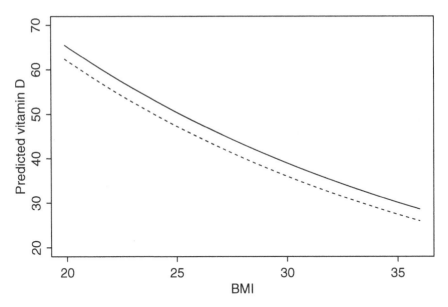

Fig. 7.3.2. Comparison of estimated relations corresponding to models in rows 3 and 5.

proximately 48, thus a CV of 38% corresponds roughly to a standard deviation of 18.24, that is,i.e. only slightly higher than for the rest of the models in Table 7.3.1.

Cardiac output example

We now turn to Example 1.11 from Section 1.1 concerned with the precision in the measurement of cardiac output. This investigation involved 80 patients, and the outcome of interest is the within-patient standard deviation based on $N = 8$ consecutive measurements for each patient.

The ultimate aim of this investigation was to make it possible to reduce the number of successive measurements (N) for each patient without losing too much information regarding the level of cardiac output. The standard deviation of the average of N successive measurements is given by $s/\sqrt{N}$, therefore we may use a smaller N if the standard deviation on single measurements s is small itself. Hence it is of interest to identify possible predictors for the size of this standard deviation. If certain covariate values predict a high standard deviation, we can react by taking more observations on these patients than on others.

In the left panel of Figure 7.3.3 the subject-specific standard deviations are plotted against the corresponding average values of cardiac output, with symbols indicating sex. The positive relation between standard deviations and levels seen in this figure suggests a constant coefficient of variation rather than a constant standard deviation, leading us to perform a logarithmic transformation of the cardiac output measurements and calculating the standard deviation on this scale instead. If we performed the analysis for the standard deviations on the original scale, we would run the risk of identifying covariates associated with the level instead of the measurement uncertainty. Gender may be such a variable. Table 7.3.2 shows medians for levels (individual averages) and standard deviations for the untransformed data, subdivided according to sex. We note that both standard deviations and levels are lower for women than for men. However, in the left panel of Figure 7.3.3 we can see that this sex difference is not the only reason for the positive association between standard deviation and level, because this association is present for both sexes separately.

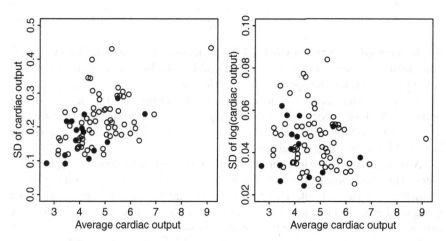

Fig. 7.3.3. Subject-specific standard deviations plotted against level of cardiac output. Left panel: SD on original scale; right panel: SD on logarithmic scale (circles: males; dots: females).

Table 7.3.2. Medians of individual cardiac output (average of $N = 8$ measurements) and standard deviations.

| | Medians | |
Gender	Average Cardiac Output	Standard Deviation
Female	4.0875	0.1852
Male	4.6125	0.2070

In the right panel of Figure 7.3.3, the standard deviations on the logarithmic scale are plotted against the levels. The positive association from the left panel is seen not to present on this scale.

The standard deviations are all obviously positive, but a few are very close to zero. Including a linear effect on such a scale may not be wise inasmuch as estimated values will run a high risk of becoming negative. However, in this example it creates no problems because the only quantitative explanatory variable is age (as shown later, this does not seem to have any effect). On the other hand, the distribution of the standard deviations is obviously skewed, with a heavy tail to the right suggesting that a logarithmic transformation may be a better idea for these data. We compare the two approaches from Equation (7.3.1) and (7.3.2), that is, models assuming the linear predictor to be either $E(\log(y_i))$ or $\log(E(y_i))$ where we let

$$y_i = \hat{s}_i^2$$

be the *squared* standard deviation (the variance) for patient i. Following this comparison, we compare with a third (and probably more realistic) model taking into account the specific distribution of $\hat{s}_i^2$.

The covariates that were believed to be of importance for the size of the standard deviation were primarily the age of the patient and whether the patient had a pacemaker. Gender was not a priori considered to be of importance but could not be ruled out either.

A preliminary investigation of the effect of age can be seen in Figure 7.3.4 where the logarithm of the SD (for logarithmic cardiac outputs) are plotted against age of the patient. This figure shows that we cannot expect any effect of age. This was confirmed in later analyses (not shown here), therefore we are not concerned with the effect of this covariate here.

We therefore look at a model including only the two categorical covariates gender and presence of pacemaker. Table 7.3.3 shows medians of logarithmic standard deviations according to these two categorical covariates. We notice that patients with a pacemaker seem to have a somewhat lower variation than patients without a pacemaker and that women tend to have a smaller variation than men. We also recognize that pacemaker and gender are related because the data include only a single woman with a pacemaker. Note, however, that in this situation the association between the covariates leads to an *enhanced* effect for each covariate when the other is also included (the difference between the pacemaker groups is larger for each of the gender groups separately than for the sexes combined). We return to a comment on this below.

The estimated contrast between the two categories for each of the two covariates is given in the first two rows of Table 7.3.4. We see that patients without a pacemaker have a somewhat higher standard deviation than patients with a pacemaker but that this difference does not reach statistical significance. If we estimate using the log-link, we have to multiply the squared SD by $\exp(0.319) = 1.38$, that is, a 38% increased squared standard deviation

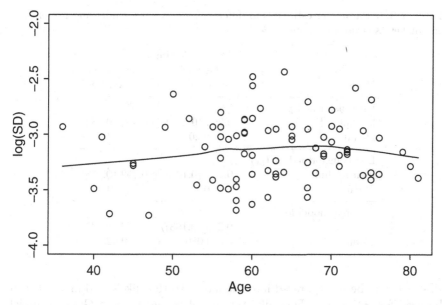

Fig. 7.3.4. Preliminary investigation of the effect of age on standard deviation.

Table 7.3.3. Median standard deviations for logarithmic cardiac output (number of subjects), according to gender and pacemaker use.

| | Pacemaker Use | | |
Gender	No	Yes	All
Female	0.0429 (14)	0.0283 (1)	0.0417 (15)
Male	0.0471 (46)	0.0410 (19)	0.0426 (65)
All	0.0455 (60)	0.0399 (20)	0.0426 (80)

for patients without pacemaker. For the log-transformed outcome, the multiplication factor is $\exp(0.252) = 1.29$, somewhat lower (precisely as we found it in the vitamin D example above).

Performing a logarithmic transformation and using the least squares method on this scale corresponds to assuming the distribution of the logarithms of the squared standard deviations to be symmetric or even Normal. In this particular situation we can do something a little closer to reality because we know that the outcome is a squared standard deviation. If we can assume the eight successive measurements (on the logarithmic scale) for each patient to be Normally distributed around some (patient-dependent) mean then it can be shown that the distribution of the quantity $7 \times \widehat{s}_i^2$ will be Chi-squared with 7 degrees of freedom and scale parameter s_i^2 (the true squared standard deviation for this patient). This distribution is a specific form of a Gamma distribution (with shape parameter $7/2$ and scale parameter s_i^2), and

Table 7.3.4. Parameter estimates in different models with gender and presence of pacemaker as covariates.

| | Estimates | |
| | Gender | Pacemaker |
Model	Male vs. Female	No vs. Yes
Untransformed y_i		
log-link	0.261 (0.203)	0.319 (0.188)
P-value	0.20	0.09
Log-transformed $\log(y_i)$		
identity link	0.248 (0.169)	0.252 (0.153)
P-value	0.15	0.10
Gamma model $\log(y_i)$		
log link	0.280 (0.163)	0.333 (0.147)
P-value	0.086	0.023

this fact may be incorporated into the model so that likelihood methods can be used for estimation. Formally, the model is said to be a Gamma model with log-link and mean value $m_i = 7s_i^2$. A linear predictor with log-link now specifies

$$\log(\mathrm{E}(7\hat{s}_i^2)) = \log(m_i) = \log(7) + \log(s_i^2) \tag{7.3.4}$$
$$= a + b_1 I(\text{patient } i \text{ is a man})$$
$$+ b_2 I(\text{patient } i \text{ has a pacemaker})$$

and the estimates from the model are added as the last row of Table 7.3.4. As mentioned, the log-transformed model in the second row of Table 7.3.4 corresponds to an assumption that the standard deviations are log-Normally distributed. Because the difference between a Gamma distribution and a log-Normal distribution is not that big, we should expect results to be rather close. It seems, however, that they are not any more similar than the other models.

We notice that the Gamma model actually makes the use of a pacemaker significant, and the estimated effect is a factor $\exp(0.333) = 1.40$ on the squared standard deviation. However, this significance is only present as long as we adjust for gender. This is due to the confounding mentioned above (i.e., that we only have a single woman with a pacemaker). Figure 7.3.5 attempts to give an illustration of this situation. We see that in the marginal pacemaker categories (labeled "All"), the "no pacemaker" category is a mixture of 46 men (with a relatively high SD) and 14 women (with a lower SD), whereas the "pacemaker" category is a mixture of 19 men and only a single woman. Hence the average of the "no pacemaker" category is lowered more than the "pacemaker" category due to the presence of relatively more women, and in

the marginal comparison, the difference between the two groups will therefore
not be quite as big as when adjusting for gender.

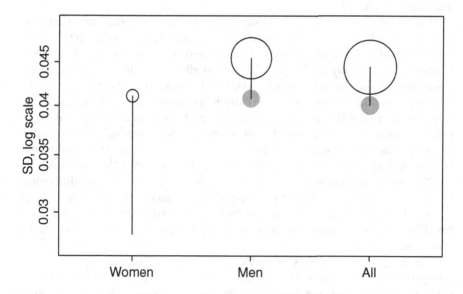

Fig. 7.3.5. Estimated means (of logarithmic standard deviation) in groups according to gender (horizontal axis) and presence of pacemaker (open circles: no pacemaker, shaded circles: pacemaker). The vertical lines illustrate the estimated effect
of a pacemaker.

7.4 Binary outcome

In previous chapters, binary data have been analyzed using the logit link
$(\log(p/(1-p)))$ when relating the mean of the binary outcome y (i.e., $p_i =$
$\mathrm{pr}(y_i = 1)$), to the linear predictor LP_i. This provided regression parameters
to be interpreted as odds ratios (or log(odds ratios)).

In Section 7.4.1 we study two classes of alternative link functions. One
class, like the logistic function, has the desirable property that estimated probabilities always stay between 0 and 1. These models have the interpretation
that the binary outcome y_i can be defined via a *latent*, that is, unobserved,
variable y_i^* such that $y_i = 1$ whenever y_i^* is below some threshold c:

$$I(y_i = 1) = I(y_i^* \leq c).$$

We mostly discuss one model of this kind, namely the *probit* model where
the latent variable has a Normal distribution. The logistic model, discussed in

earlier chapters, has a similar interpretation with a latent variable following the Logistic distribution (similar in shape to the Normal) . However, we also briefly mention the *cloglog* link and its relation to the proportional hazards model for survival data.

The second class of link functions discussed does not guarantee that predicted probabilities stay between 0 and 1. At first glance it may seem that such models are of no interest, however, as discussed in Section 3.1.2, alternatives to the log(odds ratio) are frequently used as effect measures in epidemiology when quantifying the discrepancy between the event probabilities, p_0 and p_1 in two groups. One such measure is the log(relative risk) $= \log(p_1/p_0)$, the other is the risk difference $p_1 - p_0$. Because of the simple interpretation of risk ratios and risk differences it is of interest to have methods by which one can relate them to covariates. Generally, risk ratios are easier to communicate than odds ratios and only when the outcome is "rare" can the odds ratio be interpreted as an approximate risk ratio (Figure 3.1.5). The risk difference, on the other hand, has the nice property that it immediately quantifies effects on the absolute risk scale in contrast to both the risk ratio and the odds ratio. This may be an important feature in applications in fields such as health economics.

We illustrate the models using the fever in pregnancy Example 1.2. The interpretation of regression coefficients of the models introduced is illustrated using the binary outcome fetal death as used previously. However, because fetal death is a rather rare outcome, some further aspects of the models are illustrated using a more frequent binary outcome variable for this dataset, namely *small for gestational age*, sga. This is defined as the birthweight being below the fifth percentile in the distribution of birthweights for each given gestational week. Details follow below.

In Section 7.4.2 we briefly discuss inference for binary data sampled in a *case-control study*. Here, instead of following a "cohort" of individuals and observing the binary outcome y_i, data are sampled depending on the outcome. That is, *cases* are sampled among individuals in whom $y_i = 1$ and *controls* among those where the outcome is $y_i = 0$. This is a very useful way of ascertaining individuals to a study of the relationship between covariates and disease risks when the disease outcome is rare. Whereas, for cohort data, several link functions can be applied (as discussed in Section 7.4.1), logistic regression is the only binary regression model feasible for case-control studies. Use of the other link functions (introduced below) is simply incorrect in case-control studies or requires further information in the form of selection probabilities for both cases and controls.

7.4.1 Alternatives to the logit link

To illustrate the alternative link functions we recall the fever in pregnancy Example 1.2. Table 7.4.1 shows the distribution of the binary outcome fetal death y_i in relation to smoking and to the number of fever episodes in early pregnancy. It is seen, as noted earlier, that fetal death is a very rare event occurring in only 1% of the women.

Table 7.4.1. Fever in pregnancy study: distribution of fetal death by smoking and by number of fever episodes in early pregnancy.

Category	Women	Fetal Deaths	%
No smokers	8647	81	0.94
1–10 cigarettes/day	1760	19	1.08
11+ cigarettes/day	1371	19	1.39
No fever episodes	9693	98	1.01
1 fever episode	1872	20	1.07
2 fever episodes	183	1	0.55
3+ fever episodes	30	0	0
Total	11778	119	1.01

We look at models where the linear predictor LP_i depends on each of the two categorical covariates from Table 7.4.1. The reference categories are no smokers and no fever episodes, respectively, and the four models for $p_i = pr(y_i = 1)$ considered are:

$$logit(p_i) = LP_i, \tag{7.4.1}$$
$$probit(p_i) = LP_i, \tag{7.4.2}$$
$$log(p_i) = LP_i, \tag{7.4.3}$$
$$p_i = LP_i. \tag{7.4.4}$$

In (7.4.2), $probit(p)$ denotes the pth percentile in the standard Normal distribution, that is, the value (z_p) satisfying $pr(u \le z_p) = p$ when u is a standard Normally distributed random variable. The probit function has a very similar form to the logit function, shown in Figure 1.3.3. In (7.4.3) and (7.4.4), the link functions are log and the identity function, respectively. Table 7.4.2 shows the results. For the variable smoking we can interpret the estimates in relation to the relative frequencies in the three categories shown in Table 7.4.1, 0.94%, 1.08%, and 1.39%, respectively. Thus for the logit link, the coefficients are

$$log\left(\frac{\left(\frac{0.0108}{1-0.0108}\right)}{\left(\frac{0.0094}{1-0.0094}\right)}\right) = 0.143, \quad log\left(\frac{\left(\frac{0.0139}{1-0.0139}\right)}{\left(\frac{0.0094}{1-0.0094}\right)}\right) = 0.396,$$

(as explained in earlier chapters) whereas, for the log link, they are

$$log\left(\frac{0.0108}{0.0094}\right) = 0.142, \quad log\left(\frac{0.0139}{0.0094}\right) = 0.392.$$

These two sets of parameter estimates are very close because the log(odds ratio) and the log(risk ratio) are almost identical for rare events. The intercepts are logit(0.0094) = −4.66 and log(0.0094) = −4.67 for the logit and log links, respectively. For the identity link the estimates are simply

$$0.0108 - 0.0094 = 0.0014, \quad 0.0139 - 0.0094 = 0.0045$$

and the intercept is 0.0094. For the probit link, the interpretation is as follows. As mentioned in the introduction to this section, we should imagine a latent variable y_i^* for each woman (her "health") and if this latent variable is smaller than some threshold c then the woman experiences a fetal loss. The latent variable is assumed to follow a standard Normal distribution in the reference group (no smokers) and, in the two other smoking categories, the "mean health", that is, the mean value of y_i^* is reduced by 0.053 and 0.150, respectively. In the probit model, the intercept is −2.35, the percentile in the standard Normal distribution with the property that $pr(u \le -2.35) = 0.94\%$, the relative frequency of fetal deaths in the reference group.

Table 7.4.2. Fever in pregnancy study: effects on fetal death of smoking and number of fever episodes in early pregnancy estimated using different link functions.

Link Function	Logit	Probit	Log	Identity
0 cigs/day	0 (ref)	0 (ref)	0 (ref)	0 (ref)
1–10 cigs/day	0.143 (0.256)	0.053 (0.096)	0.142 (0.254)	0.0014 0.003)
11+ cigs/day	0.396 (0.257)	0.150 (0.098)	0.392 (0.253)	0.0045 (0.003)
Intercept	−4.66 (0.11)	−2.35 (0.041)	−4.67 (0.11)	0.0094 (0.0010)
0 episodes	0 (ref)	0 (ref)	0 (ref)	0 (ref)
1 episode	0.056 (0.247)	0.0208 (0.092)	0.055 (0.244)	0.0006 (0.0026)
2 episodes	−0.620 (1.01)	−0.223 (0.350)	−0.615 (1.00)	−0.0046 (0.0056)
3+ episodes	−19.78 (35670)	−4.17 (4256)	−19.69 (34198)	−0.0101 (0.0010)
Intercept	−4.58 (0.10)	−2.32 (0.038)	−4.59 (0.10)	0.010 (0.0010)

For the number of fever episodes the interpretation of the regression coefficients are of course similar for the 1 versus 0 and 2 versus 0 comparisons. Note, however, the "strange" results for the 3+ versus 0 comparison for the logit, probit, and log links. Here, the regression coefficient is "$-\infty$" with a ridiculously large standard deviation. This is because there are no events in the 3+ category making both the odds ratio and the risk ratio 0. For the probit link the explanation is that "the value z_p for which the probability that a standard Normal variable, u is less than $p = 0$ is $-\infty$." However, as we see, the other comparisons between categories are not affected by this. This problem does not occur for the identity link because subtraction from 0 is not problematic (but analysis using this link may imply some numerical instability for other reasons).

We next study the quantitative covariate, age of the mother, which has an average of 29.6 years (SD=4.2 years). Smoking and fever episodes did not affect the risk of fetal death much, thus we fit models including only age. Models with a linear effect of age-25 gives the results shown in Table 7.4.3. It is seen that, for all link functions, the risk of fetal death increases significantly with mother's age. For the logit and log links, as above, results are very close: the odds ratio and the risk ratio are both around $\exp(0.72) \approx 2$ for every ten years of mother's age. According to the probit model, the mean of the latent variable y_i^* decreases by 0.269 for every ten years, and the model with the identity link suggests that the absolute risk of fetal death increases by 0.0059 for every ten years. This means that for mothers below 25 years of age, the predicted risk of fetal death according to the model with identity link (the "additive risk" model) is below the intercept 0.0074. Indeed, for mothers below 13 years of age, the predicted probability is negative. Because the youngest mother in the dataset was 16 years, the negative predicted risk is an unjustified extrapolation outside the range of covariate values observed. However, this finding does highlight that problems may occur when using the additive risk model.

Table 7.4.3. Fever in pregnancy study: effects on fetal death of mother's age estimated using different link functions.

Link Function	Logit	Probit	Log	Identity
Intercept	−4.967	−2.462	−4.974	0.0074
Age-25 (per 10 years)	0.726	0.269	0.718	0.0059
(SD)	(0.216)	(0.081)	(0.213)	(0.0018)

Digression. The cloglog link

Let us, finally, briefly comment on still another link function, the "complementary log–log" link, cloglog. It also has the nice property that predicted probabilities stay within the interval (0,1). This is given by

$$\mathrm{cloglog}(p) = \log(-\log(1-p)).$$

If we think of a latent "time to event" y_i^* then, as discussed above,

$$p = \mathrm{pr}(y_i = 1) = \mathrm{pr}(y_i^* \le c)$$

for some threshold c. If the latent variable follows a Cox regression model with hazard rate function $h_0(t)\exp(b_1 x_{i,1} + \cdots + b_{n_c} x_{i,n_c})$ then

$$\mathrm{pr}(y_i^* > c) = \exp\left(-H_0(t)\exp(b_1 x_{i,1} + \cdots + b_{n_c} x_{i,n_c})\right),$$

where $H_0(t)$ is the cumulative baseline hazard rate and, therefore,

$$\log(-\log(\mathrm{pr}(y_i^* > c))) = \log(H_0(c)) + b_1 x_{i,1} + \cdots + b_{n_c} x_{i,n_c}$$

showing that the cloglog link for the binary outcome variable y_i arises from a Cox proportional hazards model for the latent variable y_i^*. This motivates the use of this link function for certain applications and parameter estimates based on this model will have a log(hazard ratio) interpretation. ◇

Small for gestational age

To study multiple regression models using the alternative link functions, as mentioned above we turn to a more common outcome than fetal death, namely "small for gestational age," sga. Having a low birthweight is, generally, an unfavorable condition for the child, however, how low a birthweight should be to be considered too low will depend on the gestational age of the fetus, that is, the number of weeks elapsed from conception to birth. Sga is therefore defined as having a birthweight below a given percentile for given value of gestational age, for example, below the fifth percentile. To define sga we therefore divided the data according to gestational weeks, as follows: $\leq 31, 32, 33, \ldots, 40, \geq 41$, and identified the fifth percentile in the distribution of birthweights for each of the resulting 11 categories. The distribution of sga for given combinations of smoking and parity (number of previous births, 0 or 1+) is shown in Table 7.4.4. It is seen that the risk of sga increases with smoking and it is larger for first-time pregnancies (parity 0) than for those with previous births (parity 1+).

Table 7.4.4. Fever in pregnancy study: Distribution of small for gestational age (sga) by parity and smoking.

	\multicolumn{8}{c}{Cigarettes/Day}							
	0		1–10		11+		Total	
	Fraction	%	Fraction	%	Fraction	%	Fraction	%
Parity 0	223/3635	6.1	77/855	9.0	58/584	9.9	358/5074	7.1
Parity 1+	115/4637	02.5	42/830	5.1	59/726	8.1	216/6193	3.5
Total	338/8272	4.1	119/1685	7.1	117/1310	8.9	574/11267	5.1

We analyze models using all four link functions including these two covariates. Table 7.4.5 shows the results. It is seen that, for all four link functions, both parity and smoking affect the risk of sga quite significantly and in the expected directions based on the information in Table 7.4.4. However, when examining whether there is an interaction between the two covariates, the results differ. According to the logit, probit, and log-link models there is a significant interaction although this is not at all the case for the identity link.

This shows that *interaction is scale-dependent* (see also Section 5.2). In order to evaluate whether there is an interaction between smoking and parity, the choice of model, including a choice of link function, has to be addressed. Such a choice is based on a number of aspects, such as how well do the competing models fit judged from certain criteria and how easy are the interpretations of results from the models. For the present study, choosing the model on the basis of simplicity points to the additive risk model with the identity link because this is the model where no interaction seems to be needed. This is also the choice of link function for which the largest value of the likelihood function is achieved. However, the choice of link function is not at all easy and we would argue that model fit and convenient interpretation of parameters are the most important criteria for this choice.

Table 7.4.5. Fever in pregnancy study: effects on small for gestational age of parity and smoking estimated using different link functions.

Link Function	Logit	Probit	Log	Identity
Parity 1+ vs. 0	−0.730 (0.089)	−0.344 (0.041)	−0.683 (0.084)	−0.0357 (0.0041)
Smoking 1–10 vs. 0	0.434 (0.111)	0.253 (0.053)	0.499 (0.103)	0.0271 (0.064)
Smoking 11+ 3 vs. 0	0.836 (0.112)	0.407 (0.055)	0.768 (0.103)	0.0499 (0.0080)
LR test for	10.58	8.1	11.7	1.32
no interaction	0.005	0.017	0.003	0.52

Digression. "Biological interaction"

In the epidemiological literature, it has been argued that for risk models such as those discussed in the present section, interaction should be assessed on the risk difference scale because, for this scale, interaction can be interpreted "biologically" (Rothman and Greenland, 1998, Ch. 18). However, we do not find the arguments put forward in this literature sufficiently convincing to abandon studies of interaction for other scales. In fact, we believe that if presentation of a given effect measure is relevant then, more or less by definition, a study of how this effect measure varies between relevant subgroups will also be relevant. ⋄

7.4.2 Case-control studies

In previous examples dealing with binary data, the design has been *prospective* in the sense that individuals were selected for the study before the possible occurrence of the event of interest. This was the case in the fever in pregnancy Example 1.2 where pregnant women were ascertained and followed up for the events under study, fetal death or small for gestational age, and it was also the case in the surgery Example 1.4 where patients were recruited before operation and observed for the occurrence of postsurgery complications.

However, when the outcome is rare such a design may be costly if sufficiently many individuals are to be recruited and followed, perhaps for an extended follow-up period, before the event can be observed. In such a situation, an alternative to the prospective cohort design is a *case-control* design where typically, subjects are selected for study *retrospectively*, that is, after the possible occurrence of the event. Thus, *cases* are selected randomly among those with $y_i = 1$ and *controls* among those with $y_i = 0$. A difficulty is how to define the population from which cases and controls are selected. We do not go into detail here but refer to Clayton and Hills (1993, Ch. 16) for further discussion. However, we wish to emphasize that there are methodological advantages if both cases and controls can be selected from a well-defined "underlying cohort," leading to a *nested case-control study*. This underlying cohort could be an entire country or region if, for example, population and disease registries are available from which one may sample, for instance, all cases of a certain disease during a specific period and a random sample of disease-free individuals from the population as controls. When cases and controls are identified, covariate information must be obtained by interviews, registry data, or from other sources.

Inasmuch as researchers choose the numbers of cases and controls, one can, obviously, not estimate the absolute disease risk based on a simple relative frequency for the retrospectively ascertained cases and controls. In what follows, we explain when one, for a simple binary covariate x, may still estimate the odds ratio as a measure of association between the covariate and the binary (disease) outcome y (and, thereby, use logistic regression for analysis). The data may then be displayed in a two-by-two table just as in Table 3.1.8. See Table 7.4.6 where notation has been adapted to the current situation. The number of exposed (unexposed) cases is d_1 (d_0), and the number of exposed (unexposed) controls is c_1 (c_0).

Table 7.4.6. The basic two-by-two table for a case-control study with a single binary exposure, x.

Group	Controls $(y = 0)$	Cases $(y = 1)$
Unexposed $x = 0$	c_0	d_0
Exposed $x = 1$	c_1	d_1

Denote the probability that a diseased subject is sampled as a case by q_d and the probability that a disease-free subject is sampled as a control by q_c. The crucial assumption is that both of these sampling probabilities are *independent of exposure* x; that is, the exposure distribution among all diseased subjects in the population should be represented by the sampled cases and, similarly, the exposure distribution among all disease-free subjects in the population should be represented by the sampled controls. Our goal is to estimate the odds ratio

$$\text{OR} = \frac{\frac{p_1}{1-p_1}}{\frac{p_0}{1-p_0}},$$

where p_0 and p_1, as previously, are the disease risks given no exposure, $x = 0$, and given exposure, $x = 1$, respectively. Now, the *case-control ratio*, d_1/c_1 among exposed estimates $p_1 q_d/((1-p_1)q_c)$ and similarly, the case-control ratio among unexposed d_0/c_0 estimates $p_0 q_d/((1-p_0)q_c)$. In the ratio between these case-control ratios, the sampling probabilities q_c, q_d cancel

$$\frac{\frac{p_1 q_d}{(1-p_1)q_c}}{\frac{p_0 q_d}{(1-p_0)q_c}} = \text{OR},$$

showing that this ratio estimates OR.

This is illustrated graphically in Figure 7.4.1. Here, a population consisting of $N_0 = C_0 + D_0$ unexposed and $N_1 = C_1 + D_1$ exposed individuals is depicted. Here, one should think of both N_0 and N_1 as *large* numbers. After a certain follow-up period, $D_0 = p_0 N_0$ unexposed individuals develop the disease and $D_1 = p_1 N_1$ exposed individuals develop the disease (i.e., the split of N_0 into C_0 and D_0 is only realized after the follow-up period and similarly for N_1). The population value for the odds ratio is then OR $= (D_1/C_1)/(D_0/C_0)$. At the end of follow-up, $c_0 + c_1 = q_c(C_0 + C_1)$ controls are sampled and $d_0 + d_1 = q_d(D_0 + D_1)$ cases are sampled, and their values of exposure, that is, the splits into c_0, c_1 and d_0, d_1, are ascertained. If, as assumed, cases and controls are sampled independently of exposure, then $c_j \approx q_c C_j = q_c(1 - p_j)N_j, j = 0, 1$ and $d_j \approx q_d D_j = q_d p_j N_j$, and the "observed odds ratio" estimates OR.

Letting $b = \log(\text{OR})$ be the log(odds ratio) and $a = \log(p_0/(1 - p_0))$ the log(odds) among unexposed, the logistic regression model in the population is

$$\ell_i = a + b x_i,$$

where ℓ_i is the log(odds), and x_i the exposure for individual i. The argument shows that the log(odds) of being a case among those sampled in the case-control study $\widetilde{\ell}_i$ is

$$\widetilde{\ell}_i = \widetilde{a} + b x_i, \tag{7.4.5}$$

where the intercept is

$$\widetilde{a} = a + \log\left(\frac{q_d}{q_c}\right).$$

It follows that, under the assumption that sampling probabilities for both cases and controls do not depend on exposure, logistic regression of the case-control data allows consistent estimation of the log(odds ratio), b for exposure, but not of the intercept, a (and thereby not of the absolute risks, p_0, p_1). The argument may be extended to cover a multiple logistic regression model

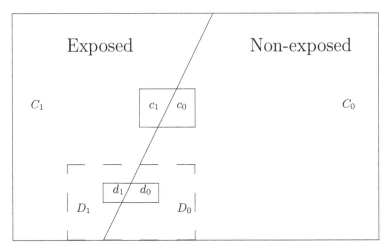

Fig. 7.4.1. Illustration of case-control sampling from a population with $C_0 + D_0$ unexposed and $C_1 + D_1$ exposed individuals.

$$\ell_i = a + b_1 x_{i,1} + \cdots + b_{n_c} x_{i,n_c},$$

where $b_1, \ldots, b_{n_c}$, but not a may be estimated consistently based on case-control data, provided that the sampling probabilities q_d, q_c for cases and controls are independent of all covariates. Note that in *matched* studies (defined below) the sampling probability for controls will depend on covariates because, in such studies, controls are selected in such a way that, for example their age distribution is the same as for cases.

If q_c and q_d are known (as may be the situation in a nested case-control study, as discussed above) then also the intercept and the absolute risks may be estimated. As a consequence, effect measures other than the odds ratio (i.e., risk ratio, risk difference) may be estimated. But for unknown sampling probabilities it is only the odds ratios that are estimable.

We use the fever in pregnancy study for illustration and create a case-control study nested in the Danish National Birth Cohort Study (see Section 1.1.1 for details). The underlying cohort here consists of women recruited to the study before April 1999. We select as cases all sga cases, that is, those with a birthweight below the fifth percentile for given gestational week, and we sample controls among those without sga. More specifically, we randomly select 15% of those without sga as controls, leading to 574 cases and 1562 controls, that is, approximately three controls per case. In general, such choices will be based on a sample size calculation as described in Section 6.3. We fit the model including smoking and parity as covariates to these case-control sampled data. Table 7.4.7 shows the case-control ratios according to these two covariates and Table 7.4.8 shows the results from fitting a model with interaction between smoking and parity to both the case-control sample and to the entire dataset.

Table 7.4.7. Fever in pregnancy study: distribution of sga cases and controls by parity and smoking: cases/controls.

	No Smokers	1–10 Cigarettes/Day	11+ Cigarettes/Day	Total
Parity 0	223/498	77/113	58/86	358/697
Parity 1+	115/668	42/114	59/83	216/865
Total	338/1166	119/227	117/169	574/1562

Table 7.4.8. Fever in pregnancy study: logistic regression models for case-control sample and for the entire dataset.

Effect	Case-Control Sample		Full Dataset	
Parity 0 vs 1+, No Smokers	0.956	(0.129)	0.944	(0.117)
Smoking 1–10 vs. 0, Parity 0	0.420	(0.168)	0.415	(0.138)
Smoking 1–10 vs. 0, Parity 1+	0.761	(0.207)	0.740	(0.184)
Smoking 11+ vs. 0, Parity 0	0.410	(0.188)	0.523	(0.155)
Smoking 11+ vs. 0, Parity 1+	1.418	(0.198)	1.247	(0.165)
Intercept	−1.76	(0.10)	−3.67	(0.094)

From Table 7.4.8 we first notice the large similarity between covariate effects estimated from the case-control sample and from the full dataset, however, with a somewhat larger SD for the case-control study. This is to be expected because the case-control data set has 574 cases and 1562 controls whereas the full dataset has 11,267 subjects out of whom 574 experienced the sga event. That is, the full dataset has the same number of cases and more noncases, however, these extra noncases do not increase precision much. The test for no interaction is highly significant, also for the case-control study: the LR test statistic is 13.85 with 2 df ($P = 0.001$). In this example, the sampling fractions are known: $q_d = 100\%$ of the diseased are sampled as cases and $q_c = 1562/(11,267 - 574) = 14.6\%$ of the disease-free as controls. This fits nicely with the two intercepts (Table 7.4.8), inasmuch as

$$\widehat{\widetilde{a}} - \widehat{a} = -1.76 + 3.67 = 1.91 \approx \log \frac{q_d}{q_c} = \log\left(\frac{1}{0.146}\right).$$

Digression. Exposure odds ratio; sample size determination

In the two by two table, Table 7.4.6, the numbers of cases $(d_0 + d_1)$ and controls $(c_0 + c_1)$ are fixed by design and it is the *exposure distribution* that varies randomly. This means that what can immediately be estimated from the case-control data is the *exposure odds ratio*

$$\frac{\mathrm{pr}(x = 1 \mid d = 1)/\mathrm{pr}(x = 0 \mid d = 1)}{\mathrm{pr}(x = 1 \mid d = 0)/\mathrm{pr}(x = 0 \mid d = 0)}$$

for which the estimate is simply $(d_1/c_1)/(d_0/c_0)$. The exposure odds ratio is not a quantity of primary interest and the crucial (and clever) feature of the case-control design is its ability to estimate the *disease odds ratio*

$$\frac{\mathrm{pr}(d = 1 \mid x = 1)/\mathrm{pr}(d = 0 \mid x = 1)}{\mathrm{pr}(d = 1 \mid x = 0)/\mathrm{pr}(d = 0 \mid x = 0)} = \frac{p_1/(1 - p_1)}{p_0/(1 - p_0)},$$

the parameter of primary interest. In fact, this will equal the exposure odds ratio under the crucial assumption that selection probabilities for cases and controls (q_d and q_c) are independent of exposure. Furthermore, case-control studies are often conducted when the disease is rare, in which case the disease odds ratio provides an excellent approximation to the easier interpretable risk ratio p_1/p_0.

However, the exposure odds ratio may be useful for planning purposes where sample size determination may be based on a prespecified value of the fraction of exposed individuals in the disease-free population and on the minimum relevant odds ratio. Suppose, for example, that a case-control study with equal numbers of cases and controls is to be planned and suppose that the exposure is present in 10% of the disease-free population (i.e. the odds of exposure is 0.1/0.9). If we want the study to be large enough to detect an odds ratio of 1.5 with 80% power, then the relevant exposure fraction among cases to consider is given by the odds

$$1.5 \cdot \frac{0.1}{0.9} = 0.167;$$

that is, the fraction $0.167/(1 + 0.167) = 0.143$. We can then use (6.3.5) with $f = 1$ (same numbers of cases and controls), $s^2 = \bar{p}(1 - \bar{p})$ (with $\bar{p} = (0.1 + 0.143)/2 = 0.1215$) and $b_0 = 0.143 - 0.1 = 0.033$ to get $n = 3074$, that is, 1537 cases and 1537 controls. ◇

Matched case-control studies

In some case-control studies, controls are not sampled randomly among all disease-free individuals but rather, to adjust for confounding, an equal distribution of, for example, age and gender, is ensured by matching controls to cases. This is known as *frequency matching*. Alternatively, to each case, one or more controls can be *individually matched* on characteristics such as family membership or neighborhood. Frequency matched case-control studies can be analyzed using standard logistic regression as indicated above. However, to ensure consistent estimates for the exposure effect, the matching variables *must* be included in the model even though matching on, for example, age prevents the age effect from being estimated (see, e.g., Clayton and Hills, 1993, Ch. 18). This is because the sampling frequencies depend on age in this situation. However, interactions between match variables and other covariates (most important exposure) *are* estimable.

If controls are matched individually to each case then we are in the same situation as described in Section 5.4 and in the simplest case of individual one-to-one matching, the ith pair consists of one case, $y_{i,1} = 1$ and one control $y_{i,2} = 0$. For a binary exposure x the relevant model to consider is (5.4.2):

$$\text{logit}(\text{pr}(y_{i,j} = 1)) = a_i + b_2 x_{i,j},$$

where the pair-specific intercept a_i can be interpreted as the joint effect of all match variables. Data can be summarized in a table such as Table 5.4.1; see Table 7.4.9.

Table 7.4.9. Data from $n = n_{0,0} + n_{1,0} + n_{0,1} + n_{1,1}$ pairs in an individually one-to-one matched case-control study with a single binary exposure, x.

	Cases	
Controls	$x = 0$	$x = 1$
$x = 0$	$n_{0,0}$	$n_{1,0}$
$x = 1$	$n_{0,1}$	$n_{1,1}$

Only the $n_{0,1} + n_{1,0}$ case-control pairs that are *discordant on exposure* contribute to the conditional likelihood and inference proceeds as described in Section 5.4 . Adjustment for confounders $x_3, x_4, \ldots$ that are not constant within pairs can be performed using conditional logistic regression by adding the relevant terms to the linear predictor leading to

$$\text{logit}(\text{pr}(y_{i,j} = 1)) = a_i + b_2 x_{i,j} + b_3 x_{3,i,j} + b_4 x_{4,i,j} \cdots \qquad (7.4.6)$$

Also, the common situation with "one-to-many" matching (one case and several matched controls) and the less common situation with "many-to-many" matching (several cases and several matched controls) can be handled using conditional logistic regression.

Model (7.4.6), analyzed using conditional logistic regression, is the appropriate technique to apply in case-control studies matched on truly individual characteristics. Examples of such characteristics could be family membership or neighborhood, that is, variables that are difficult to adjust for in a regression model (because of the large numbers of categories). The same situation arises in a nested case-control study where controls are sampled from the cohort at the specific times at which cases fail, that is, individually matched on time. However, when controls are matched to cases on "less individual" characteristics such as age and gender, we find the use of conditional logistic regression unjustified, for a number of reasons. First, efficiency may be lost because only discordant pairs provide information and inasmuch as incomplete pairs due to missing values provide no information at all. Second, standard "unconditional" logistic regression for frequency-matched case-control studies, that is, simply including the match variables such as age and gender as covariates can be used as indicated above.

7.5 Survival time outcome

When, in previous chapters, we have discussed survival analysis, focus has been on the Cox proportional hazards model

$$l_i(t) = \log(h_0(t)) + b_1 x_{i,1} + b_2 x_{i,2} + \cdots + b_{n_c} x_{i,n_c} = \mathrm{LP}_i(t), \qquad (7.5.1)$$

where the log(hazard rate) $l_i(t)$ was given by the linear predictor $\mathrm{LP}_i(t)$, that is, the link function was the cloglog. In Equation (7.5.1), the baseline hazard, $h_0(t)$ is left completely unspecified and the effect b_j of the jth covariate is the log(hazard ratio) associated with a one-unit increase for $x_{i,j}$.

In the present section we first (Section 7.5.1) look at alternative proportional hazards models where, in contrast to (7.5.1), the baseline hazard is specified as a particular function of time t. One such example is a power function leading to the *Weibull* distribution for the survival time y. Another important special case (discussed in Section 7.5.1) is the so-called *Poisson regression model* where $h_0(t)$ is a piecewise constant function of t. In Section 7.5.2 focus is on *additive* hazard models where it is the hazard rate itself that is written as the linear predictor. In these models, the interpretation of the regression coefficients b_j appearing in $\mathrm{LP}_i(t)$ is that of hazard differences, rather than $\exp(b_j)$ being hazard ratios. Finally, in Section 7.5.3, we study the *accelerated failure time model*. This provides a model for the expected survival time rather than specifying the hazard rate. However, because the survival time y_i is positive, it is the mean of the log survival time $\mathrm{E}(\log(y_i))$ that is written as the linear predictor. We return to the interpretation of the resulting regression coefficients in Section 7.5.3.

The Cox model (7.5.1) has gained a very dominating role in survival analysis but, as we show, the models discussed in the present section all have various desirable features, not all shared by (7.5.1).

7.5.1 Multiplicative hazard models

In the Cox model, the shape of the baseline hazard $h_0(t)$ is not specified and this semiparametric feature of the model has the advantage that covariate effects (hazard ratios, $\exp(b_j)$) may be estimated in the same way no matter the functional form of the survival time distribution, as long as the assumption of proportional hazards is reasonable. However, for purposes of, for example, prediction and simulation, the nonparametric $h_0(t)$ is a drawback. Also, if a given parametric shape of the baseline hazard fits the data well, then, using this information for inference may provide estimates of the hazard ratios associated with the explanatory variables with (slightly) smaller standard deviations. In the present section we briefly study a number of parametric proportional hazards models.

The simplest such model is one where the baseline hazard is constant, for example, $\log(h_0(t)) = a$. The resulting survival distribution is known as the *Exponential* distribution and is the simplest of all possible models for survival data. Being a very simple model, the Exponential model is also quite restrictive and two important extensions are considered in the following. One is the *Weibull* distribution given by

$$\log(h_0(t)) = a + (c - 1)\log(t), \tag{7.5.2}$$

or equivalently, the baseline hazard is a power function of time, $h_0(t) = \exp(a)t^{c-1}$. In (7.5.2) the Exponential model is the special case where the shape parameter c is equal to 1 making the dependence on t disappear. For $c > 1$ the hazard rate increases with time whereas, for $c < 1$ it decreases. Another important extension of the simple Exponential model is the piecewise Exponential model also known as the *Poisson* regression model (for reasons explained in a digression below) . Here it is assumed that there exist a number of time intervals $[t_{j-1}, t_j), j = 1, 2, \ldots, k$, given by interval endpoints $0 = t_0 < t_1 < \ldots < t_k = \infty$, such that the baseline hazard rate is constant within each interval:

$$\log(h_0(t)) = a_j \quad \text{when} \quad t_{j-1} \leq t < t_j.$$

The Exponential model is the special case corresponding to only $k = 1$ time interval (from $t_0 = 0$ to $t_1 = \infty$).

We illustrate these parametric proportional hazards models using the malignant melanoma data, Example 1.10. For comparison we first study a standard Cox model (as discussed in earlier chapters) for these data. Table 7.5.1 shows parameter estimates, log(hazard ratios) $\widehat{b}$, with corresponding SD in a model including the four covariates; gender (male= 1, female= 0), tumor thickness (mm), ulceration (absent= 0, present= 1), and age (per 10 years). The quantitative covariates were centered by subtracting 3 mm from tumor thickness and 50 years from age to obtain an intercept (baseline hazard) with a sensible interpretation (women without ulceration with age 50 and thickness 3). Proportional hazards and linearity of the two quantitative covariates were examined as exemplified in earlier chapters and found not to be clearly violated. It is seen that males have an insignificantly higher hazard rate than females when adjusting for the other covariates and thickness, ulceration, and age are highly significant with effects in the expected directions; that is, the hazard rate increases with both age and tumor thickness and patients with ulceration have a higher hazard rate than those without.

Table 7.5.1. Results from fitting a Cox regression model to the malignant melanoma survival data.

Covariate	$\hat{b}$	SD	$(\hat{b}/\text{SD})^2$	P
Gender	0.413	0.240	2.96	0.09
Tumor thickness	0.0994	0.0345	8.32	0.004
Ulceration	0.952	0.268	12.62	0.0004
Age	0.218	0.0775	7.94	0.005

Weibull models

To evaluate whether a Weibull model with log(hazard rate)

$$l_i(t) = a + (c-1)\log(t) + b_1 x_{i,1} + b_2 x_{i,2} + \cdots + b_{n_c} x_{i,n_c} \qquad (7.5.3)$$

fits the melanoma data we consider the Cox model just fitted and its estimated cumulative baseline hazard. If $h_0(t) = \exp(a)t^{c-1}$, the cumulative baseline hazard is

$$H_0(t) = \int_0^t h_0(s)ds = \frac{\exp(a)}{c}t^c$$

and it follows that the log(cumulative hazard), $\log(H_0(t))$ is linear in $\log(t)$ (Appendix B). To evaluate the Weibull model, Figure 7.5.1 shows a plot of $\log(\widehat{H}_0(t))$ against $\log(t)$ (with 95% confidence limits). It is seen that the curve is roughly linear, thereby not contradicting the Weibull model. In fact, an Exponential distribution seems to provide a good fit to these data because the slope c is close to 1. Table 7.5.2 shows the results from fitting both Weibull and Exponential regression models including the same four explanatory variables as above. It is seen that both estimates and standard deviations are close to what we saw in Table 7.5.1. The LR test for the Exponential model, that is, the hypothesis $H_0 : c = 1$, is 1.10 ($P = 0.29$).

Table 7.5.2. Results from fitting Weibull and Exponential regression models to the malignant melanoma survival data.

Covariate	Weibull $\hat{b}$	SD	Exponential $\hat{b}$	SD
Gender	0.397	0.240	0.395	0.240
Tumor thickness	0.0967	0.0346	0.0932	0.0344
Ulceration	0.969	0.269	0.953	0.269
Age	0.231	0.0758	0.216	0.0741
Intercept ($\hat{a}$)	−4.724	0.463	−4.963	0.460
Shape parameter ($\hat{c}$)	1.119	0.118	1	(fixed)

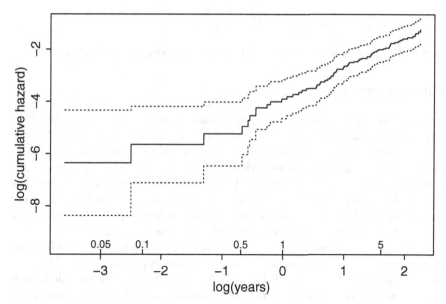

Fig. 7.5.1. Melanoma data: log(cumulative baseline hazard) plotted against log(time). The upper scale for the horizontal axis is time in years.

For a parametric model such as (7.5.3) it is simple to predict the survival probability, $S(t)$ for all values of t and for given covariates as this is simply given by

$$S(t) = \exp(-H_0(t)\exp(b_1 x_1 + b_2 x_2 + \cdots + b_{n_c} x_{n_c}))$$
$$= \exp(-\frac{\exp(a)}{c} t^c \exp(b_1 x_1 + b_2 x_2 + \cdots + b_{n_c} x_{n_c})).$$

In fact, the expected failure time may also be estimated from estimates of $a, b_1, \ldots, b_{n_c}, c$. For the Exponential model ($c = 1$) this is particularly simple:

$$\mathrm{E}(y_i) = \frac{1}{\exp(a + b_1 x_1 + b_2 x_2 + \cdots + b_{n_c} x_{n_c})}.$$

Also for the general Weibull distribution ($c \neq 1$) this may be done. This is because the parametric model also predicts the behavior of the hazard rate for "large" values of t, even beyond the range of the available data. This may be considered an advantage of the parametric models because such predictions are not possible to perform based on a Cox regression model. However, we recommend not to put too much emphasis on model predictions beyond the range of the observed data. Often, it is more relevant to consider median survival time than mean survival time inasmuch as the median is not sensitive to the right tail of the distribution. For the Exponential model with constant hazard rate h, the median survival time is simply

$$M = \frac{\log(2)}{h},$$

an equation which was useful for sample size determination, Section 6.3.

Poisson regression

Poisson regression relies on a choice of timeintervals in which the baseline hazard rate is assumed to be constant. That is, compared to the Cox model, the baseline hazard is approximated by a piecewise constant function. The choice of intervals may not always be obvious and results may, to some extent, vary according to this choice. In general, however, results from Poisson regression tend to be rather robust to "sensible" choices of intervals and, at the same time, they tend to be similar to results from analysis of a Cox regression model. We now illustrate these points using the melanoma data.

Two choices of intervals are studied: one with cutpoints at 2.5 and 5 years, and one with a single cutpoint at 4 years; both choices provide reasonable numbers of deaths in all intervals. Table 7.5.3 shows the results. It is seen that, once again, these are very similar to those from the Cox (and Weibull/Exponential) model. For both choices of cutpoints, the LR test for reducing to the simple Exponential model is clearly insignificant (0.36, 2 d.f., $P = 0.83$ and 0.55, 1 d.f., $P = 0.46$, respectively).

Table 7.5.3. Results from fitting piecewise Exponential (Poisson) regression models to the malignant melanoma survival data. Two choices of time intervals are studied: 3 intervals with cutpoints at 2.5 and 5 years, and 2 intervals with cutpoint at 4 years.

	3 intervals		2 intervals	
Covariate	$\hat{b}$	SD	$\hat{b}$	SD
Gender	0.396	0.240	0.395	0.240
Tumor thickness	0.0964	0.0346	0.0950	0.0346
Ulceration	0.960	0.269	0.962	0.269
Age	0.222	0.0763	0.227	0.0757
Intercept $(\hat{a}_1)$	−5.093	0.523	−5.107	0.503
Intercept $(\hat{a}_2)$	−4.936	0.506	−4.919	0.464
Intercept $(\hat{a}_3)$	−4.963	0.476		

Thus, for the melanoma data the choice of intervals has little influence on results. However, in this example the hazard is nearly constant, and in cases with a less regular hazard rate, sensitivity to the choice of intervals may be greater. General advice is to choose few (and thereby fairly wide) intervals in areas where the hazard rate is expected to vary slowly and more (and narrower) intervals where the hazard rate varies more rapidly.

Due to the potential dependence on the arbitrary choice of cutpoints one may well ask why one should consider using Poisson regression instead of the Cox model where choice of intervals is not an issue. Poisson regression has a great advantage (of technical character) over the Cox model in the case where all covariates are categorical. Even though (as we show in a moment) this advantage is most apparent for large datasets, it is illustrated using the melanoma data. For the purpose of illustration, we consider a Poisson model for these data with the two covariates tumor thickness, categorized into the intervals $[0, 2mm)$, $[2mm, 5mm)$ and from 5 mm and up, and ulceration. Time is categorized as in the example above, with cutpoints at 2.5 and 5 years. Table 7.5.4 shows the number of deaths and the number of person-years at risk according to the two categorical covariates and time. The advantage is that the information in these two tables is sufficient to estimate the parameters in the Poisson model. This means that, instead of having to work with the entire melanoma dataset and its $n = 205$ records, it is possible first to preprocess the data by computing the tables of failure counts and person-years, here two $3 \times 3 \times 2$ tables.

Table 7.5.4. Failure counts/person-years at risk for the malignant melanoma survival data according to tumor thickness, ulceration, and three time intervals.

Time < 2.5 years	Tumor thickness		
Ulceration	0–2 mm	2–5 mm	5+ mm
Absent	1/53.47	11/96.12	12/47.12
Present	3/212.30	3/50.00	0/17.50

Time 2.5–5 years	Tumor thickness		
Ulceration	0–2 mm	2–5 mm	5+ mm
Absent	4/47.13	9/64.54	4/26.91
Present	4/193.60	2/42.88	1/15.35

Time ≥ 5 years	Tumor thickness		
Ulceration	0–2 mm	2–5 mm	5+ mm
Absent	1/44.88	6/38.87	0/28.88
Present	7/151.97	2/59.44	1/17.32

For the melanoma data, this is not a great data reduction. However, in large cohort studies the entire dataset may contain hundreds of thousands of records and the sufficient tables (like those illustrated in Table 7.5.4) be considerably smaller. This will provide important savings of computing time compared to using the Cox model when analyzing survival data from large cohorts. Another nice feature of the Poisson regression model is that it works directly with the "epidemiological rate," that is, the ratio between cases and person-years at risk for a group of subjects. These are exactly the numbers presented in Table 7.5.4 which thus represent thickness-, ulceration-, and time-specific mortality rates for the melanoma patients. The multiplicative Poisson model describes how such rates vary according to factors depending on the explanatory variables.

Digression. The name "Poisson" regression

Readers may wonder why the model with a piecewise constant baseline hazard rate is called Poisson regression inasmuch as we nowhere mentioned the Poisson distribution (Section 2.1.3). The reason for the name is that the likelihood function (Section 2.3.4) derived from the piecewise Exponential model is proportional to the likelihood one would obtain if the failure counts (as those in Table 7.5.4) were formally treated as independent and Poisson distributed with a mean that is the product of the person-years (from that same table) and the hazard rate. The intuition is as follows. In each cell (j_1, j_2, j_3) in the table, the log(rate) is written as a sum of terms

$$\log \left(\frac{\text{cases}_{(j_1,j_2,j_3)}}{\text{pyrs}_{(j_1,j_2,j_3)}} \right) \approx a + b_{1,j_1} I(\text{time-interval} = j_1)$$
$$+ b_{2,j_2} I(\text{thickness category} = j_2) + b_{3,j_3} I(\text{ulceration} = j_3).$$

This means that $\text{cases}_{(j_1,j_2,j_3)}$ are linked to the linear predictor and to $\log(\text{pyrs}_{(j_1,j_2,j_3)})$ via the logarithmic function. It has the pleasant consequence that the model may be analyzed using software for the Poisson distribution including log(person-years) as an "offset" (e.g., McCullagh and Nelder, 1989, Ch. 6). In Section 7.2, we studied Poisson regression for truly Poisson distributed count data. ◇

7.5.2 Additive hazard models

The class of multiplicative hazard models discussed in the previous section is the natural choice for a hazard regression model because, as already noted in Section 1.3, taking the exponential function of the linear predictor ensures positivity. However, as we already saw for binary data in Section 7.4.1, other link functions may be considered to obtain regression parameters with alternative interpretations. One of the models studied for binary data in Section 7.4 was the additive risk model where the link is "the identity function," that is, $\text{pr}(y_i = 1) = \text{LP}_i$. Regression parameters in that model are risk differences.

In a similar vein, we now briefly look at additive hazard models and thereby obtain parameters that are hazard rate differences. A simple such model, directly inspired by the Cox model, is

$$h_i(t) = h_0(t) + b_1 x_{i,1} + \cdots + b_{n_c} x_{i,n_c} = \text{LP}_i(t), \qquad (7.5.4)$$

where the hazard rate $h_i(t)$ for individual i is written directly as the linear predictor. In (7.5.4), the regression coefficient b_j associated with the jth covariate $x_{i,j}$ is the difference between the hazard rates for two subjects differing one unit for their values for covariate j and having identical values for all other covariates in the model. This means that if only a single binary covariate x_i is included in (7.5.4) then the hazard rate would be equal to the baseline hazard $h_0(t)$ if $x_i = 0$, and equal to $h_0(t) + b$ when $x_i = 1$. It is seen that the "standard" proportional hazards assumption from the Cox model is replaced by a "time-constant hazard difference" assumption.

It is possible to estimate the parameters in (7.5.4) using the likelihood principle. However, one may quite simply handle a quite flexible extension of that model, namely *Aalen's nonparametric additive hazard model* given by

$$h_i(t) = h_0(t) + b_1(t)x_{i,1} + \cdots + b_{n_c}(t)x_{i,n_c}. \qquad (7.5.5)$$

In (7.5.5) the regression parameters, $b_1(t), \ldots, b_{n_c}(t)$ are unspecified functions of time t and one may estimate the cumulative regression functions

$$B_j(t) = \int_0^t b_j(s)ds, j = 1, \ldots, n_c.$$

These are then typically plotted against time to see how the effect of each covariate varies over time. The steepness of the estimate $\widehat{B}_j(t)$ around time point t indicates the influence of the corresponding covariate on the hazard rate at that timepoint. If $\widehat{B}_j(t)$ is roughly linear then this signals that the effect is time-constant and, therefore, the regression function $b_j(t)$ may be replaced by a constant b_j as in (7.5.4). In fact, inference in (7.5.5) may result in a model "intermediate between (7.5.4) and (7.5.5)" where some, but not necessarily all, regression functions are replaced by constants. This will typically result in reduced standard deviations for the parameter estimates.

For the malignant melanoma survival data, Example 1.10, Table 7.5.5 shows results from fitting a model of the form (7.5.4) including the same four covariates as in the previous section: gender, tumor thickness, ulceration, and age. The direction of the effects are, obviously, the same as seen for the multiplicative models in the previous section. The interpretation, however, is different. Thus, for ulceration the coefficient $\widehat{b} = 0.0592$ tells us that if we observe a group of patients with ulceration for, say, a total of 100 years then we would expect to see $100\widehat{b} = 5.9$ more deaths compared to observing a group of patients without ulceration for 100 years (if other covariates do not differ between the two groups). This interpretation in absolute numbers of failures is useful from, for example, public health or health economics perspectives (cf. the discussion in Section 7.4).

Figure 7.5.2 shows the cumulative baseline hazard from model (7.5.4) (with 95% confidence limits). It is seen that, in accordance with the analyses of multiplicative hazard models, the baseline hazard seems to be roughly constant (the cumulative baseline hazard is close to linear as we also noted in connection with Figure 7.5.1).

We further fitted the nonparametric Aalen model (7.5.5). The estimated cumulative baseline hazard and the cumulative regression coefficients are

Table 7.5.5. Results from fitting an additive hazard regression model to the malignant melanoma survival data.

Covariate	$\widehat{b}$	SD	$(\widehat{b}/\text{SD})^2$	P
Gender	0.0241	0.0162	2.22	0.14
Tumor thickness	0.00954	0.00436	4.80	0.03
Ulceration	0.0592	0.0173	9.42	0.002
Age	0.0127	0.00502	6.36	0.01

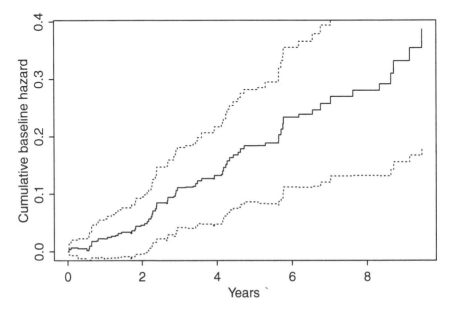

Fig. 7.5.2. Melanoma data: cumulative baseline hazard from additive model.

shown in Figures 7.5.3 and 7.5.4, respectively (with 95% confidence limits). The cumulative baseline hazard is close to that from model (7.5.4) (see Figure 7.5.2), and the cumulative regression coefficients seem to indicate that, at least for gender, age, and ulceration, the effects are roughly time-constant on the additive hazard scale (close to linear curves). For tumor thickness, the effect (the slope of the cumulative curve) tends to decrease after more than five years of follow-up time. These tendencies are confirmed by formal tests for constant effects; see Table 7.5.6. As a result, one may consider fitting a model with time-constant effects of gender, ulceration, and age and a time-varying effect of tumor thickness.

Let us add a few comments to Aalen's model. The model attempts to extract more information from the data in the sense that, instead of providing constant regression coefficients, the model gives functions to describe the covariate effects. This results, as we can see in Figure 7.5.4, in very wide confidence limits. The way to interpret the estimated functions is by thinking of smoothed versions of the curves in that figure. Also, in Figure 7.5.3 it is seen that the rough estimate is not always increasing in time which makes the interpretation as a cumulative hazard difficult. Therefore, one should again think of adding a smooth curve.

Table 7.5.6. Results from fitting Aalen's additive hazard regression model to the malignant melanoma survival data.

Covariate	P: No Effect	Time-Constant Effect
Gender	0.19	0.58
Tumor thickness	0.008	0.03
Ulceration	0.006	0.83
Age	0.05	0.33

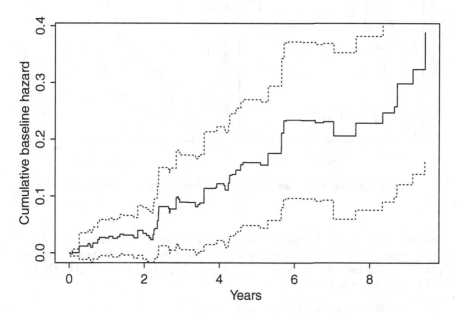

Fig. 7.5.3. Melanoma data: cumulative baseline hazard from Aalen's additive model.

Digression. Additive Poisson models

The "multiplicative Poisson model" studied in Section 7.5.1 is the most often used model with a piecewise constant hazard rate. However, *additive* Poisson models may also be studied. Because this is most often done in situations with categorical

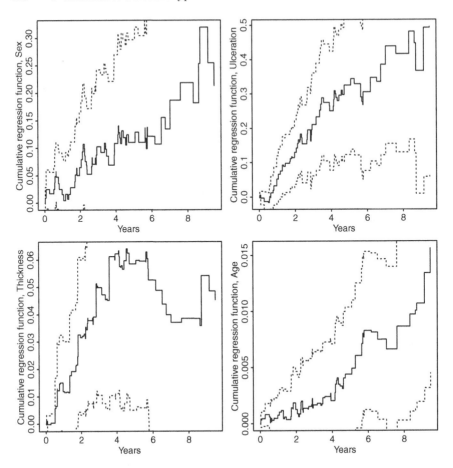

Fig. 7.5.4. Melanoma data: cumulative regression functions from Aalen's additive model.

covariates we exemplify additive Poisson regression using the tabulated melanoma data and the two categorical covariates ulceration and (categorized) tumor thickness, Table 7.5.4. The intuition is, as follows. In each cell (j_1, j_2, j_3) in the table, the rate is written as a sum of terms

$$\frac{\text{cases}_{(j_1,j_2,j_3)}}{\text{pyrs}_{(j_1,j_2,j_3)}} \approx a + b_{1,j_1} I(\text{time-interval} = j_1)$$
$$+ b_{2,j_2} I(\text{thickness category} = j_2) + b_{3,j_3} I(\text{ulceration} = j_3).$$

The model can then be fitted treating $\text{cases}_{(j_1,j_2,j_3)}$ as independent Poisson variates with mean given by the linear predictor

$$\text{pyrs}_{(j_1,j_2,j_3)}(a + b_{1,j_1} I(\text{time-interval} = j_1)$$
$$+ b_{2,j_2} I(\text{thickness category} = j_2) + b_{3,j_3} I(\text{ulceration} = j_3)).$$

◇

In conclusion, additive hazard models with time-constant effects have regression coefficients with quite simple interpretations. Furthermore, Aalen's nonparametric model (7.5.5) provides a flexible extension of the simple additive hazard model (7.5.4) by means of which one can get an idea (on the additive hazard scale) of how covariate effects may change over time. However, the curves tend to be rather variable and, due to a hazard rate being nonnegative, the identity link function is not the most "natural" one to use, inasmuch as predictions from an additive hazard model may become meaninglessly negative. More details on additive hazard model are provided by Martinussen and Scheike (2006, Ch. 5).

7.5.3 Accelerated failure time models

Formally, survival data are nothing but nonnegative quantitative outcomes but, as discussed in previous chapters, the inevitable presence of censored observations has the consequence that special methods are needed for survival analysis. This has also led to using special models for survival data. However, in principle, one could also build on ideas for quantitative outcome variables and study a linear model

$$E(\log(y_i)) = a + b_1 x_{i,1} + \cdots + b_{n_c} x_{i,n_c} \qquad (7.5.6)$$

for the mean of the logarithm of the survival time y_i.

If the survival function for a subject with all covariates equal to 0 is $S_0(t)$ then it can be shown that, according to model (7.5.6), the survival function for a subject with covariates $x_{i,1}, \ldots, x_{i,n_c}$ is given by

$$S_i(t) = S_0(t \exp(-b_1 x_{i,1} - \cdots - b_{n_c} x_{i,n_c})).$$

If (7.5.6), therefore, includes only a single binary covariate x, then subjects with $x = 1$ have the survival function $S_0(t \exp(-b))$; that is, time is *accelerated* by a factor $\exp(-b)$ compared to the reference group ($x = 0$). Hence the name, the *accelerated failure time model*. It has been argued (e.g., Kalbfleisch and Prentice, 2002, Ch. 7) that this interpretation of the regression coefficients in (7.5.6) is simpler than that of the hazard ratios obtained from the Cox proportional hazards model and, furthermore, model (7.5.6) may be used in cases where the proportional hazards assumption of the Cox model is not reasonably fulfilled. It should be realized, however, that in the accelerated failure time model this assumption is replaced by another model assumption, namely linearity on the mean log(survival time) scale.

Even though (7.5.6) is the well-known multiple linear regression model for $\log(y_i)$, estimation of the parameters $a, b_1, \ldots, b_{n_c}$ cannot be performed using the ordinary least squares method (e.g., Section 4.1.1) due to the presence of censored observations. The model is specified as having the mean (7.5.6) equal to the linear predicto LP_i and a specified "error" distribution around that mean. This complete model specification allows parameters to be estimated using the likelihood principle as in Section 7.3. Frequent choices for the error distribution are

- The *Normal* distribution
- The *Logistic* distribution (briefly mentioned in Section 7.4)
- The *Extreme Value* distribution (leading to a Weibull distribution for y_i)

We illustrate accelerated failure time models for the malignant melanoma survival data, Example 1.10. Table 7.5.7 shows parameter estimates and associated SD from models with Normal and Extreme Value error distributions including the same four covariates as in the previous two sections: gender, ulceration, tumor thickness, and age. It is seen that the results using the two different error distributions are numerically similar and qualitatively they are quite similar: effects are in the same directions and of similar significance. It is seen that, according to the interpretation explained above, the estimated acceleration factor for ulceration is $\exp(1.001) = 2.7$ according to the Normal model and $\exp(0.866) = 2.4$ according to the Extreme Value model.

Table 7.5.7. Results from fitting accelerated failure time regression models to the malignant melanoma survival data.

Error Distribution	Normal		Extreme Value		Buckley–James	
Covariate	$\widehat{b}$	SD	$\widehat{b}$	SD	$\widehat{b}$	SD
Gender	−0.522	0.262	−0.355	0.218	−0.504	0.269
Tumor thickness	−0.103	0.0438	−0.0864	0.0314	−0.0947	0.0407
Ulceration	−1.001	0.285	−0.866	0.252	−0.911	0.299
Age	−0.194	0.0786	−0.206	0.0669	−0.174	0.0794
SD parameter ($\widehat{s}$)	1.463	0.134	0.893	0.0939	1.112	

As mentioned above, choosing an Extreme Value distribution for the error term is completely equivalent to fitting a Weibull proportional hazards model. In fact, the relation between the estimates in Table 7.5.7 and those in Table 7.5.2 is as follows.

$$\widehat{c} = 1.119 = \frac{1}{\widehat{s}} = \frac{1}{0.893}$$

and for all regression effects

$$\widehat{b}_{\text{WeibullPH}} = -\frac{\widehat{b}_{\text{ExtremeValueAFT}}}{\widehat{s}},$$

for example, for ulceration

$$0.969 = -\frac{-0.866}{0.893}.$$

The Extreme Value error distribution is the only distribution with this property; that is, for other distributions no equivalent proportional hazards model exists.

Because of the censored observations it is difficult to define residuals to study how a given error distribution fits the data. It is, therefore, of interest to consider whether the regression parameters $b_1, \ldots, b_{n_c}$ in (7.5.6) may be estimated without having to provide a parametric specification of the shape of the error distribution. Estimation algorithms (not based on the likelihood principle, but generalizing ordinary least squares) for this purpose have been developed, one such procedure leading to the so-called Buckley–James estimator (e.g., Kalbfleisch and Prentice, 2002, Ch. 7). Table 7.5.7, last columns, shows the results which are seen to be comparable with those based on either Normal or Extreme Value errors, however, with a tendency to larger standard deviations.

Accelerated failure time models are in a way the most "natural" regression models for survival data if the aim is to generalize methods for uncensored quantitative outcome variables and they give easily interpretable parameter estimates. However, the models do specify the mean of a distribution, the tail of which is not observed because of censoring and, therefore, it is difficult to assess how well such a model fits a given set of survival data.

7.6 Exercises

Exercise 7.1. Draw a model diagram for the fibrosis Example 1.9, corresponding to the analyses as presented in Section 7.1.1.

Exercise 7.2. Baseline tryptase is considered elevated if it is above 11.4. Use the tryptase dataset 2 from Example 1.12 for investigating the relation between the probability of this event (during the suspected allergic reaction) and age of the patient.

1. In Exercise 4.7 the odds ratio for the occurrence was studied as a function of age. If you have not done this exercise, do it now.
2. Compare the result of the above question with an analysis using instead a logarithmic link, or an identity link.

Exercise 7.3. Use the tryptase dataset 2 from Example 1.12 and look at the patients that have been subjected to a test for allergy following the surgery (tested= 1).

1. Relate the probability of a positive test result to the value of the reaction tryptase, using a logit link and a linear effect of logarithmic tryptase value.
2. Compare to Exercise 4.3 from Chapter 4 where reaction tryptase was used on the untransformed scale.

3. Show that problems arise if we try to use instead a log link or an identity link.
4. Make a scatterplot of the test result (converted into a binary variable) against reaction tryptase and explain the problems encountered in the previous question.

Exercise 7.4. Use data from the fever in pregnancy Example 1.2 to study the number of fever episodes in pregnancy.

1. Make a Poisson regression for the number of fever episodes, as a function of alcohol habits and parity, using a log link.
2. Compare the results from using an identity link.

Exercise 7.5. Use data from the study of malignant melanoma Example 1.10 to perform a model check of a Cox regression model of time to death.

Exercise 7.6. Use data from the PBC-3 Example 1.3 to evaluate the treatment effect using alternative models for time to treatment failure.

1. Fit an accelerated failure time model assuming a log-Normal distribution with inclusion of
   • Only treatment
   • The covariates from Model 1 in Table 6.2.18
2. Do the same for a Poisson regression model assuming the baseline hazard to be constant in the three timeintervals 0–2, 2–4 and 4–6 years.

8

Further topics

In this final chapter we briefly mention a number of topics related to the general class of regression models with a linear predictor. This chapter is mainly meant as a precaution because some of the assumptions made throughout earlier chapters are now relaxed. Section 8.1 discusses the situation where responses are multivariate, often as a consequence of having several response variables observed in the same subjects. In such cases, the assumption of independence between all the responses needs to be relaxed, because observations from the same subject tend to be more alike than observations from different subjects and this intrasubject correlation must be accounted for to obtain valid inference. Another assumption from all previous chapters is that, although responses are considered random, the covariates have been assumed to be observed "precisely" (i.e. with no error). Section 8.2 discusses the situation where covariates are, indeed observed with error. We discuss consequences of this and ways to adjust for it.

This chapter is only meant as a brief introduction to these topics, a thorough discussion of which goes beyond the scope of the book.

8.1 Multivariate outcome

An important assumption from previous chapters is *independence* between outcome variables $y_1, \ldots, y_n$. However, frequently situations are met where such an assumption is not justified. These include both *clustered data* (that is, data on related individuals such as siblings, patients treated by the same general practitioner, or students from the same class, and longitudinal data where the same experimental unit gives rise to a series of measurements of the response variables, typically over time ("repeated measurements"). A special case is *paired* observations (see also Section 5.4) where the same response variable is recorded, for example, before and after an intervention. A final situation is simultaneous measurement of different, and possibly correlated, outcomes

in the same individuals, such as serum albumin and serum bilirubin in patients with liver cirrhosis. For notation, let $y_{i,j}, i = 1, \ldots, n, j = 1, \ldots, N_i$ be
the observations of the response, where i refers to the independent individuals
or clusters, N_i is the size of the ith cluster, and $j = 1, \ldots, N_i$ refers to observations within the ith cluster. The important feature is that, within cluster i,
the observations $y_{i,1}, \ldots, y_{i,N_i}$ cannot reasonably be considered independent.
Such data are denoted *multivariate* meaning that the outcome for each of the
experimental units (subject, cluster, $\cdots$) is more-than-one-dimensional.

Digression. Nomenclature

Note the difference between the notion of "multivariate", (high-dimensional *outcome*), and that of "multiple" regression, used in earlier chapters (high-dimensional
covariates). This is our preferred terminology although multivariate in some texts is
taken to mean more-than-one-dimensional covariates and although the name "multivariable" has been proposed to mean exactly the same as "multiple". For that
reason, we find the attempts to introduce the notion "multivariable" an unnecessary reinvention of the wheel! ◇

One approach to the problem with multivariate outcomes was discussed in
Section 5.4 where an intercept parameter for each cluster was introduced into
the linear predictor. For quantitative outcomes these cluster-specific intercepts
were estimated jointly with the other parameters in the linear predictor and,
for binary and survival time outcomes, the cluster-specific intercepts were
eliminated when estimating the remaining parameters using a conditional or
a partial likelihood, respectively.

However, because these cluster-specific, "fixed" effects parameters are usually of no interest, it seems reasonable to consider models for multivariate
responses that avoid introducing them altogether. Furthermore, when one is
interested in studying effects of between-cluster covariates, it is necessary to
go beyond the fixed effects models. In this section, two such approaches for
handling the within-cluster dependence: *random effects models* and *marginal
models* are briefly discussed. For linear models for a quantitative outcome
(and for other models with an identity link) these two approaches are equivalent. However, for logistic regression and other models with a nonlinear link
function they generally estimate different parameters.

In Section 8.1.1 we study random effects models ("variance component
models"), a special case of which is also known as "multilevel models". Compared to the models studied in Section 5.4, the fixed, cluster-specific intercept
a_i is replaced by a common fixed intercept a plus a zero-mean unobserved random variable r_i. This random effect shared by all members of cluster i creates
a (nonnegative) within-cluster dependence and by assuming that $r_1, \ldots, r_n$
follow some distribution, likelihood methods may often be applied for parameter estimation. In Section 8.1.2 we consider marginal models where focus in
on the marginal distribution of $y_{i,j}$. Here, parameters are estimated by solving
generalized estimating equations (GEE) that allow for the interdependence of

observations from the same cluster when assessing the effects and their SD. Finally, Section 8.1.3 treats the situation of longitudinal data where individuals are observed over time. Special attention is paid to life history data (or "generalized survival analysis") where the outcome consists of events occurring at random points in time.

8.1.1 Random effects models

In this section we briefly consider random effects models for the multivariate outcomes $y_{i,j}, i = 1, \ldots, n, j = 1, \ldots, N_i$. Most attention is devoted to the situation where the outcome is quantitative but we also add comments on binary and survival time outcomes.

Quantitative responses

We assume that observations from different clusters are independent. Furthermore, the unobserved random effects $r_i, i = 1, \ldots, n$ are assumed to be independent and to follow the same distribution with $E(r_i) = 0$ and $SD(r_i) = v$. Conditionally on the random effects, the relation between the expected value and the linear predictor is written as

$$E(y_{i,j} \mid r_i) = LP_{i,j} + r_i = a + b_1 x_{i,j,1} + \cdots + b_{n_c} x_{i,j,n_c} + r_i. \qquad (8.1.1)$$

The idea is that the random effect r_i *shared* by all subjects from cluster i explicitly creates a (positive) within-cluster dependence because, for example, for a large r_i, all responses from that cluster $(y_{i,j}, j = 1, \ldots, N_i)$ will tend to be large. By taking expectation over the distribution of the random effects in (8.1.1), it follows that the *marginal mean* of $y_{i,j}$ is simply

$$E(y_{i,j}) = LP_{i,j}$$

and if the residual SD for $y_{i,j}$ for given r_i is denoted s, then the *marginal* SD of $y_{i,j}$ is

$$SD(y_{i,j}) = \sqrt{v^2 + s^2}.$$

For different clusters, i_1 and i_2, y_{i_1,j_1} and y_{i_2,j_2} are independent whereas the correlation between observations y_{i,j_1} and y_{i,j_2} from the same cluster i is

$$ICC = \frac{v^2}{v^2 + s^2}. \qquad (8.1.2)$$

This *intraclass correlation* coefficient, ICC, gives the fraction of the total variation $v^2 + s^2$ which stems from the variation v^2 between clusters. Inasmuch as this is the same for all pairs of observations from the same cluster, the correlation structure is called *exchangeable* or *compound symmetric*. The coefficient b for a given covariate in the linear predictor has the interpretation that $b = \mathrm{E}(y_{i_1,j_1} - y_{i_2,j_2})$ if subjects i_1, j_1 and i_2, j_2 have values for that co-variate that differ by one unit and have identical values for all other covariates in the linear predictor; that is, the interpretation of b is exactly the same as discussed in earlier chapters. This interpretation holds no matter whether the two subjects come from the same cluster ($i_1 = i_2$) or not. This is because of the linear model (8.1.1) (i.e., the use of the identity link) and, as we show below, the interpretation of b for a nonlinear link is different. Often both $y_{i,j}$ and r_i are assumed to be Normally distributed.

We now study the simple 2-sample situation in more detail; first when the mean value is constant within clusters but differs between clusters (a between-cluster covariate) and next when all clusters have size $N_i = 2$ (that is, when data are paired) and one member of the pair has mean a and the other $a + b$. An example of the first situation could be a cluster-randomized study among general practitioners, where clusters (general practices) were randomly sampled and all patients from a given cluster randomized to the same group and the latter situation is what was studied for matched or paired data in Section 5.4 (e.g., a situation where the same subject is measured before and after treatment).

For simplicity we assume that all clusters have the same size $N_i = N$ and that, in clusters $i = 1, \ldots, n_0$, we have $\mathrm{E}(y_{i,j}) = a$ whereas, for clusters $i = n_0 + 1, \ldots, n = n_0 + n_1$, we have $\mathrm{E}(y_{i,j}) = a + b$. In other words, we have a single binary covariate $x_{i,j}$ taking the value 0 in the first n_0 clusters and 1 in the last n_1, so the covariate varies between clusters whereas it is constant within clusters. If there were no clustering at all then we would be in the simple 2-sample situation studied in Section 3.1.1. As in that section we estimate b as the difference between the averages

$$\bar{y}_0 = \frac{1}{n_0 N} \sum_{i=1}^{n_0} \sum_{j=1}^{N} y_{i,j}, \quad \bar{y}_1 = \frac{1}{n_1 N} \sum_{i=n_0+1}^{n_0+n_1} \sum_{j=1}^{N} y_{i,j}.$$

A simple calculation now shows that for $\hat{b} = \bar{y}_1 - \bar{y}_0$ we have

$$\mathrm{SD}(\hat{b})^2 = \left(\frac{1}{n_0 N} + \frac{1}{n_1 N} \right) \mathrm{SD}(y)^2 \left(1 + \mathrm{ICC}(N - 1) \right)$$

with ICC given by (8.1.2). If all observations were independent (Section 3.1.1), we would have ICC$= 0$ and

$$\mathrm{SD}(\hat{b})^2 = \left(\frac{1}{n_0 N} + \frac{1}{n_1 N} \right) \mathrm{SD}(y)^2$$

showing that

$$\mathrm{VIF} = 1 + \mathrm{ICC}(N - 1) \tag{8.1.3}$$

is a *variance inflation factor* arising from the within-cluster correlation. Equation (8.1.3) shows that VIF increases with both ICC and with N; that is, larger clusters and/or a larger intraclass correlation will lead to a relatively larger SD for the estimated effect $\widehat{b}$ of the between-cluster, binary covariate x. The intuition for the example is that adding a new patient from a practice that is already included in the study does not give rise to as much extra information as when a patient from a new practice is added.

This has important consequences for inference on clustered data and the precision of parameter estimates will be overestimated if the effect of clustering is not properly accounted for, not only for a 2-sample situation but also more generally for other between-cluster covariates. Note that inference for the random effects model (8.1.1) will consist in estimating both the mean value parameters in the linear predictor and the *variance components* s^2, v^2 (and thereby ICC). Also note that, for sample size calculations (Section 6.3), an estimate of the intraclass correlation is needed to adjust the computations performed for independent observations.

Let us next look at a situation where the binary covariate is no longer constant within clusters (a within-cluster covariate). An example is paired data, that is, all $N_i = 2$ where, for all pairs, i, $E(y_{i,1}) = a$ and $E(y_{i,2}) = a + b$. This is the situation studied in Section 5.4. The effect b of the binary covariate with values $x_{i,1} = 0, x_{i,2} = 1$ is estimated as the average of the differences:

$$\widehat{b} = \frac{1}{n} \sum_{i=1}^{n} (y_{i,2} - y_{i,1}) = \bar{y}_2 - \bar{y}_1$$

(which is also the difference between the averages $\bar{y}_j, j = 1, 2$). Now

$$\text{SD}(\widehat{b}) = \sqrt{\frac{2}{n}} s$$

only depends on the residual (within-cluster) SD, s and not on the variation between clusters v. This means that if v is considerably larger than s then the paired design will be efficient; see also Section 6.3. Note that the argument leads to the paired t-test studied in Section 5.4 which is then seen to be valid both for the fixed effects model studied there and for the random effects model

In general, more levels of clustering could be relevant (e.g., students in classes in schools in districts), and *hierarchical* models could be of interest with variance components associated with each level of the clustering. Also, covariates could refer to different levels (e.g., some covariates could be student-specific, some could be school-specific, etc.). Such *multilevel models* are beyond the scope of this book but it is worth noticing that, because of the shared random effects, the (intraclass) correlation between subjects from the same cluster is explicitly modeled. Random effects models may be more general than multilevel models, for example, allowing for random interactions or random effects of quantitative covariates. If all random effects (and the residual variation) are assumed to be Normally distributed then parameter estimates may be obtained using (restricted) maximum likelihood (Diggle et al., 2002, Ch. 4).

Binary responses and survival data

For multivariate binary data, $y_{i,j}, i = 1, \ldots, n, j = 1, \ldots, N_i$ from independent clusters the linear predictor, conditionally on the random effects, may be written in a way similar to (8.1.1); that is,

$$\text{logit}(\text{pr}(y_{i,j} = 1 \mid r_i)) = \text{LP}_{i,j} + r_i. \tag{8.1.4}$$

Again, the random effects r_i follow some distribution with $\text{E}(r_i) = 0$ and $\text{SD}(r_i) = v$ across the population. Expressed on the probability scale we have:

$$\text{pr}(y_{i,j} = 1 \mid r_i) = \frac{\exp(\text{LP}_{i,j} + r_i)}{1 + \exp(\text{LP}_{i,j} + r_i)}; \tag{8.1.5}$$

see also (1.3.13) and (4.1.15). The marginal distribution of $y_{ij,}$, that is, the un-conditional probability $\text{pr}(y_{i,j} = 1)$, is now the expectation of the probabilities in (8.1.5) taken over the distribution of the random effects r_i. This marginal probability no longer follows a logistic regression model. Figure 8.1.1 illustrates the situation. The model is (8.1.4) with a single quantitative covariate, x with an effect $b = 1$, and an intercept $a = 0$. The r_i are standard Normal; that is, $v = 1$. The conditional probabilities given the random effects are logit curves with "slope" parameter $b = 1$ and the marginal probability is a curve with a smaller slope. This is the population-averaged value of the conditional probabilities given r where the average is taken over the standard Normal distribution of r. This is not a logit curve (although the approximation may be close as we show in Section 8.1.2).

It follows that, as a consequence of the nonlinear logit link, we need to make within-cluster comparisons when interpreting the parameters. For the coefficient b for a given covariate in the linear predictor we, therefore, consider the conditional probabilities given the random effects. That is, we look at y_{i,j_1} and y_{i,j_2} from *the same cluster*, i such that subjects i, j_1 and i, j_2 have values for that covariate which differ by one unit and have identical values for all other covariates in the linear predictor. For such a comparison the random effect r_i cancels out and the odds ratio between these two subjects is $\exp(b)$ leading to a within-cluster interpretation for b.

A similar situation arises for survival data models. Here, the log(hazard rate) $l_{i,j}(t)$, conditionally on the random effect is typically written

$$l_{i,j}(t \mid r_i) = \text{LP}_{i,j}(t) + r_i \tag{8.1.6}$$

where, most often, the random effects are assumed to follow some distribution with $\text{E}(\exp(r_i)) = 1$ across the population. For survival data, the random effect $\exp(r_i)$ is often denoted the "frailty". For mathematical convenience, a

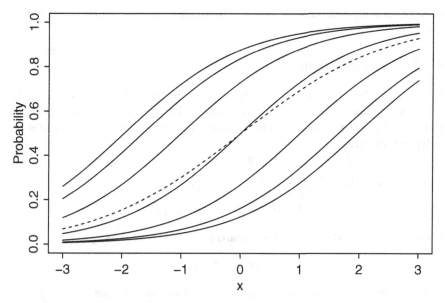

Fig. 8.1.1. Conditional probabilities that $y_{i,j} = 1$ given random effects of $\pm 1.96, \pm 1.645, \pm 1, 0$ plotted against the covariate x (solid curves) and population-averaged, marginal probability (dashed curve).

Gamma distribution with mean 1 is often assumed for the frailty but also a log-Normal distribution; that is, a Normal distribution for r_i has been studied (e.g., Duchateau and Janssen, 2008, Ch. 4). In this model, parameters in $LP_{ij}(t)$ are again *conditional* on r_i: they compare individuals from the same cluster. This is because the marginal hazard is no longer log-linear in covariates. In fact, if the conditional hazard given r_i, following (8.1.6) is

$$h_{i,j}(t \mid r_i) = h_0(t)\exp(bx_{i,j} + r_i)$$

then the marginal hazard, if r_i is Gamma distributed with mean 1 and SD $= v$, is given by

$$\frac{h_0(t)\exp(bx_{i,j})}{1 + v^2 H_0(t)\exp(bx_{i,j})},$$

where $H_0(t)$ denotes the cumulative (conditional) baseline hazard. That is, the marginal distribution of $y_{i,j}$ does not follow a proportional hazards model.

As for quantitative data, failure to account for the within-cluster correlation will lead to an underestimation of the variability, $SD(\widehat{b})^2$, of a between-cluster covariate by a factor of the form

$$\text{VIF} = 1 + \text{ICC}(\bar{N} - 1),$$

where $\bar{N}$ is the average cluster size and ICC an intraclass correlation coefficient. Ways of estimating ICC for simple situations with binary outcome data (e.g., the 2-sample situation), were discussed by Fleiss, Levin, and Paik (2003, Ch. 15).

8.1.2 Marginal models

Marginal models for clustered multivariate outcomes $y_{i,j}, i = 1, \ldots, n, j = 1, \ldots, N_i$ are specified via the linear predictor in exactly the same way as we have seen for independent data in previous chapters. That is, for quantitative outcomes we write

$$\mathrm{E}(y_{i,j}) = \mathrm{LP}_{i,j}$$

and for binary data the log(odds) is

$$\mathrm{logit}(\mathrm{pr}(y_{i,j} = 1)) = \mathrm{LP}_{i,j}.$$

Finally, for survival data the log(hazard rate) is specified as

$$l_{i,j}(t) = \mathrm{LP}_{i,j}(t).$$

The new feature of the models is that when estimating the parameters in the linear predictor and assessing their SD, allowance is made for the non-independence between observations from the same cluster. This is done via generalized estimating equations and robust SD estimation as briefly explained below.

In marginal models, parameters in LP_{ij} have a marginal interpretation; that is, they compare subpopulations defined by specific covariate patterns. In particular, the coefficient b for a given covariate in the linear predictor for a quantitative outcome has the interpretation that $b = \mathrm{E}(y_{i_1,j_1} - y_{i_2,j_2})$ if subjects i_1, j_1 and i_2, j_2 have values for that covariate which differ by one unit and have identical values for all other covariates in the linear predictor. Note that this interpretation holds no matter whether the two subjects come from the same cluster ($i_1 = i_2$) or not and, thus, for a linear model for quantitative data, parameters have the same interpretation in random effects models as in marginal models. For binary data and survival data, interpretations of parameters in the marginal models are similar to those for quantitative outcomes and for the models considered in all previous chapters, that is, they are marginal log(odds ratios) and log(hazard ratios), respectively. Thereby the interpretation differs from that seen in random effects models, the magnitude of the difference depending on the effect of the clustering. Thus, under independence they are identical, and, for binary data, the two sets of parameters (b_{cond} for the random effects model and b_{marg} for the marginal model) are approximately related as

$$b_{\mathrm{cond}} \approx b_{\mathrm{marg}} \sqrt{0.346 v^2 + 1} \qquad (8.1.7)$$

when random effects are Normally distributed with SD $= v$ (Diggle et al., 2002, Ch. 9). This is exactly the relation we saw in Figure 8.1.1. Figure 8.1.2

shows the same relationship, now in logit scale (and now with $v = 3$). Note that, because the conditional model is logistic, the corresponding curves are straight lines, however, the marginal model is not logistic and the relationship (8.1.7) between the two sets of parameters is only approximate. The approximation with a straight line will be better for smaller values of v. The logit-transform of the marginal probability in Figure 8.1.2 is seen to be close to a straight line. The slope of this is approximately 0.47, in nice accordance with (8.1.7) which for $v = 3$ gives the ratio $1/\sqrt{0.346 \cdot 9 + 1} = 0.49$ between b_{marg} and $b_{\text{cond}} = 1$.

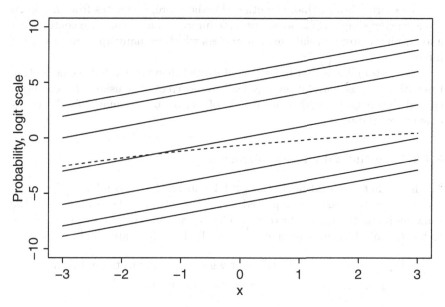

Fig. 8.1.2. Conditional probabilities that $y_{i,j} = 1$ given random effects of $\pm v \cdot 1.96, \pm v \cdot 1.645, \pm v, 0$ plotted against the covariate, x (solid lines) and population-averaged, marginal probability (dashed curve); logit scale. The distribution of the random effects is Normal with mean 0 and $SD = v = 3$.

The situation is similar for survival data where, except for special choices of the frailty distribution, we typically do not have proportional hazards both conditionally and marginally.

For marginal models the full distribution of data is often not specified and, in such situations, parameters cannot be estimated via maximum likelihood. Instead, they are estimated by solving *unbiased generalized estimating equations* (GEE). Often, the equations are those that one would have obtained from the likelihood function if all observations were independent, in which case the GEE are said to be derived under "a working independence assumption." However, other working correlations may increase efficiency if they are closer to the true correlation structure. The SD for the parameter estimates are obtained via "robust" (or "sandwich") estimators. Thus, GEE and sandwich SDs work in spite of the within-cluster correlation and without specifying this correlation which is treated as a "nuisance". This is in contrast to the random effects models where the correlation structure follows from the specification of the random effects. It has, therefore, been argued (e.g., Lin, 1994) that marginal models are more robust than random effects models and, indeed, estimation procedures are simpler, relying on fewer approximations, and software tends to be more reliable. However, it should be kept in mind that, for nonlinear links, different parameters are estimated from the two classes of models and, for some applications, one set of parameters may be more relevant than the other. Furthermore, estimates from marginal models using simple GEE do not provide information on variance components and within-cluster correlations, parameters which in many applications are of interest.

The bottom line is that if data are clustered then naive inference neglecting the within-cluster correlation may lead to incorrect conclusions, for example, caused by an underestimation of SDs of parameter estimates for between-cluster covariates.

8.1.3 Longitudinal and life history data

Much of what was said in Sections 8.1.1 and 8.1.2 is also relevant for *longitudinal data*, that is, when repeated measurements are taken over time in the same individuals. Here, "clusters" i refer to individuals and $j = 1, \ldots, N_i$ to times, $t_{i,j}$ at which measurements are made. Data for individual i consist of

$$t_{i,1} < \cdots < t_{i,N_i} : \text{ the times at which measurements are taken,}$$

$$y_{i,1}, \ldots, y_{i,N_i} : \text{ the outcome measurements,}$$

and

$$(x_{i,1,u}, u = 1, \ldots, n_c), \ldots, (x_{i,N_i,u}, u = 1, \ldots, n_c) : \text{ covariates.}$$

The covariates are allowed to depend on time, in fact, often the values of the timepoints $t_{i,j}$ are taken to be part of the covariates. The clustering structure imposed by a shared random effect will, as mentioned in Section 8.1.1 make all pairs of observations within each cluster equally correlated (the so-called *exchangeable* or *compound symmetry* situation). For longitudinal data, the temporal aspects will typically call for alternative correlation structures: observations in the same subject made closer in time should be more closely correlated than measurements taken farther apart. This leads to studying various *autoregressive* correlation structures where, for example, $y_{i,1}$ and $y_{i,2}$ are allowed to be more closely correlated than $y_{i,1}$ and $y_{i,3}$. A consequence of the longitudinal structure is the possible existence of a baseline value observed before any intervention. It is often advisable to include such a baseline value as a covariate rather than studying it as a part of the outcome. A simple approach to longitudinal data is often to base analysis on summary features of the data for each subject, (e.g., individually estimated slopes; Crowder and Hand, 1990, Ch. 2; Matthews et al., 1990).

In longitudinal studies it is a crucial assumption that the times, $t_{i,j}$ of measurements are independent of the measurements themselves: measurements should not be taken when individuals are particularly ill or the opposite. Otherwise, parameter estimates are likely to be biased. When planning longitudinal studies, attempts are therefore made to examine all individuals at the same inspection times ($t_{i,j} = t_j$ for all i). This will also produce clusters of the same size and structure. However, *drop-out* often complicates analysis; that is, individuals may leave the study before its planned time of termination. In this case, joint models for the repeated measurements and the drop-out mechanism are needed if the drop-out mechanism depends on the outcomes. Such a joint analysis is often based on a model where subject-specific random effects affect both the repeated measurements and the drop-out mechanism. In fact, marginal models are likely to provide inconsistent estimates when the drop-out mechanism is not "completely random." The topic of joint modeling was briefly touched upon in Section 6.2.3 in connection with discussion of time-dependent covariates in survival analysis but a detailed account goes beyond the scope of this book (see, e.g., Diggle et al., 2002, Ch. 13 for further information). In addition to dropping out completely, individuals may skip intermediate planned examinations and/or show up for unscheduled visits. In such cases, one should be suspicious about the assumption of independence between times and values of measurements and, at any rate, it is always advisable in the dataset to keep track of which measurements are taken at a planned follow-up visit and which are not.

Life history analysis

A slightly different situation occurs in *life history analysis* (or *event* history analysis) where, again, individuals are followed over time but where the responses are the times at which events occur for the individuals. That is, data consist of the times of events (y) and the type of event ($d(y)$) occurring at y: $(y_{i,1}, d(y_{i,1})) \ldots, (y_{i,N_i}, d(y_{i,N_i}))$ for subject i. In addition, covariates may be observed. In simple situations, the covariates could be *time-fixed*, $x_{i,u}, u = 1, \ldots, n_c$, but also models allowing for *time-dependent* covariates $x_{i,u}(t), u = 1, \ldots, n_c$ may be studied.

The simplest example of event history data is encountered in survival analysis as discussed in earlier chapters where only a single type of event, failure (death) is studied. In this case, $N_i = 1$ time of observation y_i is seen for subject i, either corresponding to a failure ($d(y_i) = 1$) or a censoring time ($d(y_i) = 0$) and most often (see, however Section 6.2.3) only time-fixed covariates, recorded at "time zero" are available.

This example illustrates that incomplete observation of the life histories in the form of *censoring* must be accounted for. In life history analysis, other kinds of data-incompleteness may be relevant. Sometimes, individuals are not observed from "time zero" but only from some later point in time, leading to *delayed entry* (or *left-truncation*). It is then a crucial assumption that censoring and truncation are *independent* in the sense discussed in Section 3.1.3. This means that selection out of the sample (censoring) and into the sample (left-truncation) at any time t should be unbiased in such a way that the available sample at all times should be representative of the underlying, potentially completely observed population. Whether there is delayed entry may depend on the time variable chosen for the analysis. In a study of mortality among diabetics there would be no delayed entry if the survival time y were taken to mean the disease duration at death and if all diabetics in the study were ascertained at the time of diagnosis. On the other hand, had y been taken to be the age at death then individuals would not be at risk of dying as a diabetic before their age at diagnosis and the survival time would be left-truncated at age at diagnosis.

It is seen that in life history analysis it is important to keep track of when each subject is at risk for each type of event and one way of depicting this is to look at life history analysis via *multistate models*. The simple survival data situation may be represented as the two-state model shown in Figure 8.1.3. The idea is that an individual is in state 0 "Alive" when recruited to the study and followed over time. The event, death is a *transition* from state 0 to state 1 "Dead" and the rate or *intensity* at which such transitions occur is given by the hazard rate, $h(t) = h_{01}(t)$ which is a function of a chosen time variable t. Recall from Section 3.1.3 that the interpretation of a hazard rate is the instantaneous rate of mortality

$$h_{01}(t)dt \approx \mathrm{pr}(t < y < t + dt \mid y > t)$$

which, using the notation from Figure 8.1.3, may be rewritten as

$$h_{01}(t)dt \approx \mathrm{pr}(\text{state 1 at time } t + dt \mid \text{state 0 at time } t).$$

The individual is at risk for a $0 \rightarrow 1$ transition whereas in state 0 and if recruitment takes place at time 0 then there is no delayed entry. If, when last seen, the individual is still in state 0, then the time of transition to state 1 is censored.

A simple extension of the survival model from Figure 8.1.3 is the *competing risks* model; see Figure 8.1.4. This is a model for several (here: two) causes of failure and, again, individuals are recruited to the study in state 0 "Alive" and followed over time. There are now two types of event, one for each cause of death corresponding to a transition from state 0 to either state 1, "Dead from cause 1" or to state 2, "Dead from cause 2." The rates or intensities at which transitions occur are given by the hazard rates, $h_{01}(t)$ or $h_{02}(t)$, respectively. The hazard rates are here denoted *cause-specific hazards* and have interpretations similar to the hazard rate for survival data; that is,

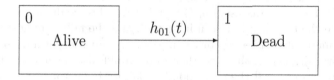

Fig. 8.1.3. The two-state model for survival data.

$$h_{01}(t)dt \approx \text{pr}(\text{state 1 at time } t + dt \mid \text{state 0 at time } t)$$

and similarly for $h_{02}(t)$. Individuals are at risk for both of the transitions, $0 \rightarrow 1$ and $0 \rightarrow 2$ while in state 0 and both censoring and delayed entry are possible. As for survival analysis, data for individual i will include a single observation time y_i and a failure indicator $d(y_i) = 1$ if failure from cause 1, $d(y_i) = 2$ if failure from cause 2, and $d(y_i) = 0$ if i was censored. Extension to more than two causes of death is obvious.

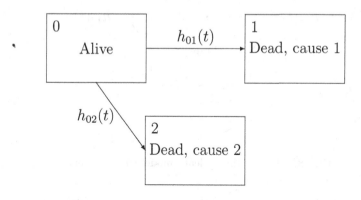

Fig. 8.1.4. The competing risks model.

Another extension of the simple model for survival data is the *illness–death* or *disability model*; see Figure 8.1.5. Here, disease-free individuals (state 0) are recruited and followed over time. Transitions to state 1 ("Diseased") or to state 2 ("Dead") may be observed and the rates at which they occur are $h_{01}(t)$ and $h_{02}(t)$, respectively. Diseased individuals, that is, those in state

1, may die with intensity $h_{12}(t)$ and, for a nonchronic disease as depicted in Figure 8.1.5, the disease may disappear with rate $h_{10}(t)$ (the "cure rate") whereas, for a chronic disease, $h_{10}(t) = 0$. For the chronic disease model, data will include the time $y_{i,0}$ last seen in state 0, and the failure indicator $d(y_{i,0})$ for that timepoint (a $0 \rightarrow 1$ transition, a $0 \rightarrow 2$ transition or a censoring). If a $0 \rightarrow 1$ transition was observed then data would also include the time $y_{i,1}$ last seen in state 1 and the corresponding failure indicator $d(y_{i,1})$ (a $1 \rightarrow 2$ transition a or censoring). If delayed entry is possible, then, in principle, an individual may be in state 1 at the time of entry into the study.

Ignoring the "Dead" state, the model may be used for describing *recurrent events*, for example, admissions to $(0 \rightarrow 1)$ and discharges from $(1 \rightarrow 0)$ hospitals. In this case, data consist of transition times and the corresponding event indicators. The number of observed transition times for different subjects will usually be random as it depends on the individual's life course.

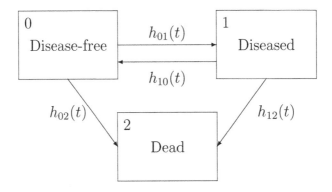

Fig. 8.1.5. The illness–death model with recovery.

Studying life history data as multistate models, the basic parameters are the transition rates. Therefore, models for life history data may be analyzed using models based on hazard rates as exemplified in previous chapters, for example, Section 7.5. Other parameters of interest are the *state occupation probabilities*. For the simple two-state model for survival data (Figure 8.1.3) the state occupation probabilities pr(state 0 at time t) and pr(state 1 at time t) are simple functions of the hazard rate. In fact, as seen in Section 3.1.3,

$$\text{pr(state 0 at time } t) = S(t) = \exp(-H(t)),$$

where $S(t)$ is the survival function and $H(t)$ the cumulative hazard whereas, obviously, pr(state 1 at time t) $= 1 - S(t)$. This means that a model for the hazard rate $h(t) = h_{01}(t)$ directly imposes a model for the state occupation probability. However, for more complicated multistate models, such a simple relationship does not exist. This has the consequence that, although transition rate models may be analyzed quite simply, it is more difficult to estimate state occupation probabilities. A thorough discussion of life history analysis based on multistate models is beyond the scope of the book (see, e.g., Andersen and Keiding, 2002, for more details) but to illustrate the concepts we have a closer look at the competing risks model (Figure 8.1.4).

Recall Example 1.10 from Section 1.5 concerning survival with malignant melanoma. Here, 205 patients were followed after operation; 57 died from the disease and 14 died from other causes. That is, we have two causes of death and, thereby, two cause-specific hazards, $h_{01}(t) = $ hazard rate of dying from malignant melanoma and $h_{02}(t) = $ hazard rate of dying from other causes. There are three state occupation probabilities, $P_j(t) = $ pr(state j at time t), $j = 0, 1, 2$. Here, $P_0(t) = S(t)$ is the survival probability, and the state occupation probabilities for states 1 and 2 are known as the *cumulative incidences*. They describe, as functions of time t, the probabilities of having died from cause 1 or 2 before time t:

$$P_1(t) = \text{pr(state 1 at time } t), \quad P_2(t) = \text{pr(state 2 at time } t).$$

It is important to note that even though $P_1(t)$ describes the probability of death from cause 1, it also depends on the cause-specific hazard rate for cause 2. The intuition is that a high cause 2 hazard rate will have the consequence that "fewer subjects are left to die from cause 1." Failure to realize this is a frequent mistake in the analysis of competing risks data and not rarely has the risk of dying from cause 1 mistakenly been estimated by "1 minus the Kaplan–Meier estimator corresponding to cause 1 events" (see, e.g., Andersen, Abildstrom, and Rosthøj, 2002b).

Digression. Cumulative incidences

The expression for the way in which a cumulative incidence depends on the cause-specific hazards is not too complicated. To die from cause 1 before time t, the failure from cause 1 must take place on some day between time 0 and time t. The probability of dying from cause 1 on a particular day u between 0 and t is the probability of surviving both causes of failure till just before day u times the conditional probability of failing from cause 1 on day u given survival till just before day u. The first factor is the survival probability

$$S(u) = \exp(-H_{01}(u) - H_{02}(u))$$

with $H_{0j}(u), j = 1, 2$ being the cumulative cause-specific hazards, and the latter, by the interpretation of a cause-specific hazard, is $h_{01}(u)du$ where $du = 1$ day. The cumulative incidence at time t is now the "sum over all days between 0 and t," that is, the integral

$$P_1(t) = \int_0^t S(u)h_{01}(u)du \tag{8.1.8}$$

which is seen, via $S(u)$ to depend also on the cause-specific hazard, $h_{02}(u)$ for the competing cause. ◇

For the melanoma data, we studied in Section 7.5 a number of models for the total hazard rate, and covariates such as age, tumor thickness, and ulceration were identified as important prognostic factors. It is to be expected that tumor-specific risk factors such as thickness and ulceration are likely to mostly affect the rate of dying from the disease whereas a covariate such as age is likely to mostly affect the rate of dying from other causes. To study such questions, separate Cox regression models for the two cause-specific hazards were fitted (although the model for the rate of dying from other causes should be interpreted with caution because of the small number of events). The model for a cause-specific hazard is fitted by only treating failures from the relevant cause as failures. The results in Table 8.1.1 support that thickness and ulceration significantly affect the cause-specific hazard of dying from the disease and age that of dying from other causes whereas gender has an insignificant effect on both cause-specific hazards. This illustrates that a study of cause-specific mortality may provide a different insight compared to modeling the total mortality. (It should be kept in mind, however, that formally all models in Table 8.1.1 cannot hold at the same time. This is because the total hazard is the *sum* of the two cause-specific hazards and "the sum of two Cox models is not a Cox model" because of the nonlinear log-link.)

Table 8.1.1. Results from fitting Cox regression models for the cause-specific hazards in the malignant melanoma study.

Covariate	All Causes		Disease		Other Causes	
	$\widehat{b}$	SD	$\widehat{b}$	SD	$\widehat{b}$	SD
Gender	0.413	0.240	0.433	0.267	0.358	0.549
Tumor thickness	0.0994	0.0345	0.109	0.0377	0.0496	0.0879
Ulceration	0.952	0.268	1.164	0.310	0.109	0.591
Age	0.218	0.0775	0.121	0.0830	0.725	0.217

Based on (e.g., Cox regression) models for the cause-specific hazards it is possible to predict the cumulative incidences. Here, it should be noted that because the cumulative incidences depend on both cause-specific hazards then, for the melanoma data, it follows that even though the hazard for death from the disease is not much affected by age, then the risk of dying from the disease will depend on age via the cause-specific hazard for other causes. The relationship between a covariate and the cumulative incidences is complicated based on Cox models for the cause-specific hazards; see Equation (8.1.8). Therefore, direct regression models for the cumulative incidences have been proposed, mostly based on the cloglog link; that is, the linear predictor is $\log(-\log(1 - P_1(t)))$, the "Fine–Gray model" (Fine and Gray, 1999).

8.2 Errors in covariates

In all of the preceding chapters, we have tacitly assumed that explanatory variables are measured without error. This is of course not correct in a strict sense inasmuch as almost all measuring processes involve some kind of measurement uncertainty, exceptions being demographic data such as gender, age, and education. Such a contamination will most often, although not always, lead to a less pronounced effect of the relevant covariate.

In Chapter 4 we related the vitamin D status of 41 Irish women to their body mass index (BMI), using traditional linear regression. This model assumes that for a fixed body mass index, the distribution of vitamin D status has a mean value linearly related to body mass index, and a standard deviation which is constant (i.e., independent of body mass index). This variation seen in vitamin D concentration for women with identical body mass index was interpreted as biological variation and it reflects that other (measured as well as unmeasured) explanatory variables may be relevant to explain the vitamin D status of an individual woman. However, some of the variation may also be due to uncertainty in the measuring process itself. Assessment of vitamin D status involves measuring the concentration of 25OHD in some form of assay and several sources of uncertainty may enter this process, giving a somewhat imprecise measurement. Traditionally, such an imprecision is assumed to be very small compared to the true biological variation but the important fact is that the presence of measurement error in the outcome variable does not induce bias in the estimates, although it will increase the standard deviation of all estimated effects and may therefore make us overlook weak effects. If the measurement error on the outcome is substantial, we may consider taking double or even triple measurements of the same quantity (if possible) and use the average or median of these in the subsequent analysis.

For regression models, inference is made conditional upon fixed true values of the explanatory variable and consequently, a measurement error in an explanatory variable is assumed to be nonexistent. In the vitamin D example, the assessment of body mass index involves measurement of height and weight, both of which are probably subject to small errors. As a matter of fact, we should be concerned not only with the pure measurement errors for body mass index but also with short-term fluctuations, because there will typically be a time gap between the measurement of body mass index and the measurement of vitamin D status or between the time of measurement and the time of effect. Such an "error" in body mass index cannot just be absorbed in the biological variation of body mass index between individuals inasmuch as this variation does not enter the model at all.

In contrast to measurement errors in the outcome, the presence of such errors (combined measurement errors and short-term fluctuations) in explanatory variables does in general induce bias in the estimated parameters. As mentioned, this bias will usually be towards zero so that the effect of the explanatory variable will be underestimated. In multiple regression, however, the relations between the covariates may reverse the effect, so that we may experience an overestimated effect of some covariates.

Most often, such a measurement error is not taken into account in the literature. The reasoning behind this neglect of possible problems is twofold:

- The magnitude is believed to be small in comparison with the biological variation in the explanatory variable and therefore of minor influence on the results (as appears from Equation (8.2.3) below).
- The magnitude of the error/uncertainty is most often not known and repeated observations required to give an estimate may not be available and/or hard to obtain.

A third argument for disregarding errors in the covariates is often given, namely that the model is intended for prediction purposes only. In this case, the uncertainties in the explanatory variables are expected to be of the same magnitude when the model is to be used for prediction of an unmeasured outcome of a new subject and it can be shown that the resulting prediction will therefore be unaffected by this uncertainty, in the sense that the prediction disregarding the errors in the covariates is still valid. The main focus of this book is not prediction, thus this argument is, however, not so relevant here.

It should be stressed that even if the uncertainties in the explanatory variables are often too small to be of any importance, there may also be situations in which they play an important role and may be a potential threat to the validity of the conclusions by producing serious bias in the estimates. Therefore, a thorough analysis should at least consider the potential problem and make a qualified (theoretical) guess concerning the importance.

In the vitamin D example, we have looked at covariates such as country, body mass index, vitamin D intake, and sun habits (see Section 6.2.1). Surely, country is measured without error and body mass index with a small error. The vitamin D intake, however, is based on the reporting of food items eaten over some period of time and will probably be subject to a considerable amount of error. Likewise, the covariate "sun habits" with three levels ("avoiding sun", "sometimes in sun", "prefer sun") may contain an appreciable amount of error due to individual interpretations of the categories. For such a categorical variable the measurement error is referred to as a classification error.

A full treatment of methods for correcting for measurement errors in covariates is beyond the scope of this book. We only give a sketch here of two possible approaches and illustrate using the vitamin D example. We also concentrate on quantitative covariates and only comment briefly on categorical covariates in the end of the section.

8.2.1 Regression dilution

For ease of reading we need some notation that is not quite identical to what we have used in the previous sections and chapters. This is because we need to distinguish between covariates measured with error (denoted x) and those measured without error (denoted z).

Furthermore, we assume that the relationship between the observed x_i for subject i and the corresponding true (error-free, but unobservable) value x_i^* is given by adding an error term e_i to x_i^*; that is,

$$x_i = x_i^* + e_i. \tag{8.2.1}$$

We assume this error e_i to have mean zero and standard deviation s_e and to be independent of both the true value x_i^* and the error-free covariate value z_i. We further assume that the outcome y_i can be described through a linear predictor depending upon the explanatory variables x_i^* and z_i, as described in the previous chapters in this book although here with a notation that explicitly refers to either an error-prone covariate (b_x^*) or an error-free covariate (b_z):

$$\mathrm{LP}_i = a + b_x^* x_i^* + b_z z_i. \tag{8.2.2}$$

Note that we could have several x^*s as well as several zs but for notational convenience we stick to the simple notation of one of each.

Digression. Latent variable models

The true unobserved values x_i^* are also denoted *latent variables* and the models are called latent variable models if distributional assumptions are imposed on these latent variables. $\diamond$

We take as example the simple linear regression of vitamin D (transformed with the base 10 logarithm) for the 41 Irish women, with body mass index as explanatory variable. In this case we have only a single x^* and no z. If we include also vitamin D intake as an explanatory variable, we have two x^*s and still no z but if we include women from all countries, we have country as an example of a z.

For the surgery example from Section 6.2.2, the zs would be type of surgery, age, and type of neuromuscular agent, whereas the x^*s would be duration of anesthesia and TOF-ratio.

For a quantitative outcome y, such as vitamin D concentration, and a single explanatory variable, an explicit formula for the estimated slope exists (see (4.1.4) in Section 4.1.1). If b_x^* (as above) denotes the true slope in the linear relation between the outcome and the hypothetical error-free values x_i^* of the covariate (body mass index), it can be shown that the slope calculated using the error-prone covariate x_i (the so-called *naive model*) will instead be b_x, given by

$$b_x = \frac{s_x^2 - s_e^2}{s_x^2} b_x^* = r_x b_x^*, \tag{8.2.3}$$

where s_x denotes the standard deviation of the observed covariate x and r_x is the *reliability coefficient* for the covariate x, defined as

$$r_x = \frac{s_x^2 - s_e^2}{s_x^2} < 1. \tag{8.2.4}$$

Because the reliability coefficient r_x from Equation (8.2.4) is always less than 1, we conclude that the slope will always be downward biased, so that it will be closer to zero than the true value, and more so, if the reliability coefficient is small, that is, if the uncertainty s_e is large compared to the natural biological variation for the unobserved x^* (the quantity $\sqrt{s_x^2 - s_e^2}$). This downward bias in (8.2.3) is called *regression dilution* or *regression attenuation*.

Even if the estimated slope is biased due to the presence of measurement error, it should be noted that the test for "no relation" between vitamin D and body mass index (the Wald test for $H_0 : b = 0$) remains valid. This is because the standard deviation of the estimated slope is biased towards zero by the same amount, leaving the test statistic unchanged.

Let us look a little closer at the example with body mass index as an explanatory variable for vitamin D concentration for the 41 Irish women. The observed body mass index has a standard deviation $\widehat{s}_x = 4.10$. We have no validation datasets (no true values of body mass index and no repetitions) but we may use common knowledge to come up with a guess at the size of the error involved in this variable. Body mass index is calculated as a height-corrected measure of weight,

$$\mathrm{BMI} = \frac{\text{weight in kg}}{\text{height in m, squared}}.$$

Weight is most often measured with an error within 50–100 g and height within 0.5–1 cm. It can be shown that this will result in a standard deviation of up to approximately 0.3 in body mass index. However, as explained above, these estimates concern the pure measurement error and do not take into account the natural variation over the course of the day or even a time span of a week or month which may be a more relevant time horizon considering that weight measurements are often collected only through a questionnaire. Taking this into account, the relevant figures are more likely to be variations of 1 kg in weight and maybe 1–2 cm in height, giving absolute deviations on body mass index up to approximately 0.7. Hence (assuming that the error distribution is approximately Normal) we may guess that a reasonable value for s_e is $\widehat{s}_e = 0.35$. This gives us an estimated reliability coefficient of

$$\widehat{r}_x = \frac{4.10^2 - 0.35^2}{4.10^2} = 0.993, \tag{8.2.5}$$

corresponding to a downward bias in slope of less than one percent.

Because of the small error involved in measurements of body mass index, the regression attenuation is only slight. If vitamin D intake were to be included in the model, the bias in the corresponding estimated regression coefficient would be larger. If we assume the error of the vitamin D intake to be up to a factor 2, corresponding to a standard deviation of the logarithmic (base 10) vitamin D uptake of $\frac{1}{2}\log_{10}(2) = 0.15$, we would get the reliability coefficient $(0.36^2 - 0.15^2)/0.36^2 = 0.82$, a downward bias of 18% (assuming the error in body mass index to be negligible).

If we consider the model with one single error-prone covariate x and one single error-free covariate z, the bias in the estimated regression coefficient for x will be given as

$$b_x = r_{x|z}b_x^*, \tag{8.2.6}$$

which is similar to (8.2.3), only with the reliability coefficient r_x replaced by the reliability coefficient in the conditional distribution given the error-free covariate z

$$r_{x|z} = \frac{s_{x|z}^2 - s_e^2}{s_{x|z}^2}, \tag{8.2.7}$$

where $s_{x|z}$ denotes the standard deviation in the conditional distribution of x given z. Because $s_{x|z} \leq s_x$ (z will explain some of the variation in x if they are related), the conditional reliability coefficient $r_{x|z}$ will be smaller than or equal to r_x and the consequence of the error in x will therefore be larger in the presence of z in the model.

Moreover, the estimate $\widehat{b}_z$ for the coefficient of the error-free covariate z will also be biased

$$E(\widehat{b}_z) = b_z + (1 - r_{x|z})b_{x|z}b_x^*. \tag{8.2.8}$$

Equation (8.2.8) shows that the estimated regression coefficient for the error-free covariate has been augmented by a fraction of the indirect effect of z (the effect of z on the outcome y passing through x in the model diagram of Figure 8.2.1). This means that the effect of an increasing measurement error in x will be to transfer more and more of the "explanatory ability" onto z and in the limit, the coefficient for z will be more or less identical to what we would get by eliminating x from the model altogether. This means of course that error in x may change b_z in either direction and by any magnitude, depending on the specific problem. Only if x and z are unrelated, will there be no bias in the estimated effect of z.

In multiple regression situations, with several error-prone covariates and several error-free covariates, it is impossible in general to predict the consequences of the errors, because this will depend strongly on the interdependencies among the various covariates.

When the outcome variable is not quantitative, the effect of measurement error in a covariate is more difficult to ascertain. In the case of a single explanatory variable, the typical effect will still be an attenuation of the relationship between the covariate and the outcome but no explicit formulas such as (8.2.6) and (8.2.8) exist.

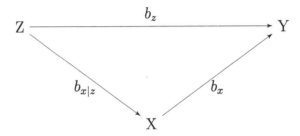

Fig. 8.2.1. Model diagram for outcome y and two covariates x and z.

Digression. Berkson model

In some situations the roles of the error-free covariate x^* and the error-prone covariate x are *reversed*, in the sense that we aim at a covariate value x_i (controlled by the investigator, e.g., a concentration of a drug) but we do not quite obtain that value. Instead, we obtain x_i^* which we cannot observe. The equation (8.2.1) is therefore replaced by

$$x_i^* = x_i + e_i. \tag{8.2.9}$$

Note that even if this relation between latent and observed variables may look quite similar to (8.2.1), the assumption of independence now applies to x_i and e_i instead of between x_i^* and e_i. This has consequences for the way of correcting for the error, but a treatment of this situation is beyond the scope of this book; see Carroll et al. (2006, Ch. 2). ◇

8.2.2 Correction for measurement error in covariates

Basically, there exist two approaches for handling this problem of error in covariate values, the regression calibration method and the Simex (simulation and extrapolation method); see Carroll et al. (2006, Ch. 4–5).

Regression calibration

The idea in regression calibration is to replace the error-prone covariate values x_i by predictions of the true (but unobserved) covariate values x_i^*. More specifically, the predicted covariate value for a single subject is taken to be the estimated conditional mean of x_i^* given x_i and z_i, that is,

$$\widehat{x}_i^* = \mathrm{E}(x_i^* | x_i, z_i) \tag{8.2.10}$$

and we therefore need to specify the joint distribution of (x_i, x_i^*, z_i). This requires additional information, either in the form of a reliability study (a study measuring the covariates x_i and z_i repeatedly in order to obtain information on their joint distribution) or a validation study (a study with joint measurements of all quantities (x_i, z_i) as well as x_i^*). Such studies may involve a subsample of the present sample (internal validation) or a sample of different subjects (external validation) and it will usually be much smaller because of the extra cost involved.

In the special case with only a single error-prone covariate x and no error-free covariates, Equation (8.2.10) gives an explicit expression

$$\hat{x}_i^* = E(x_i^* | x_i) \qquad (8.2.11)$$
$$= (1 - \hat{r}_x)\bar{x} + \hat{r}_x x_i,$$

where $\hat{r}_x$ is the estimated reliability coefficient from (8.2.4). Equation (8.2.11) shows that the predicted true covariate value is slightly shrunk in the direction of the overall average value. Inserting the estimated values $\hat{x}_i^*$ of body mass index into the formula (4.1.4) for the slope of the simple linear regression we get a correction formula for the slope that precisely corresponds to eliminating the bias from Equation (8.2.3):

$$\hat{b}_x^* = \hat{b}_x \frac{\hat{s}_x^2}{\hat{s}_x^2 - \hat{s}_e^2} = \frac{\hat{b}_x}{\hat{r}_x}, \qquad (8.2.12)$$

which is an unbiased estimate of the true regression coefficient b_x^* and therefore here denoted $\hat{b}_x^*$. In the vitamin D example we have estimated the effect of the error-prone body mass index as $\hat{b}_x = -0.0237$ so the effect of the error-free body mass index is estimated as $\hat{b}_x^* = \hat{b}_x / 0.993 = -0.0238$.

Returning to the general situation that may involve several error-prone covariates x and several error-free covariates z, the proposed method of correction for measurement errors was to substitute the estimated conditional means (8.2.10) for the error-prone values x_i. When doing so, the estimated standard deviation on the resulting parameter estimates will be too small. This may be dealt with using resampling methods such as the Bootstrap or the Jackknife but a discussion of this is beyond the scope of this book.

The Simex procedure

In the Simex method the trick is to impose further measurement error on the error-prone covariates (x), the *simulation step*, to study the consequences of this in the form of new estimates for the regression coefficients and use these estimates to extrapolate back (the *extrapolation step*) to the situation with error-free covariates. The method requires knowledge of the magnitude of the errors in the error-prone covariates so that additional error may be simulated.

For simplicity of notation, we again consider only one covariate x, measured with error (having a standard deviation s_e). Now suppose that we simulate a large number of new datasets (e.g., 1000) where we add extra error to x with a squared standard deviation (a variance) of λs_e^2 so that the total variance of the measurement error in x is now $(1+\lambda)s_e^2$. (For several covariates measured with error, the λ above refer to the same factor for each of these variables.) From each of the simulated datasets, we estimate the parameters in the model and we then compute the average over all 1000 simulations.

This is repeated for several values of λ (e.g., $\lambda = 0.5, 1, 1.5, 2$), each resulting in an average of 1000 estimated regression coefficients. Note that for $\lambda = 0$ we have the estimates from the original data and that we are seeking estimates for the value $\lambda = -1$ corresponding to the unobserved situation with error-free covariates.

In the extrapolation steps, these averages for the different λs ($\lambda = 0, 0.5, 1, 1.5, 2$) are related to λ using, for example, quadratic regression. Extrapolating back to $\lambda = -1$ yields the desired estimate. The result will of course depend on the way in which the extrapolation is carried out.

The standard deviation of the resulting estimate requires resampling, typically by means of a Jackknife procedure, but we consider a detailed description of this to be beyond the scope of this book and again refer the reader to Carroll et al. (2006, Ch. 5).

We illustrate the Simex procedure with the vitamin D concentration for the 41 Irish women, including both body mass index and intake of vitamin D as covariates, both with errors. Following the results in Section 6.2.1 we take the logarithm (base 10) of the vitamin D concentration (the outcome) as well as of the vitamin D intake. The standard deviations for the errors in the covariates are taken as described above: 0.3 for body mass index and 0.35 for logarithmic vitamin D intake.

Choosing the factors for the squared standard deviations of the measurement error to be $(1 + \lambda)$ with $\lambda = 0.5, 1, 1.5, 2$ we get the results presented in Figure 8.2.2. Here, the average of the estimated parameters (intercept as well as estimated effects of body mass index and logarithmic intake of vitamin D) are plotted against the factor $(1 + \lambda)$, that is, the ratio of the current measurement error and the measurement error in the original data. Superimposed on the graphs are the quadratic curves used for back-extrapolation to the situation where both covariates are error-free.

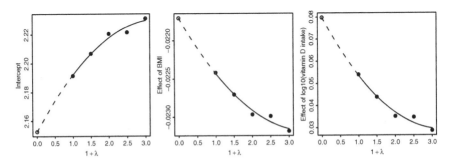

Fig. 8.2.2. Effects of error in vitamin D intake as well as in body mass index.

In Table 8.2.1 the estimated effects of the two covariates are presented, for the naive model using the error-prone covariates and for the corrected model, where the extrapolation is carried back to the error-free situation corresponding to $\lambda = -1$. We note that the effect of body mass index is only slightly corrected, from –0.0224 to –0.0217, and the estimated effect of vitamin D intake is corrected much more, from 0.0540 to 0.0798 (i.e., almost a 50% increase). Note also that the slight correction of the estimated effect of body mass index is actually towards zero. This can only happen because we have two covariates measured with error and because body mass index is virtually error-free (at least seen in comparison with vitamin D intake), such that the bias in b_x is here more along the lines of that of an error-free covariate (8.2.8).

Note also from Table 8.2.1 that the estimated standard deviations for the two estimated regression coefficients are corrected to an extent that closely resembles that of the regression coefficients themselves, leaving the Wald tests approximately unchanged.

Table 8.2.1. Estimated regression coefficients for the naive model ($\lambda = 0$) and the corrected model ($\lambda = -1$).

| Model | Covariate | | | |
| | Body Mass Index | | $\log_{10}$(Vitamin D Intake) | |
	Estimated Effect	Wald Test	Estimated Effect	Wald Test
Naive model	–0.0224 (0.0067)	11.15	0.0540 (0.0754)	0.52
Corrected model	–0.0217 (0.0072)	9.06	0.0798 (0.1159)	0.48

For a binary outcome such as the occurrence of complications in the surgery Example 1.4 we could also apply the Simex method, provided that we could come up with reasonable estimates of the standard deviation of the measurement error in one or more covariates. In Section 6.2.2 we found the important explanatory variables to be type of surgery, age, duration of anesthesia, and an interaction between the TOF-ratio and the neuromuscular blocking agent (in a dichotomized form indicating whether the agent was of a long-acting type). Out of these covariates, there is likely a small measurement error in the duration of anesthesia and perhaps a somewhat larger error in the TOF-ratio. We do not pursue this example any further here.

If the explanatory variable is categorical, measurement error amounts to *misclassification* of the subjects into wrong categories, in general with the effect of making the categories look more alike, that is, with a bias towards zero in the estimate of group differences, much as in the above simple linear regression situation. The situation can be handled by the Simex procedure by specifying the classification errors. These have to be estimated from additional information precisely as for quantitative covariates.

A

Appendix: Notation

Greek letters

Writing a text using mathematical symbols requires a certain amount of notation. As mentioned in the preface, we have striven to avoid the use of Greek letters and have succeeded, with the following exceptions.

α	level of significance (or the type I error rate), usually set to 0.05
β	type II error rate that is, $1 - \beta$ is the power
$\chi^2(df)$	Chi-squared distribution with df degrees of freedom
λ	multiple of error variance in SIMEX procedure
π	3.1415926535...
$\prod$	product symbol
$\sum$	sum symbol

Having abandoned Greek letters, our notation then uses the Roman alphabet. This resulted in some letters being used as symbols for the same concepts throughout the book, but the Roman alphabet is not sufficiently rich to avoid that some letters were used for different purposes in different sections. Below, we present the list of letters that have been used as symbols, indicating whether they have been used for different purposes in different sections.

Parameter estimates

The estimate of a parameter a, b, or $S(t)$ is typically denoted $\widehat{a}, \widehat{b}, \widehat{S}(t)$. Occasionally, when different estimators for the same parameters are discussed, the alternative estimators may be denoted $\widetilde{a}, \widetilde{b}$, and so on.

List of symbols

Symbol	Section	
a		intercept in a linear predictor; if more than one intercept is needed, it is indexed by i or j
A	4.2.3	amplitude of harmonic function
	6.3	length of accrual period
b		regression coefficient, b_j is the regression coefficient for covariate j; coefficients with a double index, e.g., $b_{1,0}$, are occasionally used
$B(t)$		cumulative regression function at time t
c	2.1.2–2.1.3, 7.2	count parameter in Binomial distribution
	3.1.3, 3.2.3	hazard ratio
	3.2	c_j characteristic of outcome in group j
	4.1.1	parameter in discussion of pseudo-observations
	4.2	parameter for Gompertz curve
	7.4	threshold for latent variable
	7.4.2	number of controls in case-control study
	7.5.1	Weibull shape parameter
	App. B	base for logarithmic function
C		number of disease-free in population
d		number of cases in case-control study
$d(y)$		number of events at time y in survival analysis
dt		length of a (small) time interval when defining the hazard rate
D		total number of failure times in survival analysis
	7.4.2	number of diseased in population
e		error term for covariate
$e(t)$		expected number at time t in logrank test
E		expected number of events/failures
$\mathrm{E}(y)$		expected value of y
f	4.2.3	phase of harmonic function
	6.3	ratio between sample sizes
$f(\cdot)$		some function of covariate x, outcome y or time t
F		length of follow-up period
g		value of categorical variable
h		discrete hazard
$h(t)$		hazard rate at time t
$H(t)$		cumulative hazard rate at time t
H_0		hypothesis to be tested

List of symbols (ctd.)

Symbol	Section	
i		indexes (independent) individuals (or clusters)
$I(...)$		indicator function, i.e., $I(...) = 1$ if ... is true and $I(...) = 0$ if ... is false
j		indexes something other than independent individuals
k		$k + 1$ is the number of categories for a categorical variable
K		number of (multiple) comparisons
l	2.3.4	log(likelihood function)
$l(t)$	All other chapters	log(hazard rate) at time t
l'		derivative of log(likelihood function)
ℓ		log(odds), i.e., $\ell = \log(p/(1 - p))$ where p is the probability
ℓ_L, ℓ_U		confidence limits for log(odds)
L	2.3.4, 3.1.2, 3.2.2	likelihood function
	4.1.2, 4.1.3	test statistic for linearity
$L(t)$		lower confidence limit for log(cumulative hazard)
m		mean value, e.g., $m = E(y)$ is the mean value of y
M		median
n		number of (independent) individuals (or clusters)
		$n \to \infty$ means "n tends to infinity," grows larger and larger
n_a, n_b etc.	3.1.2	observed number in a cell in the 2×2-table
	5.1.1	observed number in a cell for the Mantel–Haenszel test
n_c	All other chapters	number of covariates in a multiple regression model
$n_{0,1}$ etc.		number of pairs in matched pair study
N	3.1.3, 3.2.3	number of distinct times of observation in survival analysis
	5.4, 7.3, 8.1	number of observations in matched set, cluster, etc.
	7.4.2	size of population
O		observed number of events/failures

List of symbols (ctd.)

Symbol	Section	
p		probability: p_j is the probability of an event in group j
		p_i is the probability of an event for individual i
	7.1.1	$p_{i,j}$ probability of outcome category j for individual i
P		P-value when testing a hypothesis
$P(t)$		state occupation probability at time t
q	4.2.2	power for fractional polynomial
	6.3	average failure probability
	7.4.2	selection probability in case-control study
	7.1.1	cumulative probability for ordered outcome
Q		Q or $-2 \log Q$ is a likelihood ratio test statistic
r	2.3.2, 3.1.1, 3.2.1, 7.1	residual, i.e., "observed – predicted value"
	4.1.1	correlation coefficient
	4.2.1, 6.2.3	cutpoint for intervals
	5.1.2, 5.2.2	number of nonlinear functions
	6.3	multiple correlation coefficient
	8.1	random effect
	8.2	reliability coefficient
$R(t)$		number of subjects at risk at time t in survival analysis
s		standard deviation, e.g., $s = \text{SD}(y)$ is the standard deviation of y
	4.1.1	s_{xy} covariance between x and y, $s_{y|x}$ residual SD
$s(x)$		score attached to individual with covariate x
S	2.3.4, 3.1.2	sum of observations
$S(t)$		survival function, i.e. $S(t) = \text{pr}(y > t)$ for a survival time outcome y
t	3.1.1, 6.3	t-test statistic
	7.5.1	cutpoint for time in Poisson regression
	8.1.3	timepoint of measurement
	All other chapters	timepoint in survival analysis
T	2.3.3	general test statistic
	4.1.2, 4.1.3	trend test statistic

List of symbols (ctd.)

Symbol	Section	
u	2.1	possible outcome value for variable y
	7.1.2, 8.1	index
	7.4.1	standard Normal variable
	App. B	positive number
$U(t)$		upper confidence limit for log(cumulative hazard)
v	App. B	positive number
		between-cluster SD
V		variance in logrank test
w		index
W		Wald test statistic
x		covariate (explanatory variable), x_i is its value for individual i;
		$x_{i,j}$ is covariate j for individual i (multiple regression)
$\bar{x}$		average covariate value
x^+		spline function for covariate x ($x^+ = (x - r)I(x > r)$)
x^*	4.1.3	transformed covariate
	8.2	true (unobserved) covariate value
X	3.1.3, 3.2.3, 5.1.1	X^2 is the logrank or Mantel–Haenszel test statistic
y		outcome (response) variable, y_i is its value for individual i
	5.4, 8.1	$y_{i,j}$ is the jth response variable for individual (cluster) i
$\bar{y}$		average outcome value
y^*	3.1.1	transformed outcome
	7.4	latent variable
z	3.1.2, 3.2.2	z^2 is the chi-square test in 2×2-table
	6.3, 7.4.1	quantile in standard Normal distribution
	8.2	error-free covariate
Z		Z-score

Abbreviations

In addition to the separate symbols, a number of abbreviations are used.

AIC	Akaike's information criterion
CI	confidence interval
cloglog	$\text{cloglog}(p) = \log(-\log(1-p))$ for a probability p
CLT	Central Limit Theorem
Cook	Cook's distance
CV	coefficient of variation
DAG	directed acyclic graph
$\text{dev}(b)_i$	deviation diagnostic when deleting the ith observation
df	degrees of freedom
EERC	experimentwise error rate under the complete null hypothesis
EPV	events per variable
exp	exponential function
$F(df1, df2)$	the F-distribution with $df1$ and $df2$ degrees of freedom
ICC	intraclass correlation
IQR	interquartile range
log	the natural logarithm $(\log_e)$
$\log_c$	the logarithm with base c, e.g., $c = 2$ or 10
logit	$\text{logit}(p) = \log(p/(1-p))$ for a probability p
LP	linear predictor
LR-test	likelihood ratio test
MEER	maximum experimentwise error rate
MIREDIF	minimum relevant difference
MS	mean square
$N(m, s^2)$	the Normal distribution with mean m and standard deviation s
OR	odds ratio
pr	$\text{pr}(\ldots)$ is the probability of $\ldots$, $\text{pr}(A \mid B)$ is the probability of A given B
probit	$\text{probit}(p)$ is another name for the pth percentile in the standard Normal distribution
R^2	the coefficient of determination
RR	relative risk
RSS	residual sum of squares
SD	standard deviation
SS	sum of squares
$t(df)$	the "Student-"t distribution with df degrees of freedom
Var	variance
VIF	variance inflation factor
$\pm$	$A \pm B$ is the interval from $A - B$ to $A + B$

B

Appendix: Use of logarithms

Throughout this book, logarithms have been applied in various contexts and with different purposes. We review these uses after a brief introduction to the logarithmic functions and their inverses, the exponential functions.

The logarithmic functions were originally introduced in order to ease the task of multiplication and division by translating it into addition and subtraction, respectively. The demand was that the functions should satisfy the equations

$$\log(1) = 0 \tag{B.1}$$
$$\log(uv) = \log(u) + \log(v)$$

for arbitrary positive numbers u and v.

It can be shown that Equation (B.1) has a continuum of solutions, called logarithmic functions, each with a different (positive) *base c*, characterized as the argument giving the logarithmic value 1. If we write the base explicitly as a subscript, we thus have $\log_c(c) = 1$ for all choices of $c > 0$.

The definition in Equation (B.1) leads to a few more important equalities

$$\log_c(uc) = \log_c(u) + \log_c(c) = \log_c(u) + 1$$
$$\log_c(uc^v) = \log_c(u) + \log_c(c^v) = \log_c(u) + v$$
$$\log_c(\frac{u}{v}) = \log_c(u) - \log_c(v) \tag{B.2}$$
$$\log_c(u^v) = v \log_c(u).$$

In particular, the last equation in (B.2) implies that for powers of the base, we have

$$\log_c(c^u) = u \log_c(c) = u. \tag{B.3}$$

For instance, $\log_{10}(100) = 2, \log_{10}(1000) = 3$ whereas $\log_2(4) = 2, \log_2(8) = 3$. Thus, for a number u, the logarithm with base c returns the power that we have to raise c to in order to get the value u; that is,

$$c^{\log_c(u)} = u. \tag{B.4}$$

Figure B.1 shows the logarithms with base values 2 and 10, respectively. Furthermore, the figure also shows *the natural logarithm*, with base equal to $e \approx 2.718$ (sometimes called Euler's number, not to be confused with Euler's constant). This logarithm has nice mathematical features (its derivative is the reciprocal function $1/x$) and it is the standard choice of logarithm in mathematics where it is often denoted $\ln(\cdot)$. However, we have followed the common practice from statistics and computer terminology and denote it simply as $\log(\cdot)$ without an explicit reference to the base e.

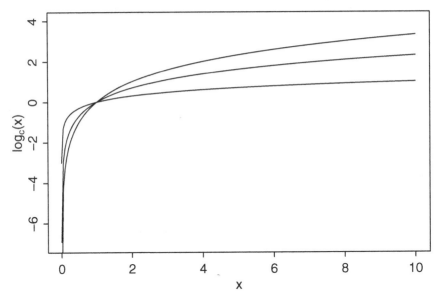

Fig. B.1. Functional form of logarithmic functions, for a selection of base values: 2, $e = 2.718$ and 10.

As mentioned, the logarithms are defined only on the positive axis, but take on values in the entire range from minus to plus infinity (see Figure B.1). All logarithmic functions are proportional, because we have the relation

$$\log_c(u) = \frac{\log_{10}(u)}{\log_{10}(c)}. \tag{B.5}$$

This means that modeling is invariant to the choice of base, in the sense that it does not matter which logarithm we choose when transforming the variables of the model or choosing a logarithm as link function. The estimates will of course depend on this choice but we can always make calculations back and forth and get the same answer. However, in certain situations, the choice has been made for us (built-in link functions in statistical software typically use the natural logarithm) and for some purposes, a specific choice of base value may facilitate interpretation of the results on the original scale.

The inverse of a logarithmic function is a function of exponential type, taht is, a function where the argument is used as the power (exponent). Such functions are defined on the entire axis but take on only positive values. For the various choices from Figure B.1, we have the corresponding relations

$$v = \log_2(u) \Leftrightarrow u = 2^v > 0 \qquad (B.6)$$
$$v = \log_{10}(u) \Leftrightarrow u = 10^v > 0$$
$$v = \log_e(u) \Leftrightarrow u = e^v = \exp(v) > 0$$

or in general, $v = \log_c(u) \Leftrightarrow u = c^v > 0$. Note that the inverse of the natural logarithm is simply called *the exponential function* and denoted $\exp(\cdot)$. The exponential functions corresponding to the logarithms in Figure B.1 are shown in Figure B.2.

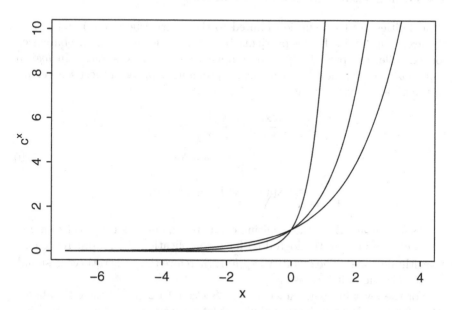

Fig. B.2. Functional form of the exponential functions, for a selection of base values: 2, e, and 10.

Equation (B.7) states the properties of the exponential functions, exemplified by the function $\exp(\cdot)$ but true in general for all choices of base value. Being the inverse functions of the logarithms, these properties are "the opposite" of the properties of the logarithmic functions.

$$
\begin{aligned}
\exp(0) &= 1 \\
\exp(u) &> 0 \\
\exp(u + v) &= \exp(u)\exp(v) \\
\exp(u - v) &= \frac{\exp(u)}{\exp(v)}.
\end{aligned}
\tag{B.7}
$$

A number of particularly interesting features for applications in model specifications and interpretation of results are

$$
\begin{aligned}
0 &< \frac{\exp(u)}{1 + \exp(u)} < 1 \\
\exp(\log(u) - \log(v)) &= \frac{u}{v} \\
\exp(u) &\approx 1 + u \quad \text{for small values of } u.
\end{aligned}
\tag{B.8}
$$

Uses of logarithms in model specifications

Probabilities are by definition limited to the interval between 0 and 1, thus the first property in (B.8) is particularly important for modeling probabilities, for example, the probability of a complication following surgery. In *logistic regression*, the relation between such a probability p_i for subject i is related to the covariate value x_i as

$$
\begin{aligned}
p_i &= \frac{\exp(a + bx_i)}{1 + \exp(a + bx_i)} \Rightarrow \\
\mathrm{LP}_i &= \log\left(\frac{p_i}{1 - p_i}\right) = a + bx_i \Rightarrow \\
\frac{p_i}{1 - p_i} &= \exp(a + bx_i) = \exp(a)\exp(b)^{x_i}.
\end{aligned}
\tag{B.9}
$$

As seen from (B.9), the resulting estimate $\widehat{b}$ quantifies the effect of a one-unit increase in x on the log(odds) for a complication (i.e., a difference on a logarithmic scale). The quantity $\exp(\widehat{b})$ is therefore the odds ratio corresponding to this one-unit increase in x.

For the fever in pregnancy example, Section 4.1.2 stated the estimate $\widehat{b} = 0.078$ for the effect on the probability of fetal death of an extra weekly drink. Because 0.078 is close to 0, this corresponds roughly to an odds ratio of 1.078 according to the last property in (B.8). More precisely, we find the odds ratio to be $\exp(\widehat{b}) = 1.081$ per weekly drink. The estimated SD of $\widehat{b}$ was 0.087, so that a 95% confidence interval is $(-0.093, 0.249)$. Transforming the endpoints of this interval with the exponential function gives us the interval for the odds ratio $(\exp(-0.093), \exp(0.249)) = (0.912, 1.282)$ so that we conclude that the increase in the odds of fetal death corresponding to an extra weekly drink may be as large as 28.2%.

Note that (B.9) involves the specific exponential function $\exp(\cdot)$ with base $e = 2.718$. This is the standard choice built into the logistic regression procedure and the subsequent transformation back to the original scale therefore also involves this particular exponential function. Because $10^x = \exp(x \log(10))$, this choice is, however, arbitrary and choosing base 10 instead of base e would only result in estimates that were scaled down by a factor $\log(10)$. Back-transformation of such estimates would give $10^{\widehat{b}/\log(10)} = \exp(\widehat{b})$, exactly the same result for the odds ratio.

For survival time outcomes, we relate the hazard rate at time t, $h(t)$ to covariates. The hazard rate is positive, therefore the natural choice is a multiplicative model (the *Cox regression model*)

$$h_i(t) = h_0(t) \exp(bx_i) \Rightarrow \qquad (B.10)$$
$$\log(h_i(t)) = \log(h_0(t)) + bx_i,.$$

where $h_0(t)$ denotes the hazard at time t when $x_i = 0$ and b is the log(hazard ratio) associated with a one-unit increase in x_i. Consequently, $\exp(b)$ is the hazard ratio between any two individuals whose x-values differ by one. For instance, in the example concerned with a randomized clinical trial of treatment of primary biliary cirrhosis (PBC) in Section 6.2.3, the regression coefficient corresponding to age in years in a Cox model (with time to treatment failure as outcome) was $\widehat{b} = 0.039$, corresponding to the hazard ratio $\exp(\widehat{b}) = \exp(0.039) = 1.040$ (i.e., a 4% increased hazard). The estimated SD of $\widehat{b}$ was 0.015, giving a 95% confidence interval for the hazard ratio of $(\exp(0.039 - 1.96 \times 0.015), \exp(0.039 + 1.96 \times 0.015)) = (1.01, 1.07)$, that is, a hazard which increases between 1% and 7% for each year of age.

Uses of logarithms for transformations

Because of the proportionality (B.5) between logarithmic functions with different base values, it does not matter which logarithm we choose when transforming the variables of the model. The estimates will of course depend on this choice but the actual relation between the outcome and the explanatory variables and therefore the conclusions do not. However, for certain purposes, a specific choice of base value may facilitate interpretation of the results on the original scale.

Basically, choosing to apply a transformation to one or more variables entering a statistical model (be it as an outcome or as an explanatory variable) has to do with trying to meet the assumptions in the model.

Logarithmic transformation of an *explanatory variable* x can be convenient in situations where the effect of x tends to level off for higher values as seen, for example for the effect of bilirubin in Section 4.1.3. The relation between outcome y and covariate x may then look like the curves in Figure B.1, corresponding to a linear predictor of the form

$$LP_i = a + b\log(x_i). \tag{B.11}$$

The interpretation of the regression coefficient b is the effect on the outcome (an increase of a mean value, a log(odds) or a log(hazard rate)) of a one unit increase in the covariate, in this case the covariate $\log(x)$. As seen from the first equation in (B.2), this corresponds to multiplying x by the base c. Therefore, when using a logarithmic transformation of an explanatory variable, it is most appropriate to choose, for example, a base 2, so that the interpretation will be the effect of a doubling of x. A base 10 logarithmic transformation will estimate the effect of a tenfold increase in x which may be outside the limit of the explanatory variable. If a doubling is also outside the limits of the explanatory variable, the base may be chosen as, for example, $c = 1.1$, leading to an estimated coefficient b corresponding to an increase in x of 10% (a factor 1.1). The *natural* base e is not particularly useful for interpretational purposes because it yields an estimate of the effect of multiplying the covariate x by 2.718. However, as pointed out previously, the choice of base is not crucial. If we have used a natural logarithm as covariate transformation and wish instead to get an estimate of the effect of a 10% increase in the covariate, this may simply be estimated as $\log(1.1)b = 0.0953b$, remembering of course to use the same multiplication factor for the SD of the estimate. We have used this in connection with analyses of the PBC-3 study.

Logarithmic transformation of a (quantitative) *outcome* may be used for several reasons:

1. To make an assumption of linearity reasonable, in the case of an exponentially increasing relation such as those in Figure B.2, that is, when $E(\log_c(y)) = a + bx$. Note that a similar effect (although not quite identical; see Section 7.3) can be obtained by using instead a log link (i.e., $\log_c(E(y)) = a + bx$). The result from the model states that a one-unit increase in x will increase $\log_c(y)$ by the amount b, which according to (B.2) corresponds to multiplying y by the factor c^b. For example, in the final model of the vitamin D example in Section 6.2.1, the effect of body mass index on $\log_{10}(y)$ yielded the estimate $-0.0096(0.0031)$. Because here $c = 10$, this means that a one-unit increase in body mass index has the effect of multiplying vitamin D level by $10^{-0.0096} \approx 0.98$, that is, a 2% reduction in vitamin D level.

2. To make a heavily (right-)tailed distribution on the positive axis more symmetric or even Normal, in order to make reference regions (regions of

"normal" values used as a reference in a clinical setting) trustworthy and comparisons more meaningful.

For such a skewed distribution the average is not the best estimate of the "central tendency" due to influential large observations. Instead, we use a geometric average. Formally, it is defined as the exponential function of the average of the logarithmic transformed observations (i.e., transform, take the average, and transform back again). In this way, the average is taken on a scale where the distribution is more symmetric and therefore avoiding the influence of extreme observations. This was used in Section 3.1.1 when comparing two groups (overweight versus normal weight Irish women) with respect to vitamin D concentration, on a logarithmic scale. Using a base 10 logarithm, we obtain an estimated difference in means (on the logarithmic scale) of –0.127, with a 95% confidence interval of (–0.245, –0.009). According to the rules of the exponential functions (B.8) such a difference transforms back to a ratio $10^{-0.127} = 0.75$ with the interpretation that overweight women have a level of S25OHD equal to 75% of the level for normal weight women, that is, a 25% lower level compared to the normal weight women. The confidence interval becomes $(10^{-0.245}, 10^{-0.009}) = (0.57, 0.98)$, indicating that our knowledge of the size of the difference is not very precise.

3. To stabilize variance in the quite common situation where the standard deviation increases proportionally to the level. When interpretation of the variation is in focus, there is an argument for using the *natural* logarithm, because it yields the approximate relation

$$SD(\log_e(y)) \approx \frac{SD(y)}{m(y)} = CV, \qquad (B.12)$$

where $m(y)$ denotes the mean value of y and CV is the *coefficient of variation* (see Section 7.3). Thus, if we estimate the standard deviation in a model for $\log_e(y)$ to, for example, 0.18, we may conclude that the CV of y (after adjusting for various explanatory variables) is 18%.

Sometimes, a logarithmic transformation is required for both outcome and explanatory variable. On the original scale, this corresponds to a power relation $y = ax^b$ (see, e.g., the Tetrahymena example analyzed in Section 4.1.1).

Why it is not cheating

Using logarithmic transformation of either outcome or explanatory variables is often thought of as cheating by nonstatisticians. We strongly stress that this is not the case. Indeed, if the assumptions in a specific model are not sufficiently accurate according to the nature of the data, it will be simply wrong not to do something about this. Transformation of one or more of the variables is a way to specify a model relying on other assumptions which may be more appropriate in the situation. Choosing another link function is an alternative option. Some typical situations are illustrated in Figures B.3 and B.4, using simulated data with clear deviations from one or more of the traditional assumptions of linearity, variance homogeneity, and Normality of residuals.

In the left panels of Figure B.3, the mean value structure is wrong (i.e., nonlinear). In the upper-left panel, the functional relation resembles that of the logarithmic functions in Figure B.1 and making a logarithmic transformation of x yields the figure to the right where all assumptions seem to be met. In the lower-left panel, the relation looks more like an exponential function (a vertically mirrored version of Figure B.2, i.e., like $\exp(-x)$) and therefore requiring a logarithmic transformation of y. Note that this transformation makes the standard deviation constant at the same time.

In Figure B.4, the assumption of constant SD is wrong in both left-hand panels, because SD is increasing proportionally to the mean, so that we have a constant coefficient of variation, requiring a logarithmic transformation of y. In the upper panel, the relation between y and x is a power function, which can be linearized by a simultaneous logarithmic transformation of y and x. The situation in the lower-left panel is more tricky because a logarithmic transformation of y will destroy the linear relationship between the untransformed y and x, no matter whether we use a logarithmic transformation of x or not. This is a situation where the sensible choice is a log-link, as discussed in Section 7.3.

Note that there may sometimes be a conflict between the three traditional requirements of linear regression: the linearity, the constant standard deviation, and the Normality. We saw an example of this in the lower-left panel of Figure B.4. In these situations, priority must be given to the linearity aspects because fitting a model with an erroneous systematic structure creates an obvious problem. The possibility of choosing between transformations and nonlinear links adds to the flexibility in this respect. With respect to conflicts between constant standard deviation and Normality, we find in practice that this is rarely the case. These assumptions concerning variation are most critical when constructing reference charts for clinical use, for example for monitoring hormone levels during pregnancy.

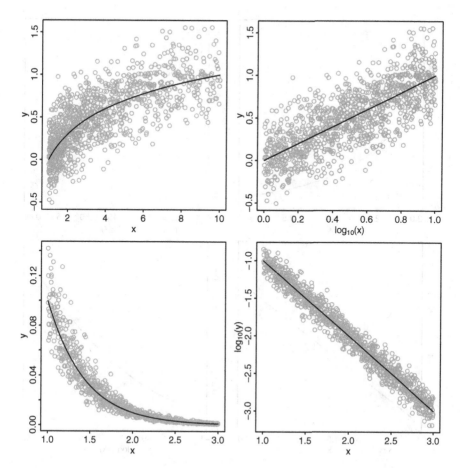

Fig. B.3. Examples of violated assumptions: upper left has nonlinear mean with constant SD, requiring a logarithmic transformation of x. Lower left has nonlinear mean and nonconstant SD, requiring logarithmic transformation of y.

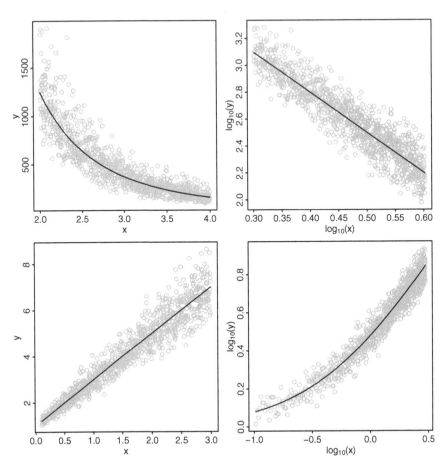

Fig. B.4. Examples of violated assumptions: upper left shows a power relation with constant CV, requiring a logarithmic transformation of both y and x. Lower left has a linear structure with constant CV and should be handled without transforming, by specifying a log-link.

C

Appendix: Some recommendations

Throughout the book we have given various recommendations which are now summarized under a number of headings. This appendix is not meant to be exhaustive, rather, it is intended to give an overview of some advice that may otherwise be "hidden" in the text. For a full discussion we refer the reader to earlier chapters.

Planning and analysis

Investigations should be planned to address one or a few simple questions, preferably comparing two groups or studying a single dose–response relationship. Thereby, difficulties in connection with multiple comparisons when testing hypotheses with many degrees of freedom are avoided (Section 3.2). Such tests also tend to lack power (Section 2.3.3). Sample size calculations should be performed for the main research question keeping in mind that the result of such a calculation should be regarded as an order of magnitude rather than an exact number of subjects to be recruited. Pilot studies may be a useful aid when assessing values of unknown quantities that appear in the calculations (Section 6.3).

It should be kept in mind that the interpretation of a covariate effect depends on which other explanatory variables are included in the model and it should, therefore, be carefully considered which covariates need to be adjusted for when addressing the primary research questions (Section 6.1). Typically, $SD(\widehat{b})$ will increase when many confounders are included, unless these are very strong predictors of the outcome and have only a moderate correlation with the exposure variable. The main analyses should concentrate on the primary research questions to reduce the amount of testing of data-generated hypotheses. However, science would not proceed if analyses of questions *not stated* in the protocol were not allowed so, obviously, new ideas generated from the data can be pursued as long as conclusions based on such additional analyses are suitably calibrated.

Selection of subjects for analysis

In regression models, there are no assumptions concerning the distribution of covariates and selecting subjects for regression analysis on the basis of their *covariate values* is perfectly valid (Section 6.1). As a consequence, it is important to realize that subjects will no longer be representative for the distribution of the response variable in the population and that this reduces the usefulness of quantities such as correlation coefficients, coefficients of determination (R^2), and Z-scores. (Sections 4.1.1 and 7.1.1).

Selection of individuals from their *outcome* variables will grossly complicate analysis and is not recommended. The only such situation that we have touched upon in the book is case-control studies. For such studies, it facilitates interpretation if both cases and controls are sampled from the same underlying cohort (a *nested case-control study*) (Section 7.4.2). When studying diagnostics (such as $\text{dev}(b)_i$ or Cook's distance) it is important to realize that large values of the diagnostics are not sufficient reason to exclude the subject from analysis (Section 4.1.1).

Reporting results

Power calculations are useful when planning studies, however, they have no role to play when reporting results (Section 6.3). Reporting should include estimates (equipped with confidence limits) for the parameters relating to the main research question. One should usually supplement with the associated P-values but it should be kept in mind that P-values quantify the strength of *evidence against* a hypothesis rather than the size of difference itself. Thus, the most useful tool when reporting results is the confidence interval. In particular, when reporting statistically insignificant results, the CI gives the limits for the group differences that are compatible with the data in spite of having too little evidence against the hypothesis of no difference. Note that the one-to-one correspondence between P-value and CI that exists for tests with one degree-of-freedom are no longer present when investigating tests with more degrees-of-freedom (Sections 2.3.3, 3.1.1).

When comparing two groups it is *incorrect* to infer from overlapping 95% confidence intervals for the levels (e.g., mean values or log(odds)) in the separate groups to nonsignificance at the 5% level of the difference between the groups. However, arguing the other way, that is, from nonoverlap of 95% confidence intervals to significant difference at 5% level between the groups, *is* correct (Sections 3.1.1, 3.1.2).

Parametrizations and choice of link function

When building the linear predictor for a regression model it should be parametrized in such a way that the intercept can be interpreted as the level of LP_i for a meaningful combination of values for the explanatory variables. The model itself is not affected, neither by this choice of parametrization, nor by the choice of reference group for a categorical covariate, only its appearance in the form of estimated coefficients (Sections 3.1.1, 3.2). When choosing the link function, the most important aspects to consider are model fit and interpretation of model parameters (e.g., Section 7.4).

Interactions

First of all, it should be recalled that the concepts of interaction and confounding have nothing in common (introduction to Chapter 5). Interactions complicate the models and only interactions that are prespecified as being of special scientific interest should be studied in the analysis (Section 6.1.7). This is particularly important for higher-order interactions (Section 5.3). Interactions should be studied by including the proper parameters in the linear predictor and not by making separate analyses in strata. Different parametrizations of LP_i are useful for *testing* for no interaction and for *presenting* results from a model including interaction terms and both types of parameters can conveniently be obtained using dummy variables (e.g., Section 5.2.1). When testing for no interaction it should be considered how to save degrees-of-freedom to obtain more powerful tests (e.g., linear-by-linear interactions may be useful for testing, whereas parameters in a model including such terms are difficult to interpret (Section 5.2.4)). In a model including interaction terms, care should be exercised if interpreting main effects (Section 5.2).

Interactions are scale-dependent and may appear or disappear with transformations and/or change of link functions (e.g., Section 7.4.1).

Importance of Normality

The 2-sample t-test compares the mean values between two independent groups, and the most important aspects are relevance of mean values and Normality of the two averages to be compared. Normality of averages is ensured in not too small samples by the Central Limit Theorem and relevance of mean values may be improved by proper transformations of the data. When reporting results obtained by carrying out the t-test on log-transformed observations it is convenient to back-transform to a ratio between medians. *Testing* for Normal distributions in the two samples is not recommended because, in small samples, Normality is rarely rejected and, in large samples, small and unimportant deviations may lead to rejection. Instead, we recommend visual inspection of residual plots (Section 3.1.1). Reference intervals should not be used based on sparse data (Section 2.2.2).

Survival analysis

To evaluate the crucial assumption of independent censoring one should always keep close track of why individuals are censored before the planned end of study (Section 3.1.3). In studies with repeated follow-up visits one should keep track of which visits are scheduled and which are not (Section 8.1.3). Although parametric models for survival data allow estimation of mean values, such extrapolation beyond the range of observed data is not recommended. Poisson regression based on a piecewise constant hazard function is a useful alternative to the Cox regression model, in particular in large samples with categorical covariates. The choice of time intervals should be based on the way in which the hazard is expected to vary with time (Section 7.5.1).

Miscellaneous

Graphical displays are extremely useful for presentation of data and evaluation of model assumptions. Smoothing of residuals is crucial for binary data and survival analysis. In linear models for a quantitative outcome, it is the distribution of the *residuals* (and not the marginals) that should be Normal (or symmetric). Tabulations of categorical data should always be studied before regression analysis (Section 5.1.1). A sharp distinction between a "standard error" of an estimate and a "standard deviation" is rarely useful and SD can be used as the generic concept thereby avoiding introduction of standard errors altogether (Section 2.3.1). In randomized studies it makes no sense to use significance tests to compare distributions of pretreatment variables between treatment groups (Section 5.1.2).

D

Programming in R, SAS and STATA.

This appendix contains a set of simple coding statements for performing a regression with a linear predictor in the three statistical packages R, SAS, and STATA.

The programs are only meant to show the most fundamental code for obtaining parameter estimates with confidence intervals and associated tests of significance, and only for simple situations where all quantitative covariates enter untransformed into the linear predictor.

Each model has a linear predictor with four covariates, two categorical and two quantitative. In all models, treatment and gender are categorical covariates, whereas age and bmi (body mass index) are quantitative covariates. If some covariates are not needed, the corresponding terms should simply be deleted from the model-statements. This may lead to simpler types of models that may also be analyzed by correspondingly simpler procedures in the three languages. For the sake of clarity, however, we have chosen to highlight the fact that even such simpler models are part of the common theme of regression and therefore also just special cases of the more general procedures.

The linear predictor built from the four covariates mentioned above is used in two ways, either without adding any interactions and with the addition of a single interaction between the categorical covariate treatment and the quantitative covariate age, to show an example of how this is done.

Three different procedures are used for each type of software, corresponding to the three different main types of outcome. We have chosen different names for the corresponding three data sets, even if we have kept the names for the covariates identical to ease the reading of the programs.

The outcome bloodpressure is quantitative (dataset quantout), complication is a binary outcome (dataset binout) and failuretime is a survival time outcome (dataset survout), with an associated variable status, indicating whether the observed timepoint is indeed a failure (status=1) or a censoring (status=0).

The names of outcomes as well as covariates are identical to those used in Tables 1.6.1 and 1.6.2. In these tables, the special names associated with simplifications of the models shown here are also given, for example, t-test, logrank test, and so on. These tables also include reference to nonlinear effects of quantitative covariates. However, this option is not part of this appendix due to the fact that it requires programming statements for construction of derived or transformed variables and therefore involves too many software details to be practical for this basic overview.

R code

Quantitative outcome

Without interaction:

```
model <- lm(bloodpressure ~ factor(gender)+factor(treatment)+
            age+bmi,data=quantout)
summary(model)
```

With interaction:

```
model <- lm(bloodpressure ~ factor(gender)+factor(treatment)+
            age+bmi+factor(treatment):age,data=quantout)
summary(model)
```

Binary outcome
Without interaction:

```
model <- glm(complication ~ factor(gender)+factor(treatment)+
             age+bmi,family=binomial(link="logit"),data=binout)
summary(model)
```

With interaction:

```
model <- glm(complication ~ factor(gender)+factor(treatment)+
             age+bmi+factor(treatment):age,
             family=binomial(link="logit"),data=binout)
summary(model)
```

Survival time outcome
Without interaction:

```
model <- coxph(Surv(failuretime, status==1) ~ factor(gender)+
               factor(treatment)+age+bmi,data=survout)
summary(model)
```

With interaction:

```
model <- coxph(Surv(failuretime, status==1) ~ factor(gender)+
               factor(treatment)+age+bmi+
               factor(treatment):age,data=survout)
summary(model)
```

SAS code

Quantitative outcome

Without interaction:

```
PROC GLM DATA=quantout;
  CLASS gender treatment;
  MODEL bloodpressure = gender treatment age bmi /
                        SOLUTION CLPARM;
RUN;
```

With interaction:

```
PROC GLM DATA=quantout;
  CLASS gender treatment;
  MODEL bloodpressure = gender treatment age bmi
        treatment*age / SOLUTION CLPARM;
RUN;
```

Binary outcome

Without interaction:

```
PROC GENMOD DATA=binout;
  CLASS gender treatment;
  MODEL complication = gender treatment age bmi
  / DIST=BINOMIAL LINK=LOGIT;
RUN;
```

With interaction:

```
PROC GENMOD DATA=binout;
  CLASS gender treatment;
  MODEL complication = gender treatment age bmi treatment*age
  / DIST=BINOMIAL LINK=LOGIT;
RUN;
```

Survival time outcome

Without interaction:

```
PROC PHREG DATA=survout;
  CLASS gender treatment;
  MODEL failuretime*status(0) = gender treatment age bmi /
                                RISKLIMITS;
RUN;
```

With interaction:

```
PROC PHREG DATA=survout;
  CLASS gender treatment;
  MODEL failuretime*status(0) = gender treatment age bmi
            treatment*age / RISKLIMITS;
RUN;
```

STATA code

Quantitative outcome

Without interaction:

```
use quantout, clear
regress bloodpressure i.gender i.treatment age bmi
```

With interaction:

```
use quantout, clear
regress bloodpressure i.gender i.treatment age bmi
                      i.treatment#c.age
```

Binary outcome

Without interaction:

```
use binout, clear
glm complication i.gender i.treatment age bmi,
                 family(binomial) link(logit)
```

With interaction:

```
use binout, clear
glm complication i.gender i.treatment age bmi i.treatment#c.age,
                 family(binomial) link(logit)
```

Survival time outcome

Without interaction:

```
use survout, clear
stset failuretime, failure(status==1)
stcox failuretime i.gender i.treatment age bmi
```

With interaction:

```
use survout, clear
stset failuretime, failure(status==1)
stcox failuretime i.gender i.treatment age bmi i.treatment#c.age
```

References

1. Altman DG (1991) Practical Statistics for Medical Research. Chapman and Hall, London
2. Altman DG, Bland JM (1983) Measurement in medicine: The analysis of method comparison studies. The Statistician 32:307–317
3. Andersen AMN, Vastrup P, Wohlfahrt J, Andersen PK, Olsen J, Melbye M (2002a) Fever in pregnancy and risk of fetal death. The Lancet 360:1552–1556
4. Andersen PK, Keiding N (2002) Multi-state models for event history analysis. Statist Meth Med Res 11:91–115
5. Andersen PK, Pohar Perme M (2010) Pseudo-observations in survival analysis. Statist Meth Med Res 19:71–99
6. Andersen PK, Borgan Ø, Gill RD, Keiding N (1993) Statistical Models Based on Counting Processes. Springer-Verlag, New York
7. Andersen PK, Abildstrom SZ, Rosthøj S (2002b) Competing risks as a multi-state model. Statist Meth Med Res 11:203–215
8. Andersen R, Molgaard C, Skovgaard LT, Brot C, Cashman KD, Chabros E, Charzewska J, Flynn A, Jakobsen J, Karkkainen M, Kiely M, Lamberg-Allardt C, Moreiras O, Natri AM, O'Brien M, Rogalska-Niedzwiedz M, Ovesen L (2005) Teenage girls and elderly women living in northern Europe have low winter vitamin D status. Eur J Clin Nutr 59:533–41
9. Armitage P, Berry G, Matthews JNS (2002) Statistical Methods in Medical Research, 4th edn. Blackwell, Malden, MA
10. Begg CB, Gray R (1984) Calculation of polychotomous logistic regression parameters using individualized regressions. Biometrika 71:11–18
11. Berg H, Viby-Mogensen J, Roed J, Mortensen CR, Engbæk J, Skovgaard LT, Krintel JJ (1997) Residual neuromuscular block is a risk factor for postoperative pulmonary complications. Acta Anaesthesiol Scand 41:1–9
12. Carroll RJ, Ruppert D, Stefanski LA, Crainiceanu CM (2006) Measurement Errors in Nonlinear Models, 2nd edn. Chapman and Hall/CRC, Boca Raton, FL
13. Clayton D, Hills M (1993) Statistical Models in Epidemiology. Oxford University Press, Oxford
14. Collett D (2003) Modeling Survival Data in Medical Research, 2nd edn. Chapman and Hall/CRC, Boca Raton, FL
15. Cook RD, Weisberg S (1982) Residuals and Influence in Regression. Chapman and Hall, New York

16. Copenhagen Study Group for Liver Diseases (1969) Effect of prednisone on the survival of patients with cirrhosis of the liver. Lancet pp. 119–121

17. Crowder MJ, Hand DJ (1990) Analysis of Repeated Measures. Chapman and Hall, London

18. Diggle PJ, Heagerty P, Liang KY, Zeger SL (2002) Analysis of Longitudinal Data, 2nd edn. Oxford University Press, Oxford

19. Dobson AJ (2002) An Introduction to Generalized Linear Models, 2nd edn. Chapman and Hall/CRC, Boca Raton, FL

20. Draper NR, Smith H (1998) Applied Regression Analysis, 3rd edn. Wiley, New York

21. Drzewiecki KT, Andersen PK (1982) Survival with malignant melanoma. A regression analysis of prognostic factors. Cancer 49:2414–2419

22. Duchateau L, Janssen P (2008) The Frailty Model. Springer-Verlag, New York

23. Efron B, Tibshirani RJ (1998) An Introduction to the Bootstrap, 2nd edn. Chapman and Hall/CRC, Boca Raton, FL

24. Farewell VT (2005) Regression. In: Armitage P, Colton T (eds.) Encyclopedia of Biostatistics, vol. 7 (2nd ed.), Wiley, New York, p. 4538

25. Fine JP, Gray RJ (1999) A proportional hazards model for the subdistribution of a competing risk. J Amer Statist Assoc 94:496–509

26. Fleiss JL, Levin B, Paik MC (2003) Statistical Models for Rates and Proportions, 3rd edn. Wiley, New York

27. Fruekilde MB, Hoy CE (2004) Lymphatic fat absorption varies among rats administered dairy products differing in physiochemical properties. J Nutr 134:1110–3

28. Gail MH, Wieand S, Piantadosi S (1984) Biased estimates of treatment effect in randomized experiments with nonlinear regressions and omitted covariates. Biometrika 71:431–444

29. Garvey LH, Bech B, Mosbech H, Krøigaard M, Belhage B, Husum B, Poulsen LK (2010a) Effect of general anesthesia and orthopedic surgery on serum tryptase. Anaesthesiology (in press)

30. Garvey LH, Belhage B, Krøigaard M, Husum B, Poulsen LK, Mosbech H (2010b) Serum tryptase in patients with suspected allergic reactions during anaesthesia - ten years experience from the Danish Anaesthesia Allergy Centre (submitted)

31. Harrell Jr FE (2001) Regression Modeling Strategies. Springer-Verlag, New York

32. Hastie T, Tibshirani R, Friedman J (2001) The Elements of Statistical Learning. Springer-Verlag, New York

33. Hastie TJ, Tibshirani RJ (1990) Generalized Additive Models. Chapman and Hall/CRC, Boca Raton, FL

34. Hellung-Larsen P, Leick V, Tommerup N, Kronborg D (1990) Chemotaxis in tetrahymena. Europ J Prostitol 25:229–233

35. Henderson R, Diggle P, Dobson A (2000) Joint modelling of longitudinal measurements and recurrent events. Biostatistics 1:465–480

36. Hoenig JM, Heisey DM (2001) The abuse of power: The pervasive fallacy of power calculation for data analysis. The Amer Statist 55:19–24

37. Holt JD, Prentice RL (1974) Survival analysis in twin studies and matched-pair experiments. Biometrika 61:17–30

38. Horn M, Vollandt R (2000) A survey of sample size formulas for pairwise and many-one multiple comparisons in the parametric, nonparametric and binomial case. Biom J 42:27–44

39. Hosmer DW, Lemeshow S (2000) Applied Logistic Regression, 2nd edn. Wiley, New York
40. Hsieh FY, Bloch DA, Larsen MD (1998) A simple method of sample size calculations for linear and logistic regression. Stat Med 17:1623–1634
41. Jewell NP (2004) Statistics for Epidemiology. Chapman and Hall/CRC, Boca Raton, FL
42. Kalbfleisch JD, Prentice RL (2002) The Statistical Analysis of Failure Time Data, 2nd edn. Wiley, New York
43. Kleinbaum DG, Klein M (2002) Logistic Regression. A Self-Learning Text, 2nd edn. Springer-Verlag, New York
44. Kleinbaum DG, Klein M (2005) Survival Analysis. A Self-Learning Text, 2nd edn. Springer-Verlag, New York
45. Lauritzen SL (1996) Graphical Models. Oxford University Press, Oxford
46. Lin DY (1994) Cox regression analysis of multivariate failure time data: the marginal approach. Stat Med 13:2233–2247
47. Lombard M, Portmann B, Neuberger J, Williams R, Tygstrup N, Ranek L, Larsen HR, Rodes J, Navasa M, Trepo C, Pape G, Schou G, Badsberg JH, Andersen PK (1993) Cyclosporin A treatment in primary biliary cirrhosis. Results of a long-term placebo controlled trial. Gastroenterology 104:519–526
48. Martinussen T, Scheike TH (2006) Dynamic Regression Models for Survival Data. Springer-Verlag, New York
49. Matthews JNS, Altman DG, Campbell MJ, Royston P (1990) Analysis of serial measurements in medical research. Br Med J 300:230–235
50. McCullagh P, Nelder JA (1989) Generalized Linear Models, 2nd edn. Chapman and Hall, London
51. Miller RG (1981) Simultaneous Statistical Inference, 2nd edn. Springer-Verlag, New York
52. Nilsson LB, Nilsson JC, Skovgaard LT, Berthelsen PG (2004) Thermodilution cardiac output. Are three injections enough? Acta Anaesthesiol Scand 48:1322–1327
53. Nøjgaard C, Johansen JS, Skovgaard PA L T Price, Becker, U for The EMALD Group (2003) Serum levels of ykl-40 and piiinp as prognostic markers in patients with alcoholic liver disease. J Hepatol 39:179–186
54. Olsen J, Melbye M, Olsen SF, Sørensen TIA, Aaby P, Andersen AMN, Taxbøl D, Hansen KD, Juhl M, Schouw TB, Sørensen HT, Andresen J, Mortensen EL, Olesen AW, Søndergaard C (2001) The Danish National Birth Cohort - Its background, structure and aim. Scand J Public Health 29:300–307
55. Panik M (2009) Regression Modeling. Methods, Theory and Computation with SAS. Chapman and Hall/CRC, Boca Raton, FL
56. Pearl J (1995) Causal diagrams for empirical research (with discussion). Biometrika 82:669–710
57. Pohar Perme M, Andersen PK (2008) Checking hazard regression models using pseudo-observations. Stat Med 27:5309–5328
58. Rothman KJ, Greenland S (1998) Modern Epidemiology, 2nd edn. Lippincott-Raven, Philadelphia, PA
59. Royston P, Altman DG (1994) Regression using fractional polynomials: Parsimonious parametric modelling (with discussion). Appl Stat 43:429–467
60. Royston P, Sauerbrei W (2008) Multivariate Model Building. A Pragmatic Approach to Regression Analysis Based on Fractional Polynomials for Modelling Continuous Variables. Wiley, Chichester

61. Rubin DB (1987) Multiple Imputation for Nonresponse in Surveys. Wiley, New York

62. Schlichting P, Christensen E, Andersen PK, Fauerholdt L, Juhl E, Poulsen H, Tygstrup, N for The Copenhagen Study Group for Liver Diseases (1983) Identification of prognostic factors in cirrhosis using Cox's regression model. Hepatology 3:889–895

63. Schoenfeld D (1983) Sample size formula for the proportional-hazards regression model. Biometrics 39:499–503

64. Seber GAF, Wild CJ (1989) Nonlinear Regression, 2nd edn. Wiley, New York

65. Secher NJ, Djursing H, Hansen PK, Lenstrup C, Eriksen PS, Thomsen BL, Keiding N (1987) Estimation of fetal weight in the third trimester by ultrasound. Europ J Obstr Gynaecol and Reprod Biol 24:1–11

66. Senn S (2002) Cross-over Trials in Clinical Research, 2nd edn. Wiley, New York

67. Therneau TM, Grambsch PM (2000) Modeling Survival Data. Extending the Cox Model. Springer-Verlag, New York

68. Vaeth M, Skovlund E (2004) A simple approach to power and sample size calculations in logistic regression and Cox regression models. Stat Med 23:1781–1792

69. Vittinghoff E, MacCulloch CE (2006) Relaxing the rule of ten events per variable in logistic and Cox regression. Amer J Epidemiol 165:710–718

70. Vittinghoff E, Glidden DV, Shiboski SC, McCullogh CE (2005) Regression Methods in Biostatistics. Linear, Logistic, Survival and Repeated Measures Models. Springer-Verlag, New York

71. Wulfsohn MS, Tsiatis AA (1997) A joint model for survival and longitudinal data measured with error. Biometrics 53:330–339

Index